Yearbook *of*
# Anesthesiology 14
2025

# Indian College of Anaesthesiologists

## Office Bearers

**Dr B Radhakrishnan**
Chief Trustee/Chairman/Vice-Chancellor

**Dr Jayashree Sood**
President

**Dr Baljit Singh**
CEO

**Dr Kanchi Muralidhar**
Dean National

**Dr Kumar Belani**
Dean International

**Dr Kirti N Saxena**
Editor-in-Chief, Journal of Indian College of Anaesthesiologists

**Dr Mukul Chandra Kapoor**
Editor, Yearbook of Anaesthesiology

**Dr Saneesh PJ**
Deputy Dean

## Board of Trustees

- Dr Manorama Mittal
- Dr B Radhakrishnan
- Dr Jayashree Sood
- Dr Baljit Singh
- Dr LD Mishra
- Dr Vijay Vohra
- Dr Kanchi Muralidhar
- Dr Roshan Lal Garg
- Dr Surinder Mohan Sharma
- Dr Bimla Sharma
- Dr Pradeep Jain
- Dr Kumar Belani
- Dr Raminder Sehgal
- Dr Naveen Malhotra
- Dr Kamal Fotedar
- Dr Manjula Sarkar
- Dr Mukul Chandra Kapoor

# Yearbook of Anesthesiology 14
## 2025

*Editors*

**Mukul Chandra Kapoor**
MD DNB MNAMS FIACTA
Chief Consultant, Professor, and Head
Department of Anesthesiology and Critical Care
Amrita Institute of Medical Sciences and Amrita Hospitals
Faridabad, Haryana, India
Chief Editor, Annals of Cardiac Anaesthesia
Director, Scientific Committee
Indian Resuscitation Council Federation (IRCF)
National Adviser, Indian Journal of Anaesthesia
Former Professor and Senior Adviser
Department of Anesthesiology and Cardiac Anesthesiology
Armed Forces Medical Services
Former President
Indian Association of Cardiovascular and Thoracic Anaesthesiologists (IACTA)

**Gaurav Kakkar**
FCARCSI CCT (UK) FSNCC
Lead Consultant
Department of Neuroanesthesia and Neurocritical Care
Amrita Institute of Medical Sciences and Amrita Hospitals
Faridabad, Haryana, India

*Foreword*
**Baljit Singh**

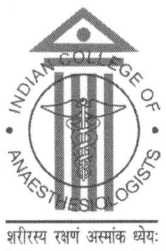

शरीरस्य रक्षणं अस्मांक ध्येय:

**Indian College of Anaesthesiologists**

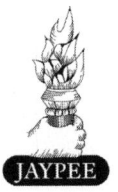

**JAYPEE BROTHERS MEDICAL PUBLISHERS**
*The Health Sciences Publisher*
New Delhi | London

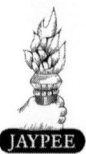 **Jaypee Brothers Medical Publishers (P) Ltd**

**Headquarters**
Jaypee Brothers Medical Publishers (P) Ltd
EMCA House, 23/23-B
Ansari Road, Daryaganj
New Delhi 110 002, India
Landline: +91-11-23272143, +91-11-23272703
+91-11-23282021, +91-11-23245672
Email: jaypee@jaypeebrothers.com

**Corporate Office**
Jaypee Brothers Medical Publishers (P) Ltd
4838/24, Ansari Road, Daryaganj
New Delhi 110 002, India
Phone: +91-11-43574357
Fax: +91-11-43574314
Email: jaypee@jaypeebrothers.com

**Overseas Office**
JP Medical Ltd.
83, Victoria Street, London
SW1H 0HW (UK)
Phone: +44 20 3170 8910
Fax: +44 (0)20 3008 6180
Email: info@jpmedpub.com

Website: www.jaypeebrothers.com
Website: www.jaypeedigital.com

© 2025, Jaypee Brothers Medical Publishers

The views and opinions expressed in this book are solely those of the original contributor(s)/author(s) and do not necessarily represent those of editor(s) or publisher of the book.

All rights reserved. No part of this publication may be reproduced, stored or transmitted in any form or by any means, electronic, mechanical, photocopying, recording or otherwise, without the prior permission in writing of the publishers.

All brand names and product names used in this book are trade names, service marks, trademarks or registered trademarks of their respective owners. The publisher is not associated with any product or vendor mentioned in this book.

Medical knowledge and practice change constantly. This book is designed to provide accurate, authoritative information about the subject matter in question. However, readers are advised to check the most current information available on procedures included and check information from the manufacturer of each product to be administered, to verify the recommended dose, formula, method and duration of administration, adverse effects and contraindications. It is the responsibility of the practitioner to take all appropriate safety precautions. Neither the publisher nor the author(s)/editor(s) assume any liability for any injury and/or damage to persons or property arising from or related to use of material in this book.

This book is sold on the understanding that the publisher is not engaged in providing professional medical services. If such advice or services are required, the services of a competent medical professional should be sought.

Every effort has been made where necessary to contact holders of copyright to obtain permission to reproduce copyright material. If any have been inadvertently overlooked, the publisher will be pleased to make the necessary arrangements at the first opportunity.

**Inquiries for bulk sales may be solicited at:** jaypee@jaypeebrothers.com

***Yearbook of Anesthesiology 14* 2025**

*First Edition:* **2025**

*Reprint:* **2025**

ISBN: 978-93-5696-626-0

*Printed in India*

**Dedicated to**

*The exceptional authors who have toiled to give this venture a distinct and remarkable shape. They have played a pivotal role in enhancing anesthesia safety through their commitment to education, mentorship, and disseminating best practices. By imparting their knowledge and expertise to the next generation of anesthesiologists, they have ensured that future practitioners are well-equipped to handle the complexities of anesthesia care. This book will enhance the competence of individual practitioners and contribute significantly to the overall safety and quality of patient care. Their influence will help shape a culture of safety that prioritizes patient well-being in all aspects of anesthesia practice.*

# Contributors

**Ali N Shariat** MD
Associate Professor
Department of Anesthesiology
Perioperative and Pain Medicine
Associate Professor
Department of Cardiovascular Surgery
Mount Sinai West and Morningside
Medical Center
New York, NY, USA

**Anju Gupta**
MBBS MD DNB IDRA MNAMS PGCCHM CEPC EDRA
Associate Professor
Department of Anesthesiology
Critical Care and Pain Medicine
All India Institute of Medical Sciences
New Delhi, India

**Anoushka M Afonso** MD FASA
Associate Professor of Clinical
Anesthesiology
Department of Anesthesiology and
Critical Care
Memorial Sloan Kettering
Cancer Center
New York, NY, USA

**Anshu Gupta** DA DNB
Director–Professor
Department of Anesthesiology
Maulana Azad Medical College
New Delhi, India

**Carolina Haylock-Loor** MD
Adjunct Assistant Professor
President-Elect, WFSA
Anesthesiologists
Critical Care Physician and
Interventional Pain Medicine
Medical Director of Interventional
Pain Unit
Hospital del Valle
San, Pedro Sula, Honduras

**Francisco Javier Escriba Alapont**
MD PHD
Pediatric Anesthetist
La Fe UiP Hospital
Valencia, Spain
Tutor, Residents of Anesthesia
Valencia University Teaching
Collaborator Chief of Anesthesia and
Intensive Care of the Virtual Simulation
Hospital of Valencia, Valencia, Spain

**Gaurav Kakkar** ARCSI CCT (UK) FSNCC
Lead Consultant
Department of Neuroanesthesia and
Neurocritical Care
Amrita Institute of Medical Sciences
and Amrita Hospitals
Faridabad, Haryana, India

**Giles Coverdale**
MBChB BSc (Hons) MACadMEd FRCA FFICM
Specialist Registrar Anesthetist
Department of Anesthesia
University Hospitals of Coventry and
Warwickshire
University Hospitals of Birmingham
Birmingham, UK

**Himani V Bhatt** DO MPA FASE FASA
Director
Division of Cardiothoracic
Anesthesiology
Mount Sinai Morningside Medical
Center, New York
Associate Professor
Department of Anesthesiology
Perioperative and Pain Medicine
Associate Professor
Department of Cardiovascular Surgery
Icahn School of Medicine
at Mount Sinai
New York, NY, USA

**Joanna Serafin** PhD
Senior Research Scientist
Memorial Sloan Kettering
Cancer Center
New York, NY, USA

**John Choi** DO
Resident
Department of Anesthesiology
Mount Sinai West and Morningside
Medical Center
New York, NY, USA

**Kara M Barnett** MD FASA SAMBA-F
Director
Department of Anesthesia Services
MSK Monmouth
Memorial Sloan Kettering
Cancer Center
Middletown, NJ, USA

**Kate Boothroyd** FRCA
Lead Consultant
Department of Anesthesia
University Hospitals of Morecambe Bay
NHS Foundation Trust
Kendal, UK

**Kelly Lebak** MD FASA SAMBA-F
Associate Professor
Department of Anesthesiology and
Pain Medicine
Case Western Reserve University
School of Medicine
Metro Health Medical Center
Cleveland, Ohio, USA

**Kishori Biradar** MD
Senior Resident
Department of Anesthesiology
ESIC Medical College and Postgraduate
Institute of Medical Sciences and
Research
Kalaburagi, Karnataka, India

**Maitree Pandey** MD
Director–Professor and Head
Department of Anesthesiology
Maulana Azad Medical College
New Delhi, India

**Manjula Sarkar** MD DNB
Professor
Department of Cardiac Anesthesia
DY Patil School of Medicine
Navi Mumbai, Maharashtra, India

**Marycarmen Flores** MD
Resident
Department of Anesthesiology and
Critical Care
Rosalind Franklin University of
Medicine and Science
North Chicago, IL, USA

**Massimiliano Meineri** FASE
Professor
Department of Anesthesiology
University of Toronto
Leitender Oberarzt, Abteilung für
Anästhesiologie und Intensivmedizin,
Herzzentrum Leipzig, Strümpellstrasse
Leipzig, Germany

**Mathew Patteril**
MBBS DA MD FFARCSI FRCA AFFICM
DipClinEdu (RCS) MBA
Consultant Anesthetist
Department of Anesthesia
University Hospitals of Coventry and
Warwickshire
Coventry, UK

**Matthew Camilleri**
MBBS DA MD FFARCSI FRCA AFFICM
DipClinEdu (RCS) MBA
Specialist Registrar Anesthetist
Department of Anesthesia
University Hospitals of Coventry and
Warwickshire, Coventry
University Hospitals of Birmingham
Birmingham, UK

**Michael J Furdyna** MD
Clinical Fellow in Obstetric
Anesthesiology
Department of Anesthesiology
Perioperative and Pain Medicine
Brigham and Women's Hospital, Boston
Instructor of Anesthesia
Harvard Medical School
Boston, MA, USA

**Michaela K Farber**
MD MS
Chief
Division of Obstetric Anesthesia
Department of Anesthesiology
Perioperative and Pain Medicine
Brigham and Women's Hospital, Boston
Associate Professor
Department of Anesthesiology
Harvard Medical School
Boston, MA, USA

**Monica Hervias Sanz** MD
Vice-President
Pediatric Section of SEDAR (Spanish
Society of Anesthesia, Reanimation
and Pain Treatment)
Chairman
Pediatric Section of the Anesthesia
Neonatal and Pediatric Anesthesia
Team and Anesthesia Simulation
Coordinator, Anesthesia, Reanimation
and Pain Treatment Service of Universal
Hospital Gregorio, Marañón
Madrid, Spain
Complutense University of Madrid
Teaching Collaborator

**Muhammad Farooq**
MBBS FRCS FC (Cardio) SA
Cardiothoracic Surgeon Charlotte
Maxeke Johannesburg Academic
Hospital
University of the Witwatersrand
Johannesburg, South Africa

**Mukul Chandra Kapoor**
MD DNB MNAMS FIACTA
Chief Consultant, Professor and Head
Department of Anesthesiology and
Critical Care
Amrita Institute of Medical Sciences
and Amrita School of Medicine
Faridabad, Haryana, India

**Nageswar Bandla** RCA FFICM EDEC
Consultant
Department of Intensive Care Medicine
King's College Hospital London
Dubai, UAE

**Natalie B Simon** MD
Resident Physician
Department of Anesthesiology
Icahn School of Medicine at Mount
Sinai, New York, NY, USA

**Neha Aeron** MD DNB
Assistant Professor
Department of Anesthesiology
Sardar Patel Medical College and
PBM Group of Hospitals
Bikaner, Rajasthan, India

**Nishant Kumar** DA DNB MNAMS
Professor
Department of Anesthesiology
Maulana Azad Medical College
New Delhi, India

**Nishkarsh Gupta** MD DNB
Professor
Department of Oncoanesthesiology
and Palliative Medicine
All India Institute of Medical Sciences
New Delhi, India

**Palesa Mogane**
MBChB DA (SA) FCA (SA) MMed (WITS)
Anesthesiologist
Department of Anesthesiology
Chris Hani Baragwanath Academic
Hospital
University of the Witwatersrand
Johannesburg, South Africa

**Palesa Motshabi Chakane**
BSc MBChB DA (SA) FCA (SA) PhD
Assistant Professor and Head
Department of Anesthesiology
University of the Witwatersrand
Johannesburg
Head of Clinical Unit, Cardiac
Anesthesia
Charlotte Maxeke Johannesburg
Academic Hospital
Parktown, Johannesburg, South Africa

**Pooja Singh** MD
Consultant Onco-Anesthesiologist
Department of Anesthesiology
BLK Max Superspeciality Hospitals
New Delhi, India

**Pradeep A Dongare** DA DNB
Assistant Professor
Department of Anesthesiology
ESIC Medical College and Postgraduate
Institute of Medical Sciences and
Research
Kalaburagi, Karnataka, India

**Praveen Kumar G** MD
Associate Staff Physician
Department of Intensive Care Medicine
Critical Care Institute
Cleveland Clinic Abu Dhabi
Abu Dhabi, UAE

**Rajiv Chawla** MD MNAMS
Director
Department of Anesthesia and
Critical Care
Rajiv Gandhi Cancer Institute and
Research Centre
New Delhi, India

**Ramprasad Matsa**
FRCP FFICM MSc (Critical Care)
Consultant
Department of Intensive Care and
Acute Medicine
Chair and Lead
Trust Strategic Sepsis Committee
Clinical Lead, Critical Care
Rehabilitation and Follow-up
University Hospitals of North
Midlands, NHS
Stoke-on-Trent, Staffordshire, UK

**Ranju Singh** MD
Director–Professor
Department of Anesthesiology
Lady Hardinge Medical College and
Associated Hospitals
New Delhi, India

**Reeta Singh** MD DNB MBA
Consultant Anesthesiologist
Department of Anesthesiology
Awali Hospital
Awali, Bahrain

**Ricardo Lopez-Betancourt**
Medical Student (Graduate Staff)
Department of Anesthesiology and
Critical Care
Memorial Sloan Kettering Cancer
Center
New York, NY, USA

**Shagun Bhatia Shah**
DA DNB Cert TEE FIMSA MNAMS FOAPAM
Senior Consultant
Department of Anesthesiology and
Critical Care
Rajiv Gandhi Cancer Institute and
Research Centre
New Delhi, India

**Shashi Kiran** DA DNB MD
Senior Professor
Department of Anesthesia
Pt BD Sharma Post Graduate Institute
of Medical Sciences
Rohtak, Haryana, India
Presently Consultant Anesthetics
University Hospitals of Morecambe Bay
NHS Foundation Trust
Kendal, UK

**Suken H Shah** MD
Director
Department of Interventional
Radiology
MSK Monmouth
Memorial Sloan Kettering Cancer
Center
Middletown, NJ, USA

**Susheela Taxak** MD DNB
Senior Professor
Department of Anesthesiology
Pt BD Sharma Post Graduate Institute
of Medical Sciences
Rohtak, Haryana, India

**Ujwal Dhundi** MD
Associate Staff Physician
Department of Intensive Care Medicine
Critical Care Institute
Cleveland Clinic Abu Dhabi
Abu Dhabi, UAE

**Uma Hariharan**
DNB MNAMS FIMSA FSNCC (Hons) DESA FICA PGDHM CCEPC
Professor
Department of Anesthesiology
Atal Bihari Vajpayee Institute of Medical
Sciences and RML Medical College
New Delhi, India

**V Bhadri Narayan** MD
Senior Professor
Department of Neuroanesthesia and
Neurocritical Care
National Institute of Mental Health and
Neurosciences (NIMHANS)
Bengaluru, Karnataka, India

**Vijayalaxmi Bellana** MBBS DNB IDCCM
Specialist
Department of Intensive Care Medicine
King's College Hospital London
Dubai, UAE

**Vivek Kakar** MD FRCA MA MPH EMBA
Director, ECMO Program
Cleveland Clinic Abu Dhabi
Abu Dhabi, UAE
Clinical Professor
Department of Anesthesiology
Lerner College of Medicine
Case Western Reserve University
Ohio, USA

# Foreword

Ensuring safe anesthesia for every patient is a daily challenge that demands not only skill in planning and execution but also a deep reservoir of knowledge. Anesthesia is more than just a job; it is a passion that requires continuous learning, refinement of skills, and the development of the art behind its administration. The *Yearbook of Anesthesiology* has been a vital source of new knowledge for over a decade. The topics are carefully selected based on current trends, emerging evidence, and their relevance to anesthesia practice. Moreover, the editors have enlisted authors with extensive experience and are recognized as experts.

Specific chapters deserve special mention, including those on anesthesia for daycare interventional radiology, nonoperating room anesthesia in children, the implications of pediatric obesity, the evolving role of artificial intelligence in airway management, and anesthesia for pediatric thoracic surgery. These topics address the increasing demand for anesthesia expertise, particularly as surgical advancements have accelerated in recent years. Additionally, issues such as burnout among anesthesiologists and the importance of mentoring are frequently discussed at academic gatherings due to their significant impact on caregivers' long-term health and performance.

The overwhelming interest and positive response to previous volumes of the Yearbook can be attributed to the diligent selection of authors, their writing prowess, and the meticulous editing process each manuscript undergoes before reaching readers. This results in an informative, clinically relevant, and user-friendly publication. Like its predecessors, this edition promises to be a well-crafted contribution to the science of anesthesiology.

**Baljit Singh**
Professor Emeritus
President Designate and CEO
Indian College of Anaesthesiologists

# Preface

*"Navigating the Evolving Landscape of Anesthesiology"*

The field of anesthesiology is a dynamic tapestry woven from physiology, pharmacology, critical care, and a deep understanding of human resilience. It is a specialty that demands constant adaptation as new technologies, procedures, and patient populations emerge. This recent edition of the *Yearbook of Anesthesiology* is an invaluable guide for navigating this ever-evolving landscape. As you delve into these pages, embrace the opportunity to expand your knowledge, refine your skills, and, ultimately, provide the best possible care for your patients.

This book tackles a broad spectrum of current concerns, from the burgeoning world of daycare anesthesia, encompassing obesity surgery and radiological interventions, to the intricacies of fluid management in the intensive care unit (ICU). It delves into the nuanced management of complex situations like peripartum cardiac arrest, geriatric cancer care, and the management of complex conditions such as tracheoesophageal fistula and traumatic brain injury.

The text ventures beyond traditional anesthesiology, addressing the challenges of high-altitude medicine and integrating cutting-edge technologies like point-of-care ultrasound (POCUS). This update does not shy away from the frontiers of technology. The inclusion of a chapter on artificial intelligence in airway management showcases the integration of these transformative tools into modern anesthesia practice.

Safety remains paramount, and this edition emphasizes its importance. The chapter on safety in anesthesia delves into strategies to mitigate risk. The discussion on periprocedural ECMO equips practitioners to manage critically ill patients requiring advanced life support. It delves into the ever-changing landscape of shock management and the importance of accurate risk assessment in emergent surgery.

In the medical profession, mentoring peers and juniors have not received due attention in most parts of the world. Including a chapter on mentoring anesthesiologists underscores the importance of fostering the next generation of practitioners. Students will find a comprehensive overview of these rapidly evolving areas, equipping them with a strong career foundation. On the other hand, clinicians will discover the latest best practices in various subspecialties, allowing them to stay current and deliver optimal patient care.

This book is not merely a compendium of topics but a roadmap for navigating the ever-changing landscape of anesthesiology. Its value extends to students seeking a foundation, clinicians refining their skills, and educators shaping the future of the field. As you delve into these pages, embrace the opportunity to expand your knowledge and elevate the care you provide to your patients. By nurturing a culture of knowledge sharing and support, we ensure the continued excellence of this vital specialty.

Anesthesiology is a rapidly evolving field with frequent advancements in techniques, medications, and technology. This update is a treasure trove for all those invested in the field. Keeping up-to-date with the latest guidelines and protocols helps enhance patient safety and minimize risks associated with anesthesia. This update encompasses these diverse topics, providing a holistic understanding of the complexities anesthesiologists face today. It empowers readers with the knowledge and tools they need to navigate the ever-shifting currents of this dynamic specialty. It will enable clinicians to deliver the highest standard of anesthesia care, ultimately improving patient outcomes and advancing the field of anesthesiology.

This book would not have been what it is without the hard work of several luminaries in the specialty of anesthesiology. We are highly indebted to these giants who toiled hard to compile this excellent collection of chapters despite their busy schedules and immense commitments. We want to conclude this preface by remembering the words of wisdom of Issac Newton, who acknowledged the role of his peers in these simple words:

*"If I have seen further, it is by standing on the shoulders of Giants"*

**Mukul Chandra Kapoor**
**Gaurav Kakkar**

# Contents

1. **Interventional Radiology Suite Within a Freestanding Ambulatory Surgery Center: Anesthetic and Quality Assurance Considerations** .................................................................. 1
   *Kara M Barnett, Joanna Serafin, Natalie B Simon, Suken H Shah*
   - Interventional Radiology Procedures Performed in the Ambulatory Surgery Center  *3*
   - Interventional Radiology Suite Design in the Ambulatory Surgery Center  *4*
   - Patient Selection Considerations  *7*
   - Anesthesia Care for Interventional Radiology in the Ambulatory Surgery Center  *9*
   - Scheduling and Efficiency Considerations  *11*
   - Postoperative Care  *12*
   - Quality Improvement Initiatives and Tracking  *13*

2. **Patients with Obesity and Obstructive Sleep Apnea in the Ambulatory Surgery Center** ................................................. 17
   *Kelly Lebak*
   - Obesity  *17*
   - Obstructive Sleep Apnea  *21*

3. **Risk Assessment in Emergency/Urgent Surgery** ........................................ 27
   *Pradeep A Dongare, Kishori Biradar*
   - Definitions  *28*
   - Need for Risk Assessment  *29*
   - Preoperative Evaluation—Estimating Perioperative Risk  *30*
   - Evolution of Risk Assessment Tools  *31*
   - American Society of Anesthesiologists  *32*
   - Scoring Systems Adapted for Emergency Surgeries  *32*
   - Scoring Systems Developed for Emergency Surgeries  *32*
   - Limitations of Scoring Systems  *37*
   - Role of Artificial Intelligence in Risk Prediction  *37*

4. **Upcoming Role of Artificial Intelligence in Airway Management** ......... 40
   *Reeta Singh, Susheela Taxak*
   - What is Artificial Intelligence?  *41*
   - Use of AI in Airway Assessment and Management  *41*
   - Use of AI in Predicting a Difficult Airway  *42*
   - Predictive Machine Learning Model Using Clinical Assessment for Difficult Airways  *43*
   - AI Used in Analysis of Radiological Images, Face Scans, and Speech for Airway Assessment  *43*
   - Role of AI in Fiberoptic Visualizing Devices Used in Intubation  *47*
   - Robotics in Airway Management  *48*
   - Challenges, Limitations, and the Future of AI in Airway Management  *48*

## 5. Maternal Cardiac Arrest .................................................................................... 54
Michael J Furdyna, Michaela K Farber
- Epidemiology  55
- Management of Maternal Cardiac Arrest  55
- Causes of Maternal Cardiac Arrest and Specific Management  59
- Postarrest Care  66
- Prevention and Preparation  66

## 6. Anesthetic Management of Tracheoesophageal Fistula ......................... 70
Anju Gupta, Manjula Sarkar, Nishkarsh Gupta
- Diagnosis and Pathophysiology  73
- Embryology  73
- Preoperative Evaluation  75
- Preoperative Preparation and Optimization  75
- Surgical Technique  76
- Anesthetic Management  77
- Postoperative Analgesia  82
- Postoperative Complications  82
- Anesthesia for Thoracoscopic Tracheoesophageal Fistula/Esophageal Atresia Repair  82

## 7. Nonoperating Room Anesthesia in Pediatrics ........................................... 88
Ranju Singh, Pooja Singh
- Patient Selection and Preoperative Assessment for Nonoperating Room Anesthesia Procedures  90
- Equipment and Resource Considerations for Nonoperating Room Anesthesia  92
- Anesthesia Techniques and Pharmacological Considerations for Pediatric Procedures  93
- Monitoring  96
- Considerations for Specific Pediatric Nonoperating Room Anesthesia Procedures  97
- Collaboration and Communication: Multidisciplinary Approach in Nonoperating Room Anesthesia  99
- Managing Emergencies and Complications in Nonoperating Room Anesthesia  99
- Postanesthesia Care and Discharge Planning for Nonoperating Room Pediatric Patients  100

## 8. Pediatric Thoracic Anesthesia ..................................................................... 104
Monica Hervias Sanz, Francisco Javier Escriba Alapont
- Pediatric Airway, Respiratory Physiology, and Ventilation  105
- One-Lung Ventilation  106
- Analgesic Techniques for Thoracic Surgery  120

## 9. Analgesia in Thoracic Surgery ..................................................................... 123
Himani V Bhatt, John Choi, Ali N Shariat
- Neuraxial Techniques in Cardiac and Thoracic Surgery  124
- Chest Wall Anatomy  125

- Techniques  *125*
- Superficial and Deep Parasternal Intercostal Plane Blocks  *129*
- Clinical Implications  *130*

## 10. Anesthesia for Pulmonary Endarterectomy .................................................. 136
*Palesa Motshabi Chakane, Muhammad Farooq, Palesa Mogane*
- Diagnosis  *137*
- Risk Prediction  *138*
- Perioperative Management  *138*

## 11. Anesthetic Considerations and Management of Traumatic Brain Injury.......................................................................................... 144
*V Bhadri Narayan*
- Consequences of Traumatic Brain Injury  *145*
- Pathophysiology  *145*
- Classification  *146*
- Pathophysiology of Traumatic Brain Injury  *147*
- Management  *150*
- Intraoperative Considerations  *153*

## 12. Remifentanil: An Update ............................................................................... 156
*Gaurav Kakkar*
- Chemical and Pharmacological Properties  *157*
- Mechanism of Action  *158*
- Clinical Applications  *161*
- Intensive Care  *161*
- Administration and Dosage  *162*
- Remifentanil in Special Populations  *163*
- Contraindications  *165*
- Strategies for Mitigation, Monitoring, and Management  *166*
- Research and Future Directions  *166*

## 13. Anesthesia for Geriatric Cancer Patients .................................................... 169
*Uma Hariharan, Rajiv Chawla, Shagun Bhatia Shah*
- Anatomical and Physiological Changes in the Elderly  *170*
- Geriatric Pharmacology  *170*
- Perioperative Concerns in the Geriatric Population  *174*
- Preoperative Assessment and Risk Stratification in Geriatric Oncological Patients  *176*
- Nutritional Assessment  *177*
- Perioperative Management  *178*
- Pain Relief and Postoperative Care in Geriatric Oncological Patients  *179*
- Geriatric Oncology in India  *181*

## 14. Perioperative POCUS..................................................................................... 185
*Massimiliano Meineri*
- Focused Cardiac Ultrasound  *186*
- Focused Intraoperative Transesophageal Echocardiography  *187*
- Lung Ultrasound  *188*

- Diaphragmatic Ultrasound  *189*
- Airway Ultrasound  *189*
- Gastric Ultrasound  *189*
- Training  *190*
- Certification and Quality Control  *190*

### 15. Fluid Stewardship in the Critically Ill .......................................................... 194
*Nishant Kumar, Anshu Gupta, Maitree Pandey*
- Fluid Stewardship  *195*
- Fluid Stewardship Team  *199*

### 16. Noninvasive Ventilation in Critical Care ..................................................... 204
*Matthew Camilleri, Giles Coverdale, Mathew Patteril*
- Noninvasive Ventilation Equipment  *205*
- Physiological Effects of Noninvasive Ventilation  *206*
- Noninvasive Ventilation to Prevent Intubation  *207*
- Noninvasive Ventilation and High-flow Nasal Oxygen Prevent Desaturation During Intubation  *211*
- Noninvasive Ventilation following Tracheal Extubation  *211*

### 17. Point-of-care Ultrasound in Critical Care .................................................. 215
*Vijayalaxmi Bellana, Nageswar Bandla*
- Ultrasound Physics  *215*
- Knobology  *219*
- Sonoanatomy  *219*
- Vascular Access  *220*
- Lung Ultrasound  *223*
- Cardiac Ultrasound  *226*
- Assessment of Volume Status  *227*

### 18. Current Concepts in the Management of Septic Shock ......................... 243
*Ramprasad Matsa*
- Pathophysiologic Principles  *244*
- Treatment and Control of Infective Process  *244*
- Shock Resuscitation  *245*
- Modulation of Host Response  *250*

### 19. Perioperative ECMO Support: A Primer for Anesthetists ...................... 256
*Ujwal Dhundi, Praveen Kumar G, Vivek Kakar*
- Extracorporeal Membrane Oxygenation Fundamentals  *257*
- Perioperative Management of ECMO Patients  *264*

### 20. High-altitude Medicine: Anesthesiology and Critical Care Challenges ............................................................................ 276
*Shagun Bhatia Shah, Rajiv Chawla, Uma Hariharan*
- Classification of Altitude Regions  *277*
- Physics at High Altitude  *277*
- Acclimatization  *279*
- High-altitude Pathophysiology  *279*
- Pregnancy and Altitude  *280*

- High-altitude Illness  *280*
- Anesthetic Challenges  *284*
- Recent Advances  *290*

## 21. Epidemiology and Management of Burnout among Anesthesiologists ........................................................................ 293
*Marycarmen Flores, Ricardo Lopez-Betancourt, Anoushka M Afonso*
- Physician Burnout  *294*
- Burnout among Anesthesiologists  *294*
- Coronavirus Disease-2019 effects on Burnout among Anesthesiologists  *296*
- Interventions for Burnout  *296*

## 22. Mentoring Anesthesiologists ........................................................................ 301
*Mukul Chandra Kapoor*
- Attributes of a Mentor  *302*
- Need for Mentorship  *302*
- Benefits of Mentorship  *303*
- Mentoring Needs Change with Time  *306*
- The Mentorship Journey  *306*
- Phases of a Mentoring Program  *307*
- Selection Process for Mentorship Program  *307*
- Monitoring of the Program  *309*
- Barriers to Successful Mentoring  *309*
- Mentorship Malpractice  *310*

## 23. Safety in Anesthesia—Global Perspective ................................................ 312
*Carolina Haylock-Loor*
- Anesthesiology, Anesthesiologists, and Safe Anesthesia  *313*
- Standardized Protocols and Guidelines  *315*
- Well-trained and Resilient Workforce  *316*
- Essential Equipment and Medications  *317*
- Safety Culture  *318*

## 24. Role of Anesthesiologist in Perioperative Patient Safety ..................... 322
*Shashi Kiran, Neha Aeron, Kate Boothroyd*
- To Err is Human  *324*
- Patient Safety—A Shared Responsibility!  *324*
- Continuous Education and Professional Development  *327*
- Patient Communication and Consent  *327*
- Patient Protection Events  *327*
- Child and Adult Safeguarding  *328*
- Teamwork  *328*
- Patient Transfers  *328*
- Medication Errors  *329*
- Airway Complications  *330*
- Healthcare-associated Infections  *330*
- Hand Hygiene  *330*

*Index* ........................................................................................................................ *335*

# CHAPTER 1

# Interventional Radiology Suite Within a Freestanding Ambulatory Surgery Center: Anesthetic and Quality Assurance Considerations

Kara M Barnett, Joanna Serafin, Natalie B Simon, Suken H Shah

## ABSTRACT

Interventional radiology (IR) is a relatively new subspecialty of radiology providing minimally invasive image-guided procedures. Compared to surgical procedures, IR procedures are less invasive and less expensive, with a shorter recovery time, making them ideal for same-day discharge and potentially increased patient satisfaction. Integrating an IR suite into an ambulatory surgery operating room area may mitigate many challenges of typical hospital-based IR programs. Design planning and program organization should involve the anesthesiology team and continue collaborating closely with the anesthesia and IR teams. We describe the design, organizational structure, and clinical protocols of IR practice in the freestanding ambulatory surgery center. We also describe anesthetic considerations, patient and procedure selection, scheduling, and postoperative care. This overview can be a template for a working care model optimized for anesthesia care within a high-volume outpatient IR practice.

**Keywords:** Interventional radiology; Ambulatory surgery center; Outpatient interventional radiology; Anesthesia for interventional radiology; Interventional radiology suite design; Patient selection for interventional radiology

## KEY POINTS

- A growing number of interventional radiology (IR) procedures can be safely performed in the freestanding outpatient setting.
- We provide a template for clinicians and administrators seeking to design a high-volume outpatient IR service with anesthesia care in a freestanding surgery center.
- The typical anesthesia for outpatient IR procedures in freestanding ambulatory surgery centers includes local injection plus sedation but may consist of regional or general anesthesia.
- Quality assurance is vital for sustaining IR services' sustained use and expansion within ambulatory surgery centers.

## ■ INTRODUCTION

Interventional radiology (IR) is a relatively recent subspecialty of radiology, providing a wide range of minimally invasive image-guided procedures. Compared to surgical procedures, IR procedures are typically less invasive and less expensive, with a shorter recovery time,[1] early discharge,[2] and potentially increasing patient satisfaction.[3] IR has recently experienced rapid growth, with one study from the

National Anesthesia Clinical Outcomes Registry (NACOR) finding a nearly threefold increase in the number of IR procedures from 2010 to 2014.[4] Similarly, the number of interventional oncology procedures has steadily increased. Estimates for the annual number of interventional oncology procedures performed in the United States range in the millions.[5] There has also been a steady increase in the number of follow-up consultations and the involvement of longitudinal patient care in interventional oncology and general IR.[3,6] According to the Cardiovascular and Interventional Radiological Society of Europe recommendations published in 2016, the value of setting up an outpatient IR clinic needs to be more appreciated and deprecated.[7]

The increase in minimally invasive procedures, including in IR, has been fueled by advancements in medical technology,[4,8] facilitating the gradual shift of many of these procedures to outpatient settings. Healthcare analysts project that by 2028, 85% of all procedures in the United States will be performed in outpatient locations.[9] The recent expansion of ambulatory surgery has also led to improved patient-centered care and reduced costs without compromising safety.[10,11] Similarly, providing IR care at ambulatory surgery centers (ASCs) promises to improve the patient experience and expand patient accessibility[12,13] while lowering costs.[11] Because of these benefits and growing demand in an aging population, there has been a steady increase in the number of consultations performed in the outpatient IR setting. Cazzato et al.[3] report that consultations increased 130% from 2011 to 2019. Moving outpatient IR procedures to freestanding ASCs may help alleviate busy hospital IR services and free up hospital beds, another benefit for patients and healthcare professionals.

Administration of anesthesia for IR procedures is typically classified as nonoperating room anesthesia (NORA), which describes anesthesia care delivered outside of a traditional operating room (OR). There has been a trend of shifting procedures from the OR into the NORA setting in the United States.[14] This trend follows the increasing demand for and volume of IR procedures.[15] NORA in the outpatient setting is projected to account for half of all anesthetics delivered in the upcoming decade in the United States.[4] Based on the NACOR data comparing NORA and OR procedures, more NORA patients are older and have an American Society of Anesthesiologists (ASA) physical status score of 3 or 4.[4] These trends have important implications, suggesting the need to continuously evaluate IR procedures to ensure NORA's growth meets quality and safety standards.[15]

Another outpatient setting for anesthesia care in IR includes office-based laboratories (OBLs). Similar to the office-based anesthesia model, in IR, OBLs are outpatient locations providing select procedures outside of the hospital and ASC settings.[16] The radiology suite has more malpractice claims than other NORA locations[17] and a higher complication and mortality rate than the OR patients.[18] The availability of imaging modalities, other resources, and patient complexity may limit procedure complexity considered at OBLs. The discussion of OBLs is outside of the scope of this chapter.

Anesthetizing patients for IR procedures presents unique challenges to anesthesia professionals. Historically, the fast-paced NORA environment has not been optimized for anesthesia care. Safety concerns include:
- Environmental, e.g., physical access to the patient and positioning of the patient
- Tools and technology-related, e.g., need for essential or unfamiliar equipment
- Task-related, e.g., team's lack of knowledge about anesthesia administration and access to anesthesia backup or support staff

- Organizational issues, e.g., need for essential or backup medications and nonstandardized workplace
- Personnel-related, e.g., need for more specific training and familiarity with procedures.[15]

Overall safety concerns exist, with the radiology suite listed as having a more significant proportion of malpractice claims than other NORA locations (Field 17) and a higher complication and mortality rate than the OR patients (Field 18). Integrating an IR suite into an operative platform with anesthesiology team input in design and organization and continued close collaboration between anesthesia and IR may mitigate many of these challenges.

We describe the design, organizational structure, and clinical protocols of IR practice in the freestanding ASC, including anesthetic considerations, IR suite design, patient and procedure selection, scheduling and efficiency, and postoperative care. This overview can be a template for a working care model optimized for anesthesia care within a high-volume outpatient IR practice.

## INTERVENTIONAL RADIOLOGY PROCEDURES PERFORMED IN THE AMBULATORY SURGERY CENTER

Many IR procedures can be successfully performed with same-day discharge, as patients can recover at home with minimal pain and postprocedural complications. Many same-day procedures are provided for cancer diagnosis, treatment, or palliative care for oncologic patients.[5] Typical outpatient oncologic IR procedures that may proceed with same-day discharge include diagnostic biopsies of lesions (e.g., soft-tissue biopsy), vascular access for treatment, or nephrostomies and drainage procedures for comfort care.[5] Additional outpatient IR procedures include peripheral arterial disease, venous disease treatments, fibroid embolization, and prostate artery embolization.

Central venous access device placement is a standard IR procedure for freestanding ASC. An estimated 8 million central venous access devices are placed annually in the United States.[19] Central venous access placement in the IR suite provides considerable cost savings compared to placement in the hospital-based OR. These procedures are safe, with a low immediate postoperative complication rate of 0.58%.[20]

Healthcare facility resources, procedural risks, and technical difficulties specific to the patient affect whether a procedure occurs in the outpatient setting. The multiple imaging modalities within the IR suite at our freestanding cancer ASC include fluoroscopy, ultrasound, and a computerized tomography (CT) angiography scanner, which enables a wide range of possible procedures. Although most sites may not have an integrated CT scanner, our facility requires this imaging modality to perform oncologic biopsies.

Patient selection and procedure risk stratification are essential for ensuring the safe performance of procedures in the outpatient setting. Low-risk procedures may not need a preoperative clinic visit and can be screened by nursing staff. Procedures with elevated risk usually require a clinic visit with a nurse practitioner or physician. The interventional radiologist should consider the specific comorbidities of each patient and procedural risk before performing a procedure in the freestanding ASC. For example, assuming the risk of bleeding associated with percutaneous liver biopsies,[21] the interventional radiologist should assess whether the lesion is sufficiently large and readily accessible to minimize the risk of adverse events in the freestanding ambulatory setting. This procedure is safe, but small lesions near major blood vessels may be more appropriate for an IR suite in a hospital.

To achieve successful procedure completion and patient recovery without increasing the risk of unanticipated transfers to a hospital, some IR procedures may be more appropriate for the hospital setting. Lung biopsies have a risk of pneumothorax, hemorrhage, and hemoptysis.[22] They may be too risky for most freestanding ASCs, especially for facilities far from the main referring or transfer hospital. Suppose a chest tube is placed for a pneumothorax. In that case, observation may be required, leading to prolonged recovery and bed utilization, which may cause a bottleneck in a minor outpatient postanesthesia care unit (PACU). Some programs have successfully performed outpatient lung biopsies with pleural vent for postoperative pneumothorax with same-day discharge and next-day office visits for follow-up.[23] **Table 1** lists a selection of procedures that may be performed in ASCs based on the facility's resources and patient risk.[24]

The IR service at our freestanding ASC has provided longitudinal cancer care for nearly 7,000 patients since opening in 2017. This has significantly expanded access to cancer care within our healthcare system and allowed the IR service at the leading hospital site to focus on more complex patients and inpatient procedures. Patients may require repeated procedures, such as exchanges of urologic stents or catheters for abscess drainage. Their initial procedure may be performed in the inpatient setting, followed by outpatient follow-up closer to home. In addition, oncology patients may require several different types of procedures during their cancer care.[5] Approximately 27% of our IR cases undergo more than one IR procedure at our location.

## INTERVENTIONAL RADIOLOGY SUITE DESIGN IN THE AMBULATORY SURGERY CENTER

Hospital NORA locations, including IR, are typically challenging anesthetizing sites compared to traditional ORs.[15] Historically, hospital IR suites were designed without considering the need for anesthesia services (e.g., suite layout is usually small and uncomfortable), making it challenging for personnel to reach the patient while maneuvering around equipment. Existing facilities may not accommodate the space needed for anesthesia machines, equipment carts, and emergency access for the patient.[25] Consequently, anesthesiologists are placed in unfamiliar positions relative to the patient and face environmental concerns of restricted patient access[4,18,26-28] and cramped workspaces.[8,25,27,29-31] The hospital IR suites may be distant from other clinical spaces and essential resources, such as the pharmacy and anesthesia personnel. For those reasons, anesthesiologists should lead the design process and plan for IR sites and services alongside interventionalists and facility managers.[8,25]

Integrating an IR suite into an ambulatory surgery OR area addresses many challenges anesthesia providers face in IR. This practical solution should also allow the anesthesiology team to participate in the design process, ensuring an ergonomic and spacious anesthesia workspace within the IR suite, allowing for ease of patient access around imaging equipment. According to the ASA Statement on NORA Services, NORA services should be located near the main OR area to enhance the safety and efficiency of anesthesia care.[32] By integrating the IR suite into the ASC, the

**TABLE 1:** List of outpatient interventional radiology procedures.

| Typical IR procedures that may be performed at freestanding ASCs | Elevated risk IR procedures that may be considered appropriate at freestanding ASCs with expanded facility resources for select patients |
|---|---|
| • Vascular access check, placement, removal, revision<br>  – Central (e.g., for cancer treatments)<br>  – Peripheral (e.g., dialysis catheter)<br>• Biopsy<br>  – Abdominal/retroperitoneal<br>  – Bone<br>  – Bone marrow<br>  – Genitourinary endoluminal<br>  – Kidney<br>  – Liver<br>  – Lymph node<br>  – Pelvic<br>  – Soft tissue<br>• Genitourinary, check, placement, exchange<br>  – Nephrostomy<br>  – Nephrouretorostomy tube<br>  – Ureteral stent<br>• Abscess procedures<br>  – Drainage<br>  – Catheter check, placement, exchange, removal<br>• Biliary, placement, removal, exchange<br>  – Drain<br>  – Catheter<br>• Cholecystostomy, check, exchange<br>• Fiducial seed placement<br>• Filter<br>  – Inferior vena cava filter, placement, exchange<br>• Gastrointestinal, check, placement, exchange, removal<br>  – Gastrostomy<br>  – Jejunostomy<br>  – Joint procedure<br>  – Aspiration<br>  – Steroid injection<br>• Lumbar puncture, may include chemotherapeutic medication injection<br>• Pain procedures<br>  – Nerve block injection<br>  – Neurolysis<br>  – Intrathecal injections<br>• Paracentesis<br>• Peritoneal catheter check, placement, exchange, removal<br>• Pleural catheter check, placement, exchange, removal<br>• Sclerosis injection<br>• Suprapubic catheter exchange, placement<br>• Thoracentesis | • Biopsy<br>  – Lung/pleural<br>• Bone<br>  – Augmentation<br>  – Ablation<br>  – Kyphoplasty and vertebral augmentation<br>• Y90 Radioembolization<br>• Varicose vein treatment |

(ASC: ambulatory surgery center; IR: interventional radiology).

IR team gains full access to the resources available to the ORs, which might not be readily accessible if the suite was located in a separate part of a hospital. This setup also has the added benefit of alleviating the increased demand for IR procedures by transferring cases from the hospital into the ASC. **Figure 1** depicts the floor plan of the IR suite, and **Figure 2** is the photograph of the IR suite at our ASC. It features an ergonomic design and spacious layout optimized for patient access for the IR proceduralist and the anesthesia provider.

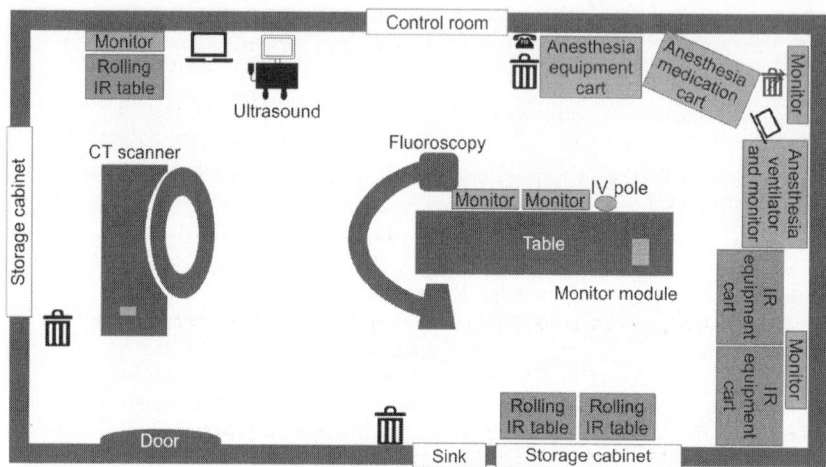

**Fig. 1:** IR suite layout with three imaging modalities. (CT: computed tomography; IR: interventional radiology)

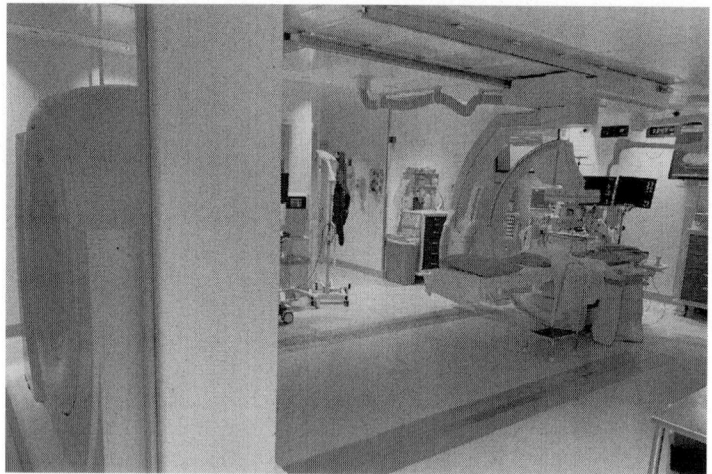

**Fig. 2:** Photograph of the interventional radiology suite at MSK Monmouth freestanding ambulatory surgery center. (MSK: Memorial Sloan Kettering Cancer Center)

The ASA Statement on Nonoperating Room Anesthesia Services includes additional pertinent considerations, including the design of the space to promote an environment of safety. Each procedure room must have adequate monitors per the ASA Standards for Basic Anesthetic Monitoring, sufficient lighting and electrical outlets, anesthetic medication, and equipment, including suction, an oxygen source, and space for equipment.[33] Emergency preparedness is also necessary, including access to essential resuscitative equipment, an emergency cart with a defibrillator, emergency medications, and difficult airway management equipment. When indicated, a malignant hyperthermia management cart with supplies should also be readily available. The protocols for a code or rapid response activation should also be protocolized. Mock code drills or procedure-specific simulations are strongly recommended to identify personnel, equipment, and logistics gaps before an emergency arises.[32]

Anesthesia providers within the IR context require protection due to the damaging effects of radiation exposure with the use of the CT scanner and fluoroscopy.[34] The ASA Statement on Nonoperating Room Anesthesia Services recommends adequate radiation protection using lead wraparound aprons, thyroid shields, and a mobile clear lead glass shield.[32] Although not included in the statement, proper eye protection should be used due to the high vulnerability of the eyes to radiation.[35] The anesthesia provider should also increase their distance from the radiation source whenever possible, as the radiation dose is calculated using inverse square law $(1/d^2)$.[35]

## ■ PATIENT SELECTION CONSIDERATIONS

A particular challenge in NORA locations is proper patient selection and optimization because these patients may present to the ASC without screening in a presurgical testing clinic, which would typically include documentation of a preanesthesia medical history and airway evaluation. One way to improve preprocedural awareness of pertinent patient comorbidities is to ensure that the patient is scheduled at the appropriate and safe IR location (hospital vs. outpatient) based on standardized electronic preprocedure screening surveys. In 2021, Memorial Sloan Kettering Cancer Center (MSKCC) implemented a pilot survey to assess patient comorbidities before their IR procedures. The survey was built into the clinical workflow and sent to the patients through a secure online portal. If a patient responded "yes" to any of the screening questions (e.g., presence of shortness of breath), a clinician would follow up with the patient and discuss potential concerns with the anesthesia and IR teams. This quality improvement initiative successfully increased preprocedure awareness of pertinent medical information, including airway concerns, before the procedure and ensured appropriate scheduling location, patient optimization, and readiness. The project also improved collaboration among the multidisciplinary team members.[36] Similar initiatives involving patient responses in the selection process have since been expanded to all procedures requiring NORA within our inpatient and outpatient healthcare system.

Patient selection guidelines vary among ambulatory settings. They consider the surgical setting, facility resources, procedure, personnel, patient comorbidities, and anesthetic requirements.[37] Some facilities may have strict exclusion criteria, such as an ASA physical status score of 3 or 4, advanced age, high body mass index (BMI), or obstructive sleep apnea (OSA) status.[38-41] Please refer to the chapter 2 discussing patients with obesity and OSA in the ASC in this book for details regarding patient selection for these particular patients. Patients with a high comorbidity burden, including ASA physical status scores of 3 and 4, have increasingly been cared for in ambulatory surgery settings.[42] Rather than using absolute criteria, a patient's comorbidity status, procedure type, and anesthetic requirements should be evaluated to determine the appropriateness of the procedure for an ASC.[43]

Anesthesia providers are trained in the perioperative management of medically complex patients. They can set the standard of patient safety for IR procedures at freestanding ASCs as increasingly medically complex patients are considered for those settings. For example, patients with considerable comorbidity burden may undergo palliative procedures, such as pleural or peritoneal catheter placements. Still, they may not be considered appropriate for other procedures (e.g., bilateral mastectomy) in the ASC setting. In addition, it may not be possible to optimize patients scheduled for procedures such as paracentesis and thoracentesis because of the pathology causing them to need that particular IR procedure. Continued collaboration between the anesthesia and IR teams is essential to ensure that high-risk patients receive their procedures safely in freestanding outpatient facilities. If the multidisciplinary team agrees that a patient is at an elevated risk for a complication, the procedure should be scheduled for an IR suite in the hospital setting.

To our knowledge, no standard patient selection guidelines exist for ambulatory IR procedures. Ambulatory surgical literature on patient selection may help deliver medically appropriate practice. A comprehensive review by Rajan et al. includes several recommendations for ambulatory surgery patients. The authors recommend that patients with an ASA physical status score of 4 with stable comorbidities, those who have a BMI >50 kg/m$^2$ without severe cardiopulmonary comorbidities, or those who are optimized while on dialysis for end-stage renal disease may be acceptable candidates for low-risk ambulatory procedures. Age alone is not recommended as an exclusion criterion. Instead, the authors suggest looking at other comorbidities, such as frailty. Patients should be screened for OSA, and positive airway pressure is encouraged whenever indicated. A multimodal analgesic approach is also encouraged for patients with OSA to minimize opioid use. Symptomatic cardiac patients or those with a recent stent, myocardial infarction, stroke, or transient ischemic attack may require optimization or a waiting period before undergoing an ambulatory procedure. Patients with severe chronic obstructive pulmonary disease or unstable metabolic conditions, such as diabetic ketoacidosis, may require exclusion.[44]

The Society for Ambulatory Anesthesia (SAMBA) Cataract Guidelines may also provide valuable criteria for scheduling patients for IR procedures in the ASC. Like outpatient IR procedures, cataract procedures usually pose a low risk of complications and have comparable anesthesia care (local anesthesia with sedation). Additionally, cataract surgery patients typically have a high comorbidity burden. The guidelines state that if a patient can tolerate the required position for the length of the procedure, then the patient may be at an acceptable risk for the ASC except for a subset of major medical issues, including cardiac, respiratory, neurologic, and diabetic issues, many of which overlap with the Rajan et al.[44] **Figure 3** lists the exclusion criteria based on the SAMBA Cataract Guidelines.[45]

Patients with known or suspected difficult airways may be candidates for an IR procedure in the ASC. If available, the anesthesiologist should collaborate with the patient's head and neck surgeon to discuss the airway, including the difficulty of intubation and mask ventilation. Complicated emergency airway equipment should be readily available per the 2022 ASA Practice Guidelines for Management of the Difficult Airway.[46] Although most outpatient IR procedures may be successful with sedation and local anesthesia injection, a backup plan is vital in case the patient requires airway protection or a deeper level of anesthesia. If a head and neck surgeon has regularly scheduled OR days at the facility, IR patients with a high-risk airway should be planned for those days. The surgeon can then serve as a qualified backup care team member in an airway emergency.

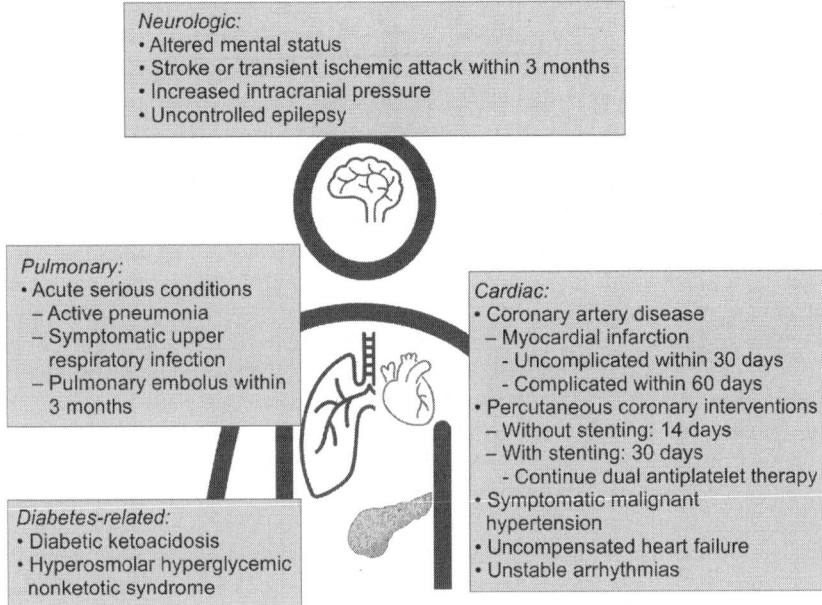

**Fig. 3:** Patient exclusion criteria for outpatient IR procedures in the ASC based on the Society for Ambulatory Anesthesia Cataract Guidelines.[45] (ASC: ambulatory surgery center; IR: interventional radiology)

The IR team should maintain separate patient selection criteria to optimize patients from the proceduralist perspective. Laboratory value requirements, such as platelets and coagulation results, and procedure bleeding risk should also be considered, primarily if the ASC is located a considerable distance from the designated transfer hospital and does not have emergency blood products. The Society of Interventional Radiology provides consensus guidelines for managing thrombotic and bleeding risk in patients undergoing percutaneous image-guided interventions.[47] However, specific outpatient risk stratification guidelines should be developed to determine the location for the procedure, either in the hospital or in the ambulatory site. For procedures involving biopsies, the location and size of the lesion must be evaluated by the interventional radiologist. Lesions with an elevated risk of bleeding should be performed in the hospital setting. As stated earlier, low-risk procedures may not require a formal clinic visit. However, for high-risk procedures or patients with significant comorbidities, a clinic visit with an interventional physician or a nurse practitioner may be needed before the scheduled procedure.

## ANESTHESIA CARE FOR INTERVENTIONAL RADIOLOGY IN THE AMBULATORY SURGERY CENTER

The goal of anesthesia care for IR in freestanding ASCs is safety with rapid recovery. Patients undergoing IR procedures may receive local, general, anxiolytic, opioid, or regional anesthesia.[48] Many patients may comfortably undergo outpatient IR procedures with a sedation anesthetic plus local or regional anesthesia because of the speed and minimally invasive nature of the outpatient IR procedures. The anesthesia care plan for a patient undergoing an IR procedure is established after the anesthesiologist and interventional radiologist discuss the level of sedation necessary for procedural success. To determine the strategy for safe anesthesia, the team should consider the patient factors such as medical condition and functional status as well as procedure-related factors, including the length of the procedure, level of procedural stimulation, positioning, need for procedural patient cooperation, and recovery.[49]

The ASA Statement on Ambulatory Anesthesia and Surgery describes the basic minimum expectations for perioperative care of the ambulatory surgical patient in all ambulatory settings in the United States. Among the guidelines, the facility must have the appropriate national accreditation and state licensure.[50] All ASCs should adhere to the ASA standards, guidelines, and policies. For example, all anesthetic practices must comply with the ASA Standards for Basic Anesthetic Monitoring.[33] According to these standards, the adequacy of ventilation should be evaluated by continual observation of qualitative clinical signs during regional anesthesia with no sedation or local anesthesia with no sedation. During moderate or deep sedation, the adequacy of ventilation should be evaluated by monitoring exhaled carbon dioxide unless precluded or invalidated by the nature of the patient, procedure, or equipment.

**Table 2** includes commonly used sedatives and possible adjuvants in the outpatient setting, along with the advantages and disadvantages of each sedative. The choice of the sedative depends on the institution (availability of the formulary), patient health, and procedure. Propofol is commonly used for sedation because of its rapid onset and offset.[51,52] Sedation medications such as midazolam or remimazolam may be preferred for patients with a recent history of cardiac disease or reduced cardiac function because of the increased risk of hypotension with propofol and dexmedetomidine; for patients with pulmonary disease or OSA, midazolam, remimazolam, and dexmedetomidine may be preferred because of the lower incidence of respiratory depression compared to propofol.[51,53,54] Dexmedetomidine may be less desirable in the ambulatory setting due to its slower onset of action and recovery;[55] instead, remimazolam and propofol are preferable because of their faster onset and offset.[53] Fentanyl is typically the opioid of choice in the ASC because of its short mechanism of action.[56] Antiemetic prophylaxis may be considered for patients who have a strong history of postoperative nausea and vomiting (PONV) or who receive a higher than standard dose of fentanyl because of the risk of PONV.[57]

General anesthesia may be required for patients who are at risk for aspiration or cannot tolerate the procedure or the required position with sedation due to pain. Regional anesthesia techniques, such as peripheral nerve blocks, are commonly used in IR procedures. Peripheral nerve blocks using short- or long-acting local anesthetics can be especially useful in patients with significant cardiac disease or those hemodynamically unstable.[8]

Depending on the IR setting, administration of sedation or analgesia may be provided by the IR physician, nurse, or licensed independent practitioner under the supervision of a physician. The Practice Parameter for Minimal and/or Moderate Sedation/Analgesia, published by the American College of Radiology and Society of Interventional Radiology, discusses the requirements for delivering sedation and analgesia by practicing interventional radiologists. Patients with an ASA physical

**TABLE 2:** Typical sedation medications for outpatient IR procedures in the freestanding ambulatory surgery center.

| Sedative Medication | Advantages of Primary Sedative | Disadvantages of Primary Sedative | Possible Adjuvant Medication |
|---|---|---|---|
| Propofol | • Rapid onset<br>• Rapid wake-up<br>• Ready to use | • Hypotension<br>• Respiratory depression<br>• No reversal agent<br>• Pain on injection | • Fentanyl<br>• Midazolam |
| Midazolam | • Anxiolytic effect<br>• Less likely to cause respiratory depression<br>• Ready to use<br>• Reversal agent available | • May have a prolonged effect<br>• Slow recovery<br>• Slower onset | Fentanyl |
| Remimazolam | • Anxiolytic effect<br>• Less likely to cause cardiovascular depression<br>• Less likely to cause respiratory depression<br>• Rapid onset<br>• Rapid wake-up<br>• Reversal agent available | • Expensive<br>• Requires reconstitution | Fentanyl |
| Dexmedetomidine | • Analgesic effect<br>• Anxiolytic effect<br>• Minimal respiratory depression | • Bradycardia<br>• Hypotension<br>• May have a prolonged recovery<br>• Slow onset | • Fentanyl<br>• Midazolam |

*Note:* Information from the table is based on references 51–54.

status score of 1 or 2 qualify for sedation or analgesia outside the OR by personnel other than anesthesiologists. Requirements for consultation with an anesthesiologist include patients with an ASA physical status score of 3 or 4 or Mallampati Class III or IV. However, the parameter states that nonanesthesiology sedation personnel should have a low threshold to consult an anesthesiologist.[58]

## ■ SCHEDULING AND EFFICIENCY CONSIDERATIONS

The ASA Statement on Nonoperating Room Anesthesia Services emphasizes the need for efficient scheduling. Cases that require anesthesia services and cases that do not should not be interspersed.[32] At our facility, nonanesthesia cases performed with local anesthesia only are scheduled after cases requiring anesthesia team care to ensure that priority is given to patients needed to fast before their procedure.

Because ASC recovery hours are limited compared to hospital-based IR suites, scheduling efficiency and practical resource utilization are necessary to avoid after-hours PACU stays. A patient-centered approach with a goal of resource efficiency should be utilized when planning the IR schedule.[59] Consider placing patients that may require longer recovery times, such as the elderly or those with OSA, earlier in the day to allow adequate recovery times during regular PACU hours. Other considerations that influence case order include high-risk procedures, such as liver biopsies, being scheduled earlier in the day. In contrast, low-risk procedures, such as central vascular access procedures, are planned for later in the day. Computerized predictive models may be developed to assist with case sequencing.[60]

## ■ POSTOPERATIVE CARE

A meaningful way to increase efficiency involves including a centralized area for all NORA patients' preoperative and postoperative care rooms.[25] The PACU should be near the IR suite.[32] Ensuring patients undergoing IR or OR procedures can recover in the same PACU optimizes using the ASC space and resources. Similar to OR patients, IR patients may require specific postoperative orders to manage adverse events, including antiemetic and pain medications. Efficient discharge prevents filling the recovery room, which causes operational holds. Ensuring efficient throughput may be a scheduling challenge if many patients require postprocedural bedrest or a prolonged recovery. Our freestanding ASC offers the integration of ORs and an IR suite into a cohesive perioperative area with cross-trained perioperative nurses, eliminating staffing redundancy and allowing beds for preoperative or postoperative care based on need. Research has shown that the flexibility of cross-trained perianesthesia nurses improves patient flow with a reduction in OR holds.[61] Additionally, our facility has a centralized nursing station to optimize accessibility for the charge nurse, perioperative pharmacist, PACU advanced practice provider, and unit assistant.

Postprocedural discharge requirements for IR patients may replicate requirements for postoperative OR patients. Postanesthesia discharge scoring tools are typically utilized to determine discharge readiness after ambulatory surgery. These tools evaluate the level of consciousness, pain, nausea, vomiting, and hemodynamic stability in the PACU. All patients undergoing anesthesia must have a care partner available and present to escort them home safely.[62] **Flowchart 1** depicts an example of a clinical workflow from the preoperative to the postoperative stage.

**Flowchart 1:** Example clinical workflow for IR procedures at a freestanding ASC.

| *Preoperative:* | *Intraoperative:* | *Postoperative:* |
|---|---|---|
| • IR and anesthesiology teams screen patients to minimize day of procedure cancellations<br>• Schedule complex procedures or patients for earlier case times<br>• Patient education and expectation setting | • Multimodal analgesia and local injection by proceduralist for pain management<br>• Antiemetic prophylaxis for patients with high-risk of nausea and vomiting<br>• Short-acting sedation medications | • Post-procedure medications as needed<br>• Discharge readiness monitoring with use of discharge tool<br>• Encourage discharge within 2 hours unless bedrest indicated<br>• Care partner present to escort patient home |

(ASC: ambulatory surgery center; IR: interventional radiology)

If, in rare cases, a patient experiences an acute issue that precludes discharge, the patient will require a transfer to a hospital. A transfer plan, including the designated transfer hospital and a protocol, should be in place for patients needing a higher level of care.[63] If a patient requires a transfer to an unaffiliated hospital, it would be prudent to develop a relationship or an agreement with the IR team at that hospital so that the IR physicians at both locations may work together to provide optimal and safe care.

## QUALITY IMPROVEMENT INITIATIVES AND TRACKING

Measuring safety and outcomes is essential for continued quality assurance for an IR program at ASC. Outcomes of interest may include rates of extended PACU stay, hospital transfer or unplanned admission, and procedure cancellation. Patient-reported outcomes are another way to assess the quality of care at ASCs. Postprocedural complaints, such as pain and PONV, can be evaluated with postprocedure phone calls and/or electronic surveys.[64] By examining quality metrics and patient-reported outcomes, the IR and anesthesiology teams may adapt their practice and improve the quality of care.

## CONCLUSION

Ambulatory surgery has been associated with increased efficiency and patient satisfaction while reducing costs. These same advantages could translate to an outpatient IR program in the freestanding ASC. In response to the growing demand for comprehensive outpatient cancer care, our freestanding ambulatory suburban facility incorporated an IR suite next to the OR location. The center was designed to accommodate anesthesia services, ensuring a spacious and intuitive layout. The IR program increases patient access and efficiency, allowing patients to undergo IR procedures close to their homes. This chapter has provided a template for clinicians and administrators seeking to design a high-volume outpatient IR service with anesthesia care in a freestanding surgery center.

## REFERENCES

1. Mashar M, Nanapragasam A, Haslam P. Interventional radiology training: where will technology take us? BJR Open. 2019;1(1):20190002.
2. Wells RD. Ambulatory care in interventional radiology: a framework for radiology daycase. Clin Radiol. 2022;77(7):489-95.
3. Cazzato RL, de Rubeis G, de Marini P, Auloge P, Dalili D, Weiss J, et al. Interventional Radiology Outpatient Clinics (IROC): Clinical Impact and Patient Satisfaction. Cardiovasc Intervent Radiol. 2021;44(1):118-26.
4. Nagrebetsky A, Gabriel RA, Dutton RP, Urman RD. Growth of Nonoperating Room Anesthesia Care in the United States: A Contemporary Trends Analysis. Anesth Analg. 2017;124(4):1261-7.
5. Schoenberg SO, Attenberger UI, Solomon SB, Weissleder R. Developing a Roadmap for Interventional Oncology. Oncologist. 2018;23(10):1162-70.
6. Zener R, Demers V, Bilodeau A, Benko AJ, Abraham RJ, Wong JK, et al. Clinical IR in Canada: The Evolution of a Revolution. J Vasc Interv Radiol. 2018;29(4):524-30.e2.
7. Tsetis D, Uberoi R, Fanelli F, Roberston I, Krokidis M, van Delden O, et al. The Provision of Interventional Radiology Services in Europe: CIRSE Recommendations. Cardiovasc Intervent Radiol. 2016;39(4):500-6.
8. Wong T, Georgiadis PL, Urman RD, Tsai MH. Non-Operating Room Anesthesia: Patient Selection and Special Considerations. Local Reg Anesth. 2020;13:1-9.

9. Ambulatory Surgery Center Association. (2020). Reducing medicare costs by migrating volume from hospital outpatient departments to ambulatory surgery centers. Available from: https://www.ascassociation.org/asca/about-ascs/savings/medicare-cost-savings/reducing-medicare-costs [Last accessed July, 2024].
10. Joshi GP. Putting patients first: ambulatory surgery facilitates patient-centered care. Curr Opin Anaesthesiol. 2021;34(6):667-71.
11. White SB. Value in Interventional Radiology: Achieving High Quality Outcomes at a Lower Cost. Radiology. 2020;297(2):482-3.
12. Doherty MG. Value of Interventional Radiology: Past, Present, and Future. Semin Intervent Radiol. 2019;36(1):26-8.
13. Irvine I, Hayden R, Greene L, Ryan AG. An Update on Patient-Reported Outcomes in Interventional Radiology: The Future Measure of Our Success. Cardiovasc Intervent Radiol. 2023;46(12):1657-61.
14. Du AL, Robbins K, Waterman RS, Urman RD, Gabriel RA. National trends in nonoperating room anesthesia: procedures, facilities, and patient characteristics. Curr Opin Anaesthesiol. 2021;34(4):464-9.
15. Herman AD, Jaruzel CB, Lawton S, Tobin CD, Reves JG, Catchpole KR, et al. Morbidity, mortality, and systems safety in non-operating room anaesthesia: a narrative review. Br J Anaesth. 2021;127(5):729-44.
16. Lee S, Srinivasa RN, Patel P, Genshaft SJ, Enzmann DR. Value of Office-Based Labs to an Interventional Radiology Practice. J Clin Interven Radiol ISVIR. 2022;07:015-9.
17. Woodward ZG, Urman RD, Domino KB. Safety of Non-Operating Room Anesthesia: A Closed Claims Update. Anesthesiol Clin. 2017;35(4):569-81.
18. Chang B, Kaye AD, Diaz JH, Westlake B, Dutton RP, Urman RD. Interventional Procedures Outside of the Operating Room: Results from the National Anesthesia Clinical Outcomes Registry. J Patient Saf. 2018;14(1):9-16.
19. Baskin KM, Durack JC, Abu-Elmagd K, Doellman D, Drews BB, Journeycake JM, et al. Chronic Central Venous Access: From Research Consensus Panel to National Multistakeholder Initiative. J Vasc Interv Radiol. 2018;29(4):461-9.
20. Machat S, Eisenhuber E, Pfarl G, Stübler J, Koelblinger C, Zacherl J, et al. Complications of central venous port systems: a pictorial review. Insights Imaging. 2019;10(1):86.
21. Neuberger J, Patel J, Caldwell H, Davies S, Hebditch V, Hollywood C, et al. Guidelines on the use of liver biopsy in clinical practice from the British Society of Gastroenterology, the Royal College of Radiologists and the Royal College of Pathology. Gut. 2020; 69(8):1382-403.
22. Anzidei M, Porfiri A, Andrani F, Di Martino M, Saba L, Catalano C, et al. Imaging-guided chest biopsies: techniques and clinical results. Insights Imaging. 2017;8(4):419-28.
23. Ball M, Babu S, Wallis A, Asciak R. Promising role for pleural vent in pneumothorax following CT-guided biopsy of lung lesions. Br J Radiol. 2022;95(1135):20210965.
24. Schenker MP, Martin R, Shyn PB, Baum RA. Interventional radiology and anesthesia. Anesthesiol Clin. 2009;27(1):87-94.
25. Boggs SD, Barnett SR, Urman RD. The future of nonoperating room anesthesia in the 21st century: emphasis on quality and safety. Curr Opin Anaesthesiol. 2017;30(6):644-51.
26. Missant C, Van de Velde M. Morbidity and mortality related to anaesthesia outside the operating room. Curr Opin Anaesthesiol. 2004;17(4):323-7.
27. Melloni C. Morbidity and mortality related to anesthesia outside the operating room. Minerva Anestesiol. 2005;71(6):325-34.
28. Metzner J, Domino KB. Risks of anesthesia or sedation outside the operating room: the role of the anesthesia care provider. Curr Opin Anaesthesiol. 2010;23(4):523-31.
29. Metzner J, Posner KL, Domino KB. The risk and safety of anesthesia at remote locations: the US closed claims analysis. Curr Opin Anaesthesiol. 2009;22(4):502-8.

30. Melloni C. Anesthesia and sedation outside the operating room: how to prevent risk and maintain good quality. Curr Opin Anaesthesiol. 2007;20(6):513-9.
31. Van De Velde M, Kuypers M, Teunkens A, Devroe S. Risk and safety of anesthesia outside the operating room. Minerva Anestesiol. 2009;75(5):345-8.
32. American Society of Anesthesiologists. (1994). Statement on Nonoperating Room Anesthesia Services. Available from: https://www.asahq.org/standards-and-practice-parameters/statement-on-nonoperating-room-anesthesia-services [Last accessed July, 2024].
33. American Society of Anesthesiologists. (2021). Standards for Basic Anesthetic Monitoring. Available from: https://www.asahq.org/standards-and-practice-parameters/standards-for-basic-anesthetic-monitoring [Last accessed July, 2024].
34. Ismail S, Khan F, Sultan N, Naqvi M. Radiation exposure to anaesthetists during interventional radiology. Anaesthesia. 2010;65(1):54-60.
35. Wang RR, Kumar AH, Tanaka P, Macario A. Occupational Radiation Exposure of Anesthesia Providers: A Summary of Key Learning Points and Resident-Led Radiation Safety Projects. Semin Cardiothorac Vasc Anesth. 2017;21(2):165-71.
36. Kotin A, Barnett KM, Liu TJ, Maresca N, Serafin J. Use of Preprocedure Questionnaire for Oncologic Interventional Radiology Patients to Enhance Patient Safety and Ensure Appropriate Procedure Scheduling and Location. American Society of Anesthesiologists Annual Meeting, San Francisco, CA, 2023.
37. Rajan N. The high-risk patient for ambulatory surgery. Curr Opin Anaesthesiol. 2020;33(6):724-31.
38. Bailey CR, Ahuja M, Bartholomew K, Bew S, Forbes L, Lipp A, et al. Guidelines for day-case surgery 2019: Guidelines from the Association of Anaesthetists and the British Association of Day Surgery. Anaesthesia. 2019;74(6):778-92.
39. Lee JH. Anesthesia for ambulatory surgery. Korean J Anesthesiol. 2017;70(4):398-406.
40. Szeto B, Vertosick EA, Ruiz K, Tokita H, Vickers A, Assel M, et al. Outcomes and Safety Among Patients With Obstructive Sleep Apnea Undergoing Cancer Surgery Procedures in a Freestanding Ambulatory Surgical Facility. Anesth Analg. 2019;129(2):360-8.
41. Vertosick EA, Assel M, Tokita HK, Zafirova Z, Vickers AJ, Simon BA, et al. Suitability of outpatient or ambulatory extended recovery cancer surgeries for obese patients. J Clin Anesth. 2019;58:111-6.
42. Walsh MT. Improving outcomes in ambulatory anesthesia by identifying high risk patients. Curr Opin Anaesthesiol. 2018;31(6):659-66.
43. Kataria T, Cutter TW, Apfelbaum JL. Patient selection in outpatient surgery. Clin Plast Surg. 2013;40(3):371-82.
44. Rajan N, Rosero EB, Joshi GP. Patient Selection for Adult Ambulatory Surgery: A Narrative Review. Anesth Analg. 2021;133(6):1415-30.
45. Sweitzer B, Rajan N, Schell D, Gayer S, Eckert S, Joshi GP. Preoperative Care for Cataract Surgery: The Society for Ambulatory Anesthesia Position Statement. Anesth Analg. 2021;133(6):1431-6.
46. Apfelbaum JL, Hagberg CA, Connis RT, Abdelmalak BB, Agarkar M, Dutton RP, et al. 2022 American Society of Anesthesiologists Practice Guidelines for Management of the Difficult Airway. Anesthesiology. 2022;136(1):31-81.
47. Patel IJ, Rahim S, Davidson JC, Hanks SE, Tam AL, Walker TG, et al. Society of Interventional Radiology Consensus Guidelines for the Periprocedural Management of Thrombotic and Bleeding Risk in Patients Undergoing Percutaneous Image-Guided Interventions-Part II: Recommendations: Endorsed by the Canadian Association for Interventional Radiology and the Cardiovascular and Interventional Radiological Society of Europe. J Vasc Interv Radiol. 2019;30(8):1168-84.e1.
48. Moran TC, Kaye AD, Mai AH, Bok LR. Sedation, analgesia, and local anesthesia: a review for general and interventional radiologists. Radiographics. 2013;33(2):E47-60.

49. Rubin D. Anesthesia for ambulatory diagnostic and therapeutic radiology procedures. Anesthesiol Clin. 2014;32(2):371-80.
50. American Society of Anesthesiologists. (2003). Statement on ambulatory anesthesia and surgery. Available from: https://www.asahq.org/standards-and-practice-parameters/statement-on-ambulatory-anesthesia-and-surgery [Last accessed July, 2024].
51. Khorsand S, Karamchandani K, Joshi GP. Sedation-analgesia techniques for nonoperating room anesthesia: an update. Curr Opin Anaesthesiol. 2022;35(4):450-6.
52. Sneyd JR, Absalom AR, Barends CRM, Jones JB. Hypotension during propofol sedation for colonoscopy: a retrospective exploratory analysis and meta-analysis. Br J Anaesth. 2022;128(4):610-22.
53. Kilpatrick GJ. Remimazolam: Non-Clinical and Clinical Profile of a New Sedative/Anesthetic Agent. Front Pharmacol. 2021;12:690875.
54. Fonseca FJ, Ferreira L, Rouxinol-Dias AL, Mourão J. Effects of dexmedetomidine in non-operating room anesthesia in adults: a systematic review with meta-analysis. Braz J Anesthesiol. 2023;73(5):641-64.
55. Mahmoud M, Mason KP. Dexmedetomidine: review, update, and future considerations of paediatric perioperative and periprocedural applications and limitations. Br J Anaesth. 2015;115(2):171-82.
56. Abebe MM, Arefayne NR, Temesgen MM, Admass BA. Evidence-based perioperative pain management protocol for day case surgery in a resource limited setting: Systematic review. Ann Med Surg (Lond). 2022;80:104322.
57. Mauermann E, Clamer D, Ruppen W, Bandschapp O. Association between intraoperative fentanyl dosing and postoperative nausea/vomiting and pain: A prospective cohort study. Eur J Anaesthesiol. 2019;36(11):871-80.
58. American College of Radiology-Society of Interventional Radiology. (2020). The practice parameter for minimal and/or moderate sedation/analgesia. Available from: https://www.acr.org/-/media/ACR/Files/Practice-Parameters/Sed-Analgesia.pdf [Last accessed July, 2024].
59. Pash J, Kadry B, Bugrara S, Macario A. Scheduling of procedures and staff in an ambulatory surgery center. Anesthesiol Clin. 2014;32(2):517-27.
60. Tully JL, Zhong W, Simpson S, Curran BP, Macias AA, Waterman RS, et al. Machine Learning Prediction Models to Reduce Length of Stay at Ambulatory Surgery Centers Through Case Resequencing. J Med Syst. 2023;47(1):71.
61. Douglas TLK, Miller TMN, Mouradjian D, Snow TM. Comprehensive Perioperative Cross-training: The Benefits of Optimizing Staffing. J PeriAnesthes Nurs. 2023;38(4):e17.
62. Rohi A, Olofsson MET, Jakobsson JG. Ambulatory anesthesia and discharge: an update around guidelines and trends. Curr Opin Anaesthesiol. 2022;35(6):691-7.
63. Twersky RS, Philip BK. Handbook of Ambulatory Anesthesia: Springer New York; 2008.
64. Glowka L, Tanella A, Hyman JB. Quality indicators and outcomes in ambulatory surgery. Curr Opin Anaesthesiol. 2023;36(6):624-9.

# CHAPTER 2

# Patients with Obesity and Obstructive Sleep Apnea in the Ambulatory Surgery Center

*Kelly Lebak*

## ABSTRACT

Patients with obesity and/or obstructive sleep apnea (OSA) are increasing in number, as are surgeries at ambulatory surgery centers (ASCs). A common belief is that these patients need to be better candidates for surgery at ASCs. There may be an increased risk for perioperative complications in certain patients with obesity and/or OSA. However, body mass index (BMI) nor OSA alone are likely the sole reasons for exclusion from surgery at an ASC. This chapter will discuss the selection of patients with obesity and OSA for surgery at ASCs.

**Keywords:** Obesity; Obstructive sleep apnea; Ambulatory surgery; Ambulatory surgery center; Patient selection

## KEY POINTS

- Body mass index (BMI) alone may not be the best reason to exclude patients from specific ambulatory surgery center (ASC) surgeries.
- Obstructive sleep apnea (OSA) alone should not be the sole reason to exclude patients from surgery at ASCs.
- Patient selection for patients with obesity and/or OSA for surgery at ASCs is a complex decision involving facility resources and capabilities, patient comorbidities and home support, proposed surgery, and anesthetic technique.

## ■ INTRODUCTION

The number of patients with obesity is increasing, with 25% of the Indian population having obesity in 2021.[1] As ambulatory surgery rises in number, it is likely that the number of patients with obesity presenting for surgery at ambulatory surgery centers (ASCs) will also increase.

This paper will describe patient selection strategies and anesthetic planning for patients with obesity and/or obstructive sleep apnea (OSA) who present for procedures in ASCs. It will address considerations of facility capabilities, surgical procedures, anesthetic techniques, and patient comorbidities.

## ■ OBESITY

Obesity has been suggested to have severe perioperative implications, including predictors of readmission and postoperative pulmonary embolus,[2] deep vein thrombosis, reintubation, myocardial infarction, septic shock, death, wound disruption,[3] and increased incidence of difficult mask ventilation.[4] Notably, Moon et al.[4] found that although patients with obesity have a higher incidence of difficult mask ventilation, they did *not* have a higher incidence of difficult *intubation*.

When deciding if patients with obesity can be done at an ASC, consider the quartet of:
- Facility type
- Surgical procedure
- Anesthetic technique
- Patient comorbidities

To the chagrin of surgeons, their schedulers, and anesthesiologists, sometimes it is a case-by-case basis to determine if a patient with obesity should proceed at an ASC as it is often a complex interplay of those four pillars. For example, can a patient with a body mass index (BMI) of 60 kg/m$^2$ with severe OSA, severe chronic obstructive pulmonary disease on 2 liters of oxygen, with a left ventricular ejection fraction of 30%, proceed with cataract surgery at a hospital-based outpatient department? If those comorbidities are optimized and the patient can lie flat for the procedure duration of 45 minutes with topical anesthesia and minimal sedation, the answer is likely yes.[5] What if a patient with a BMI of 50 kg/m$^2$ and severe OSA was scheduled for an open ventral hernia repair at a free-standing ASC? This presents a more significant challenge to answer as it depends on the facility's capabilities and equipment and the possible need for opioids postoperatively.

## Facility Type

"Ambulatory anesthesia" implies discharge within 24 hours of the procedure. Ambulatory procedures may be performed at multiple locations. The common sites are:
- Hospital-operated outpatient departments that have outpatient surgeries and procedures.
- Ambulatory extended recovery facilities with fewer than a 24-hour stay for surgeries and procedures.
- Office-based locations are not licensed as ASCs, where routine patient visits, surgeries, and procedures can occur.
- Free-standing ASCs that are often remote from an emergency room, hospital, ancillary services and/or support, including radiology, lab, or a blood bank.

For the sake of simplicity, this paper will focus primarily on free-standing ASCs.

Aside from facility *type*, the facility needs to have the appropriate equipment and resources to safely care for patients with obesity,[6] including correctly fitting stretchers, operating room (OR) tables, wheelchairs (and enough space and door widths to accommodate entry, exit, and turning), scales, gowns (to promote pulmonary excursion and prevent restrictive effects), socks (to prevent falls), blood pressure cuffs, tourniquets, needles, positioning equipment, etc. Ultrasound is ubiquitous these days, but it must be ensured that staff are comfortable using it for nerve blocks, difficult intravenous line placement, etc. Ensure that there are enough staff and/or lifting devices to move obese patients from the stretcher to and from the OR table to the stretcher to a wheelchair and personal vehicles.

Surgical equipment should be appropriately sized for patients with obesity.[6] After induction of general anesthesia, it is less than an optimal time to discover that the ASC does not have long enough scissors and speculums for a hysteroscopy and dilation and curettage. Additionally, ensure the availability of longer laparoscopic trocars, graspers, and retractors for abdominal procedures.[6]

The availability of difficult airway equipment[7] is imperative, as is its ease of accessibility and organization—an ASC with a skeleton staff encountering a difficult airway should be ready and prepared. Consider having positive airway pressure therapy and high-flow oxygen systems,[8] which many consider essential when caring for patients with obesity. Lastly, it is imperative to have transfer agreements to a hospital that can take critically-ill patients with obesity if escalation of care is required.

## Surgical Procedure

The type of surgical procedure is of utmost importance, though there is not overwhelming evidence in the literature to distinguish which methods are appropriate for an ASC. Two studies suggested a BMI cutoff for joint arthroscopy[9] and tonsillectomy,[10] but others have not concluded this.[11-17] "Surgery-specific" cutoffs have been recommended by Gabriel et al.[10] to be a better system as they found that patients with a BMI >40 kg/m$^2$ getting a tonsillectomy were at increased risk for readmission. It seems prudent for patients with obesity to undergo peripheral procedures that allow regional anesthesia (e.g., eyes, hands, or feet) or other methods that require minimal to no opioids postoperatively in an ASC. If airway surgeries or abdominal procedures (e.g., laparoscopic cholecystectomy) are proposed, one should proceed cautiously while weighing the three remaining pillars: patient comorbidities, anesthetic technique, and facility capabilities.

## Anesthetic Technique

In an ASC, optimally, the primary anesthetic consists of regional anesthesia whenever possible to avoid the cardiac and respiratory effects of anesthetics, particularly opioids.[18,19] Regional anesthesia used alone additionally avoids manipulation of the airway. If sedation is needed, the use of short-acting anesthetics is preferred. Less may be more in this population to prevent mortality and morbidity postdischarge. One newer promising anesthetic is remimazolam, which is an ultra-short-acting benzodiazepine. Like remifentanil, it is metabolized by nonspecific tissue esterases and thus has rapid offset and a short context-sensitive half-life, causing less cardiopulmonary compromise than midazolam.[20,21] Zhang et al.[22] found that its use in patients with obesity, along with esketamine, can reduce severe hypoxemia during endoscopy compared with propofol and esketamine.

Opioid-free techniques are appealing to patients with obesity. One study out of India[23] found that respiratory depression was more common in the opioid-based group and that postoperative analgesic needs and postanesthesia care unit (PACU) discharge duration were significantly less in the total intravenous anesthesia opioid-free group (using propofol, dexmedetomidine, lignocaine, and ketamine) in patients undergoing laparoscopic urological procedures.

Lastly, consider using enhanced recovery after surgery (ERAS) protocols,[24] which are multimodal care pathways designed to improve postoperative outcomes. The goal is to reduce the stress of surgery on the body and maintain or at least achieve normal physiology as soon as possible postoperatively. Pain control is one of the pillars of ERAS, with emphasis on regional anesthesia and minimalization of opioids.[25] Common components of ERAS used in ambulatory anesthesia[26] that also have an added benefit in patients with obesity include consumption of clear fluids up to 2 hours before arrival, aggressive postoperative nausea and vomiting prevention (e.g., dexamethasone, ondansetron, aprepitant, and a dopamine antagonist), and multimodal analgesia (e.g., regional anesthesia, acetaminophen, and anti-inflammatory medications or cyclooxygenase-2 specific inhibitors).

## Patient Comorbidities

In 2013, Joshi et al.[27] published a sizeable systemic review, which is considered the seminal paper on patients with obesity undergoing ambulatory surgery and anesthesia. They concluded that:
- BMI *alone* did *not* influence perioperative complications or unplanned admission after ambulatory surgery.
- BMI <40 kg/m$^2$ can proceed at an ACS if comorbid conditions are "well controlled", including hypertension, arrhythmias, right and left heart failure, cerebrovascular disease, and metabolic syndrome (see in the following text).
- BMI 40–50 kg/m$^2$ should have a detailed preoperative assessment to identify obesity-related comorbidities that *could* otherwise *exclude* the patient from surgery at an ASC, including OSA, obesity-related hypoventilation syndrome, pulmonary hypertension, uncontrolled hypertension or heart failure, and coronary artery disease.
- BMI >50 kg/m$^2$ "should be chosen carefully" as there may be a higher incidence of perioperative mortality and morbidity, as noted earlier.

At least nine studies have since examined ambulatory surgery in patients with obesity. Though all have limitations, the authors concluded that BMI alone may be a cutoff for select procedures.[9,10] But the majority concluded that BMI alone should not necessarily be used as an exclusion for surgery at an ASC[11-17] as long as comorbidities are controlled and the patients are carefully selected.

Comorbidities that are associated with obesity and thus should be controlled in patients having ambulatory surgery which include OSA, heart failure, metabolic syndrome (hypertension, hypertriglyceridemia, hypoalphalipoproteinemia, hypercholesterolemia, and diabetes),[28] pulmonary hypertension, nonalcoholic fatty liver disease, nonalcoholic steatohepatitis, gastroesophageal reflux disease,[29] arrhythmias, and coronary heart disease.[30]

Generally, *where* patients carry their weight matters more than how much they weigh or their BMI because lean muscle and body fat are not accounted for differently in the calculation of BMI.[31,32] In the "apple" body shape, most of the weight is above the waistline, and in the pear shape, most is below the waistline. Pulmonary excursion and mechanics are reduced in the apple shape, which has profound implications, particularly during anesthetic induction, emergence, and recovery.[33] Additionally, neck assessment is vital. If there is a large amount of adipose around the external neck, the chin may appear micrognathic. This is more concerning than when there is less adipose around the neck.

In summary, patients with obesity should not necessarily be excluded from surgery at ASCs, nor should there be an absolute BMI cutoff per se. Though it is more labor intensive for all involved, patients, surgeons, anesthesiologists, hospital systems, and population health should consider the whole picture when deciding if a patient with obesity can have surgery at an ASC. All four aspects of surgery location, surgery, anesthetic type, and patient comorbidities should be considered.

## ◼ OBSTRUCTIVE SLEEP APNEA

One common comorbidity in patients with obesity is OSA. The most recent prevalence estimate in India was 13.5%, equating to over 190,080,000 people. The vast majority of patients are untreated or undiagnosed.[34] The risk of OSA is increased with increasing BMI[4,35,] with up to 90% of people with a BMI over 40 kg/m$^2$ having OSA.[36,37] There is an association between patients with a high risk of OSA and adverse preoperative outcomes, including a 4-fold higher increased likelihood of postoperative complications[38] with a 3-4-fold higher risk of difficult intubation, mask ventilation, or both,[39] Still, given this, it is essential to note that it is difficult to determine *causation*.[40] It is also important to note that outcomes such as hypoxemia, oxygen desaturation, supplemental oxygen use postextubation, reintubation, etc., are mere "surrogate" outcomes and do not necessarily lead to clinically significant outcomes such as the need for readmission, surgical airway, brain injury, myocardial infarction, death, etc.[40] At least one recent study has looked at brain damage and death postoperatively in patients with OSA.[41] Most critical events occurred within the first 24 hours postoperatively, with 21% occurring at home. Additionally, vital events were more likely to happen when both opioids and sedative agents were administered within 24 hours of the event. The authors concluded that ambulatory surgery patients will "potentially be at risk for catastrophic outcomes after discharge", and thus, discharge criteria must be carefully considered for patients with OSA.

The American College of Surgeons National Surgical Quality Improvement Program (ACS-NSQIP) is a validated risk-adjusted database that quantifies 30-day surgical outcomes and includes data from 700 hospitals. This database was used to examine outcomes for patients who had surgery in an outpatient setting. Rosero and Joshi[42] found that complications and 30-day readmissions for patients with OSA are low, and there are no significant differences between inpatients and outpatients for 30-day readmissions, reoperations, or complications.

Undiagnosed OSA is common (between 60 and 90% of patients)[43] and can lead to perioperative side effects. For example, a recent study in India[44] found that the STOP-Bang questionnaire can be effectively used to predict a difficult airway with scores ≥3 having a significantly higher risk of having difficult mask ventilation, difficult intubation, and sustaining airway bleeding and pharyngeal or teeth injuries. Because underdiagnosis of OSA is common, the Society for Ambulatory Anesthesia (SAMBA)[40] and the Society of Anesthesia and Sleep Medicine (SASM)[45] recommend screening *all* patients. The SAMBA recommends the STOP-Bang screening tool as it has a high sensitivity in detecting OSA. The STOP-Bang screening questionnaire has eight criteria, each positive worth one point: snoring loudly, tiredness, observed apneas, hypertension, BMI >35 kg/m$^2$, age >50 years, neck circumference >40 cm, and male sex. Patients with a score of ≥5 are considered to have a high risk of a moderate-to-severe diagnosis of OSA and, thus, an assumed diagnosis of OSA.[46] Per the SASM, a score of >3 warrants further workup for OSA *if* the patient presents with hypoxia or uncontrolled comorbidities.[45] Thus, ambulatory surgery should likely *not* be held to get a preoperative polysomnogram if other comorbidities are optimized and any postoperative pain can be managed with minimal opioids.[40,45]

When determining if patients with OSA can or should have surgery at an ASC, the American Society of Anesthesiologists[47] recommends first determining if the surgery can be done as an outpatient. Considerations akin to those for patients with obesity in an ASC should be considered. Does the facility have the availability of:
- Difficult airway equipment
- Respiratory care equipment
- Ancillary capabilities, including radiology and laboratory facilities
- A transfer agreement with an inpatient facility

In addition, does the patient have a responsible person at home to help and observe them and get medical attention if necessary? If any of these answers are "NO", it may not be reasonable to proceed with surgery at an ASC.

There is a lack of evidence on the types of surgery a patient with OSA can undergo in an ASC. Still, as with patients with obesity, it may be prudent to assume that extremity surgery and those that do not require postoperative and postdischarge opioids are acceptable. A consensus recommendation in 2019[48] found that outpatient airway surgeries could include nasal, minimally invasive palate, or base of the tongue surgeries because significant airway swelling and hemorrhage[49] may worsen OSA complications.[40] A newer systemic review in patients with moderate to severe OSA suggested that carefully selected patients could safely undergo nasal and/or palate-pharyngeal surgery.[50,51]

The SAMBA consensus statement on preoperative selection of adult patients with OSA scheduled for ambulatory surgery[40] can determine whether patients with diagnosed or presumed OSA can proceed with surgery at an ASC. Patients should have all comorbidities optimized, be able and willing to use positive airway pressure (PAP) therapy postdischarge, and have postoperative pain controlled with mostly nonopioid medications. The crucial determination is whether comorbidities, including hypertension, arrhythmias, heart failure, cerebrovascular disease, and metabolic syndrome, are optimized or not. If not, patients may not be good candidates for ambulatory surgery. If patients are *presumed* to have OSA with controlled or optimized comorbidities *and* postoperative pain can be controlled with minimal or no opioids, then they can likely proceed. If patients *have* OSA and use PAP support, and their comorbidities are controlled, they can also likely proceed.

Patients with OSA should be encouraged to use PAP treatment before surgery as this can improve ventilatory and cardiac function, particularly in obese patients with severe OSA.[47,52,53] Patients with a mandibular advancement device should also be encouraged to use it as there is some evidence that this, like the use of PAP, improves left ventricular hypertrophy which is common in OSA patients.[54]

Patients may report that their OSA resolved with bariatric surgery and/or a large amount of weight loss, corrective surgery such as uvulo-palato-pharyngoplasty, mandibular advancement, etc. Unless they have had a polysomnogram after surgery or weight loss, they should still be considered to have OSA[47], as even with these interventions, there can still be some residual, possibly clinically significant, OSA.

The OSA alters the perception of pain and can lead to hyperalgesia through hypoxemia, sleep fragmentation, and chemoreflex dysfunction. These increase hypoxia-inducible factor 1 alpha, insulin growth factor binding protein, prostaglandin E2, tumor necrosis factor-alpha, interleukin-6, and interleukin-8 activity at the nociceptors.[55] This overexpression of opioid receptor activity also leads to the increased side effects of respiratory depression and response to opioid medications.[55] Opioid use in patients with OSA may decrease upper airway function through the hypoglossal motor nucleus, which could exacerbate OSA.[38,56] Opioids also impair the chemoreceptor responses to hypoxia and hypercarbia, thereby abolishing the normal arousal reflex.[38] At worst, this can result in respiratory arrest and death. Given this, opioids play a pivotal role in determining if a patient with OSA can safely undergo surgery at an ASC.

If surgery proceeds at an ASC, scheduling the patient with OSA early in the day is prudent due to the risk of delayed discharge.[11] Patients should be monitored "until they are no longer at risk of postoperative respiratory depression".[47] This will allow for prolonged monitoring if needed, mainly when opioids are administered, while still working within a "tight" workforce as many ASCs are staffed.

The SASM, the SAMBA, and the Society of Critical Care Anesthesiologists are working on a combined statement on guidance for patients with sleep apnea, explicitly addressing postoperative and postdischarge care. It will be evidence-based guidance to safely and efficiently care for OSA patients throughout the perioperative timeline, so stay tuned!

## ■ CONCLUSION

Patients with obesity and sleep apnea are increasing in India. As ambulatory surgery rises in number, so will the number of patients with obesity presenting for surgery at ASCs. This paper described how to determine if/when patients with obesity and/or OSA can be safely done in ASCs and safe anesthetic plans for them. Facility capabilities, surgical procedures, anesthetic techniques, and patient comorbidities must be taken into consideration, when deciding if patients with OSA and/or obesity are appropriate candidates for surgery at an ASC, not just the presence of OSA and/or a high BMI.

## ■ REFERENCES

1. International Institute for Population Sciences (IIPS) and ICF (2021). National Family Health Survey (NFHS-5), 2019-21. Available from: https://main.mohfw.gov.in/sites/default/files/NFHS-5_Phase-II_0.pdf. [Last accessed July, 2024].
2. Sloan M, Sheth N, Lee GC. Is obesity associated with increased risk of deep vein thrombosis or pulmonary embolism after hip and knee arthroplasty? a large database study. Clin Orthop Relat Res. 2019;477(3):523-32.
3. Kakarla VR, Nandipati K, Lalla M, Castro A, Merola S. Are laparoscopic bariatric procedures safe in superobese (BMI ≥50 kg/m$^2$) patients? An NSQIP data analysis. Surg Obes Relat Dis. 2011;7(4):452-8.
4. Moon TS, Joshi GP. Are morbidly obese patients suitable for ambulatory surgery? Curr Opin Anaesthesiol. 2016;29(1):141-5.
5. Sweitzer B, Rajan N, Schell D, Gayer S, Eckert S, Joshi GP. Preoperative care for cataract surgery: The Society for Ambulatory Anesthesia Position Statement. Anesth Analg. 2021;133(6):1431-6.
6. Hammond KL. Practical issues in the surgical care of the obese patient. Ochsner J. 2013;13(2):224-7.
7. Apfelbaum JL, Hagberg CA, Connis RT, Abdelmalak BB, Agarkar M, Dutton RP, et al. American Society of Anesthesiologists Practice Guidelines for Management of the Difficult Airway. Anesthesiology. 2022;136(1):31-81.

8. Liew WJ, Negar A, Singh PA. Airway management in patients suffering from morbid obesity. Saudi J Anaesth. 2022;16(3):314-21.
9. Gabriel RA, Burton BN, Ingrande J, Joshi GP, Waterman RS, Spurr KR, et al. The association of body mass index with same-day hospital admission, postoperative complications, and 30-day readmission following day-case eligible joint arthroscopy: a national registry analysis. J Clin Anesth. 2020;59:26-31.
10. Gabriel RA, Burton BN, Du AL, Waterman RS, Macias A. Should body mass index eligibility be cut off for elective airway cases in an ambulatory surgery center? A retrospective analysis of adult patients undergoing outpatient tonsillectomy. J Clin Anesth. 2021;72:110306.
11. Rosero EB, Joshi GP. Nationwide use and outcomes of ambulatory surgery in morbidly obese patients in the United States. J Clin Anesth. 2014;26(3):191-8.
12. Rosero EB, Joshi GP. Finding the body mass index cutoff for hospital readmission after ambulatory hernia surgery. Acta Anaesthesiol Scand. 2020;64(9):1270-7.
13. Barbat S, Thompson KJ, Mckillop IH, Kuwada TS, Gersin K, Nimeri A. Ambulatory bariatric surgery: does it really lead to higher rates of adverse events? Surg Obes Relat Dis. 2020;16(11):1713-20.
14. Reeves JJ, Burton BN, Broderick RC, Waterman RS, Gabriel RA. Obesity and unanticipated hospital admission following outpatient laparoscopic cholecystectomy. Surg Endosc. 2021;35(3):1348-54.
15. Hajmohamed S, Patel D, Apruzzese P, Kendall MC, De Oliveira G. Early postoperative outcomes of super morbid obese compared to morbid obese patients after ambulatory surgery under general anesthesia: a propensity-matched analysis of a national database. Anesth Analg. 2021;133(6):1366-73.
16. Tumminello ME, Hogan MG, Leonardi C, Barton JS, Cook MW, Davis KG. Morbid obesity not a risk for serious complications following outpatient surgery. Am Surg. 2023;89(6):2608-17.
17. Vertosick EA, Assel M, Tokita HK, Zafirova Z, Vickers AJ, Simon BA, et al. Suitability of outpatient or ambulatory extended recovery cancer surgeries for obese patients. J Clin Anesth. 2019;58:111-6.
18. Joshi GP. Enhanced recovery pathways for ambulatory surgery. Curr Opin Anaesthesiol. 2020;33(6):711-7.
19. Memtsoudis SG, Cozowicz C, Nagappa M, Wong J, Joshi GP, Wong DT, et al. Society of anesthesia and sleep medicine guideline on intraoperative management of adult patients with obstructive sleep apnea. Anesth Analg. 2018;127(4):967-87.
20. Rex DK, Bhandari R, Desta T, DeMicco MP, Schaeffer C, Etzkorn K, et al. A phase III study evaluating the efficacy and safety of remimazolam (CNS 7056) compared with placebo and midazolam in patients undergoing colonoscopy. Gastrointest Endosc. 2018;88(3):427-37.
21. Doi M, Morita K, Takeda J, Sakamoto A, Yamakage M, Suzuki T. Efficacy and safety of remimazolam versus propofol for general anesthesia: a multicenter, single-blind, randomized, parallel-group, phase IIb/III trial. J Anesth. 2020;34(4):543-3.
22. Zhang K, Bao Y, Han X, Zhai W, Yang Y, Luo M, et al. Effects of opioid-free propofol or remimazolam balanced anesthesia on hypoxemia incidence in patients with obesity during gastrointestinal endoscopy: a prospective, randomized clinical trial. Front Med (Lausanne). 2023;10:1124743.
23. Bhardwaj S, Garg K, Devgan S. Comparison of opioid-based and opioid-free TIVA for laparoscopic urological procedures in obese patients. J Anaesthesiol Clin Pharmacol. 2019;35(4):481-6.
24. Azizad O, Joshi G. Day-surgery adult patients with obesity and obstructive sleep apnea: Current controversies and concerns. Best Pract Res Clin Anaesthesiol. 2023;37(3):317-30.

25. Mehdiratta L, Mishra SK, Vinayagam S, Nair A. Enhanced recovery after surgery (ERAS) still a distant speck on the horizon! Indian J Anaesth. 2021;65(2):93-6.
26. Afonso AM, McCormick PJ, Assel MJ, Rieth E, Barnett K, Tokita HK, et al. Enhanced Recovery Programs in an Ambulatory Surgical Oncology Center. Anesth Analg. 2022;134(5):e32.
27. Joshi GP, Ahmad S, Riad W, Eckert S, Chung F. Selection of obese patients undergoing ambulatory surgery: a systematic review of the literature. Anesth Analg. 2013;117(5):1082-91.
28. Ortiz VE, Kwo J. Obesity: physiologic changes and implications for preoperative management. BMC Anesthesiol. 2015;15:97.
29. Sharma S, Arora L. Anesthesia for the morbidly obese patient. Anesthesiol Clin. 2020;38(1):197-212.
30. Jin J. JAMA patient page. Obesity and the heart. JAMA. 2013;310(19):2113.
31. Gurunathan U, Myles PS. Limitations of body mass index as an obesity measure of perioperative risk. Br J Anaesth. 2016;116(3):319-21.
32. Cornier MA, Després JP, Davis N, Grossniklaus DA, Klein S, Lamarche B, et al. American Heart Association Obesity Committee of the Council on Nutrition; Physical Activity and Metabolism; Council on Arteriosclerosis; Thrombosis and Vascular Biology; Council on Cardiovascular Disease in the Young; Council on Cardiovascular Radiology and Intervention; Council on Cardiovascular Nursing, Council on Epidemiology and Prevention; Council on the Kidney in Cardiovascular Disease, and Stroke Council. Assessing adiposity: a scientific statement from the American Heart Association. Circulation. 2011;124(18):1996-2019.
33. Dixon AE, Peters U. The effect of obesity on lung function. Expert Rev Respir Med. 2018;12(9):755-67.
34. Sharma SK, Kumpawat S, Banga A, Goel A. Prevalence and risk factors of obstructive sleep apnea syndrome in a population of Delhi, India. Chest. 2006;130(1):149-56.
35. Young T, Evans L, Finn L, Palta M. Estimation of the clinically diagnosed proportion of sleep apnea syndrome in middle-aged men and women. Sleep. 1997;20(9):705-6.
36. Sareli AE, Cantor CR, Williams NN, Korus G, Raper SE, Pien G, et al. Obstructive sleep apnea in patients undergoing bariatric surgery—a tertiary center experience. Obes Surg. 2011;21(3):316-27.
37. Frey WC, Pilcher J. Obstructive sleep-related breathing disorders in patients evaluated for bariatric surgery. Obes Surg.2003;13:676-83.
38. Nagappa M, Patra J, Wong J, Subramani Y, Singh M, Ho G, et al. Association of STOP-Bang questionnaire as a screening tool for sleep apnea and postoperative complications: a systematic review and bayesian meta-analysis of prospective and retrospective cohort studies. Anesth Analg. 2017;125(4):1301-8.
39. Nagappa M, Wong DT, Cozowicz C, Ramachandran SK, Memtsoudis SG, Chung F. Is obstructive sleep apnea associated with difficult airway? Evidence from a systematic review and meta-analysis of prospective and retrospective cohort studies. PLoS One. 2018;13(10):e0204904.
40. Joshi GP, Ankichetty SP, Gan TJ, Chung F. Society for Ambulatory Anesthesia consensus statement on preoperative selection of adult patients with obstructive sleep apnea scheduled for ambulatory surgery. Anesth Analg. 2012;115(5):1060-8.
41. Bolden N, Posner KL, Domino KB, Auckley D, Benumof JL, Herway ST, et al. Postoperative critical events associated with obstructive sleep apnea: Results from the society of anesthesia and sleep medicine obstructive sleep apnea registry. Anesth Analg. 2020;131(4):1032-41.
42. Rosero EB, Joshi GP. Outcomes of sleep apnea surgery in outpatient and inpatient settings. Anesth Analg. 2021;132(5):1215-22.

43. Singh M, Liao P, Kobah S, Wijeysundera DN, Shapiro C, Chung F. Proportion of surgical patients with undiagnosed obstructive sleep apnoea. Br J Anaesth. 2013;110(4):629-36.
44. Thammaiah SH, Sreenath RH, Kumararadhya GB, Babu N, Archana KN. Preoperative STOP-BANG questionnaire to predict difficult airway in undiagnosed obstructive sleep apnea patients undergoing elective gynecological surgeries under general endotracheal anesthesia: A prospective observational study. Ann Afr Med. 2023;22(4):520-5.
45. Chung F, Memtsoudis SG, Ramachandran SK, Nagappa M, Opperer M, Cozowicz C, et al. Society of Anesthesia and Sleep Medicine Guidelines on preoperative screening and assessment of adult patients with obstructive sleep apnea. Anesth Analg. 2016;123(2):452-73.
46. Chung F, Subramanyam R, Liao P, Sasaki E, Shapiro C, Sun Y. High STOP-Bang score indicates a high probability of obstructive sleep apnoea. Br J Anaesth. 2012;108(5):768-75.
47. American Society of Anesthesiologists Task Force on Perioperative Management of patients with obstructive sleep apnea. Practice guidelines for the perioperative management of patients with obstructive sleep apnea: an updated report by the American Society of Anesthesiologists Task Force on Perioperative Management of patients with obstructive sleep apnea. Anesthesiology. 2014;120(2):268-86.
48. Ravesloot MJL, de Raaff CAL, van de Beek MJ, Benoist LBL, Beyers J, Corso RM, et al. Perioperative care of patients with obstructive sleep apnea undergoing upper airway surgery: a review and consensus recommendations [published correction appears in JAMA Otolaryngol Head Neck Surg. 2019;145(8):770.
49. Rajan N, Rosero EB, Joshi GP. Patient selection for adult ambulatory surgery: a narrative review. Anesth Analg. 2021;133(6):1415-30.
50. Tan ET, Leong W, Edafe O, Mirza S. A systematic review of the feasibility and safety of day case nasal and/or palatopharyngeal surgery in patients with obstructive sleep apnoea. Clin Otolaryngol. 2022;47(6):620-7.
51. Rosero EB, Joshi GP. Outcomes of sleep apnea surgery in outpatient and inpatient settings. Anesth Analg. 2021;132(5):1215-22.
52. Redhu S, Prakash PS, Jain V, Dash HH. Morbidly obese patient with obstructive sleep apnoea for major spine surgery: An anaesthetic challenge. Indian J Anaesth. 2016;60(6):420-3.
53. Romero-Corral A, Caples SM, Lopez-Jimenez F, Somers VK. Interactions between obesity and obstructive sleep apnea: implications for treatment. Chest. 2010;137(3):711-9.
54. Dieltjens M, Vanderveken OM, Shivalkar B, Van Haesendonck G, Kastoer C, Heidbuchel H, et al. Mandibular advancement device treatment and reverse left ventricular hypertrophic remodeling in patients with obstructive sleep apnea. J Clin Sleep Med. 2022;18(3):903-9.
55. Kaczmarski P, Karuga FF, Szmyd B, Sochal M, Białasiewicz P, Strzelecki D, et al. The role of inflammation, hypoxia, and opioid receptor expression in pain modulation in patients suffering from obstructive sleep apnea. Int J Mol Sci. 2022;23(16):9080.
56. Hajiha M, Dubord MA, Liu H, Horner RL. Opioid receptor mechanisms at the hypoglossal motor pool and effects on tongue muscle activity in vivo. J Physiol. 2009;587 (Pt 11):2677-92.

# CHAPTER 3

# Risk Assessment in Emergency/Urgent Surgery

*Pradeep A Dongare, Kishori Biradar*

## ABSTRACT

Emergency/urgent surgeries are not risk free. These unplanned surgeries are associated with events in the perioperative period, complications, morbidity, readmissions, or mortality. These risks must be quantified and managed comprehensively to prevent adverse surgical outcomes. National guidance states that all emergency surgery patients should have a mortality risk assessment calculated on admission. In earlier days, clinical decision-making was based on the clinician's experience and gut feeling, which is subjective and unrealistic. Various perioperative risk assessment tools have been developed to calculate mortality and morbidity and categorize high-risk patients who can receive the appropriate levels of care. The Royal College must provide clear instructions regarding which assessment tool should be used. The most frequently studied general tools are ASA-PS, POS SUM, P-POSSUM, APACHE II, CCI and CACI, ESAS, PESAS, SORT, SRS, and ACS-NSQIP. Without accurate risk assessment, there is a higher incidence of adverse postoperative outcomes. These risk assessment tools represent the most practical means of predicting risk in emergency surgery patients, helping improve quality and prevent adverse outcomes.

**Keywords:** Emergency surgery; Risk assessment; Scoring system

## KEY POINTS

- Emergency/urgent surgeries are performed when life or limb is threatened.
- In clinical terms, risk means the possibility of unwanted outcomes.
- Scoring systems have been explicitly developed to quantify risk in emergency surgeries.
- Most of these systems predict postoperative mortality up to 30 days.

## ■ INTRODUCTION

Risk management is a method of dealing with uncertainty. Risk management includes five stages: Risk awareness, identification, assessment, and re-evaluation. After the identification of a particular risk, the magnitude of the risk has to be assessed to bring the risk within acceptable limits. Risk in surgery includes a complex interaction of many factors. These factors are classified into patient, disease, system, and surgery-related factors.[1,2] The type of surgery (high risk, intermediate risk, and low risk) contributes independently to the risk. If the surgery is performed on an emergency/urgent basis, the risk increases with it.[3]

Surgery can be elective or emergency. Emergency/urgent surgeries are performed when life or limb is threatened. The National Confidential Enquiry into Patient Outcome and Death (NCEPOD) has defined immediate, urgent, expedited, and elective surgeries. Subsequently, the timing for acute care surgery (new TACS) classification recommends the timing that surgeries need to be conducted, including a color-coded system.[4] The classification also highlights that a large portion of the workload is unplanned or has a short duration concerning anesthetic and surgical care planning. Surgery is always associated with risk, but its prediction is more recent. Stewart et al. found that the global disease burden for emergency surgeries was relatively high. The mortality rate overall was 24.3 per 100,000 people in high-income countries and 10.6 per 100,000 people in low- and medium-income countries. The number of years of life lost, disability-adjusted life years, and per capita spending are also higher in the high-income countries compared to low- and middle-income countries.[5] A literature search using the words emergency surgery, disease burden, and India yielded emergency care results but did not yield specific data on emergency surgeries. In 2017, Mullen et al. conducted a retrospective study comparing 30-day mortality and morbidity. They found that the risk of mortality and morbidity doubled if the surgery was an urgent/emergency surgery.[6] This chapter aims to assess the risks associated with perioperative patients, which helps to measure outcomes after surgery.

## ■ DEFINITIONS

### National Confidential Enquiry into Patient Outcome and Death Classification[7]

- *Emergency:* Immediate life, limb, or organ-saving intervention within the operation decision, e.g., fracture with a significant neurovascular deficit.
- *Urgency:* Intervention for acute onset that may threaten the survival of a limb or organ within hours of the operation decision, e.g., compound fractures
- *Expedited:* Patients requiring early treatment, which is not an immediate threat to life, limb, or organ within days of the decision to operate, e.g., tendon and nerve injuries.
- *Elective:* Interventions planned or booked in advance. Delay in surgery has no ill effects, e.g., joint replacements.

### Timing of Acute Care Surgery Classification

The new Timing of Acute Care Surgery (new TACS) classification is a simple, straightforward, color-coded, and easily adaptable triage system that describes the ideal times for deciding on surgery with appropriate examples.[3] **Box 1** shows the new TACS classification system for acute care surgery.

*Risks:* In clinical terms, risk means the possibility of unwanted outcomes. The risks in the perioperative period in patients undergoing emergency surgery may be anesthesia or surgery related.

Anesthetic unwanted outcomes can range from temporary discomfort, such as nausea in the recovery room, to permanent disability or death. Surgical risk can be defined as a cumulative risk of death, development of a new disease or medical

**BOX 1:** New Timing of Acute Care Surgery (new TACS) classification for acute care surgery.

- Immediate, bleeding patients, life-saving, and resuscitative surgeries, e.g., aortic aneurysmal rupture
- Within an hour, surgery after resuscitation, e.g., diffuse peritonitis, limb infection with sepsis
- Within 6 hours, administration of antibiotics without delay, e.g., soft tissue infection without sepsis
- Within 12 hours, administration of antibiotics without delay, e.g., local peritonitis, cholecystitis
- Within 24–48 hours, schedule earlier during daytime, e.g., second look laparotomy

**BOX 2:** List of postoperative and other complications.

*Common complications:*
- Surgical wound infection (superficial or deep)
- Perioperative bleeding requiring transfusion
- Cardiac arrest
- Acute kidney injury
- Sepsis
- Ventilator requirement for >48 hours
- Myocardial infarction
- Wound dehiscence
- Cardiac arrhythmia

*Other complications:*
- Liver failure
- Acute cholangitis
- Pancreatitis
- Pleural effusion
- Pneumothorax
- Peripheral nerve injury
- Paralytic ileus

condition, or deterioration of a previously existing medical condition that develops in the early or late postoperative period and can be directly associated with surgical treatment.

A list of postoperative and other complications[6] is shown in **Box 2**.

# ■ NEED FOR RISK ASSESSMENT

The Royal College of Surgeons of England has recommended that surgical procedures with predicted mortality >10% should be managed in critical care postoperatively.[2] Thus, accurate risk stratification identifies patients who could benefit from targeted interventions such as goal-directed fluid therapy, postoperative respiratory support, and admission to critical care. Identifying high-risk patients who could benefit from these interventions is vital to improve outcomes and effectively allocate resources. These tools help clinicians to calculate perioperative risk and facilitate meaningful informed consent. Accurate risk prediction is essential for safe training, treatment planning, and shared decision-making.

# PREOPERATIVE EVALUATION—ESTIMATING PERIOPERATIVE RISK

Preoperative evaluation in an emergency must involve a primary and secondary survey. The complete review should take as short a time as possible. The assessment must be multidisciplinary, involving the surgeon and anesthesiologist. The *ABCDE* protocol (*A*irway, *B*reathing, *C*irculation, *D*isability, and *E*xposure) has to be implemented by both the surgeon and anesthesiologist. Once the surgeon decides that performing surgery would make a difference to the outcome, a quick history related to *A*llergies, *M*edication, *L*ast meal, and *E*vents is obtained. Low Glasgow Coma Scale (GCS), obstruction to the airway due to injury, or other reasons may be the main reasons for airway compromise. Preoperative oxygenation and ventilation may need to be instituted to stabilize these patients.[8] Rapid sequence induction and intubation are standard techniques, as most patients are considered to have full stomachs. Those presenting with shock should be assessed using the Advanced Trauma Life Support (ATLS) classification, as shown in **Table 1**, and corrective measures should be taken.[9]

The usefulness of this scoring system has been questioned, and it has been recommended that a base deficit be added to decide whether there is no shock, mild, moderate, or severe shock. Bonanno et al.[10] have proposed a physiological classification for hemorrhagic shock **(Table 2)**.

**TABLE 1:** Advanced Trauma Life Support classification for assessing hypovolemic shock.

|  | Class I | Class II | Class III | Class IV |
|---|---|---|---|---|
| Blood loss in % | <15 | 15–30 | 30–40 | >40 |
| Pulse rate (beats/min) | <100 | 100–120 | 120–140 | >140 |
| Blood pressure | Normal | Normal | ↓ | ↓ |
| Pulse pressure | Normal | ↓ | ↓ | ↓ |
| Respiratory rate (breaths/min) | 14–20 | 20–30 | 30–40 | >35 |
| Mental status | Slightly anxious | Mildly anxious | Anxious, confused | Confused, lethargic |
| Urine output (mL/h) | >30 | 20–30 | 5–15 | Minimal |

**TABLE 2:** Physiological classification of hemorrhagic shock.

| Critical hemorrhagic shock | Shock with heart and brain involvement or >40% loss of total blood volume (impending collapse)—stand-by surgery to control the hemorrhage |
|---|---|
| Severe hemorrhagic shock | Shock with hypotension not responding to blood/fluid loading—rapid surgery to control the hemorrhage |
| Moderate hemorrhagic shock | Hypotensive shock responding with normotension and reversal of tachycardia on blood/fluid loading |
| Mild hemorrhagic shock | Normotensive tachycardia—investigate, consider surgery, interventional radiology/nonoperative intervention |

*Source:* Adapted from Bonanno FG.[10]

Based on the estimated blood loss and vital signs, the ATLS classification of hypovolemic shock is the most accepted classification worldwide. However, its validation has been questioned, and a large study has found that it must accurately reflect the clinical reality.[11]

Point-of-care (POC) investigations may be the only feasible investigations that can be performed.

The requirement of preoperative intensive care for optimization is usually a part of the preoperative assessment. The preoperative risks in patients coming for emergency or urgent surgery are the triad of hypothermia, coagulopathy, and acidosis. Correction of shock, electrolyte imbalances, blood transfusion, and maintenance of oxygenation and ventilation become the focus. The early warning scoring system was developed for monitoring these patients in the ward and indicating the requirement of intensive care is the Modified Early Warning Scoring (MEWS) system, as shown in **Table 3**.

*Risk prediction:* To identify high-risk patients, several scoring systems have been developed to predict and manage complications objectively.

## ■ EVOLUTION OF RISK ASSESSMENT TOOLS

Earlier postoperative outcomes prediction was based on the gut feeling of the surgeon.[11] The results of such assessments were subjective and depended on the surgeon's experience. There should be an objective parameter to quantify risks accurately. Subjective tools are traditional and less valued than evidence-based, objective scoring systems. Many objective scoring systems have been developed over the last quarter of a century. The disadvantage was that software was expensive to purchase and difficult to calculate. Many prediction tools are available, which are simple to complete and easily accessible in the hospital via free internet resources, for example, www.riskprediction.org.uk.

**TABLE 3:** Modified Early Warning Scoring (MEWS) system.[12]

| Score | 3 | 2 | 1 | 0 | 1 | 2 | 3 |
|---|---|---|---|---|---|---|---|
| Respiratory rate (breaths/min) | | <8 | | 9–14 | 15–20 | 21–29 | >29 |
| Heart rate (beats/min) | | <40 | 40–50 | 51–100 | 101–110 | 111–129 | >129 |
| Systolic blood pressure (mm Hg) | <70 | 71–80 | 81–100 | 101–149 | | ≥200 | |
| Urine output (mL/h) | Nil | <0.5 | | | | | |
| Temperature (°C) | | <35 | 35.1–36 | 36.1–38 | 38.1–38.5 | ≥38.6 | |
| Neurological | | | | Alert | Reacting to voice | Reacting to pain | Unresponsive |

*Source:* Adapted from Gardner-Thorpe, et al.[12]

## AMERICAN SOCIETY OF ANESTHESIOLOGISTS

In 1940, the concept of physical status classification was suggested and proposed six categories.[13] Additionally, emergency cases are designated by adding E to the classification number. The classification includes one of six categories based on the presence or absence of mild to life-threatening severe systemic disease. The advantage of this system is it is simple to use. A high American Society of Anesthesiologists (ASA) score predicts mortality and postoperative complications after surgery. This system helps anesthesiologists to identify patients who require escalated perioperative care. Physiological variables are not included in this system. The disadvantage of this system is that it is subjective. This system does not include preoperative optimization or the level of postoperative care. The ASA Physical Status classification[14] is shown in **Table 4**.

## SCORING SYSTEMS ADAPTED FOR EMERGENCY SURGERIES

Many early scoring tools are used to estimate the risk of mortality and morbidity in intensive care settings. These scoring systems have been speculated and used to assess risk in emergency surgery patients. They have been investigated and are described here.

### Physiological and Operative Severity Score for the Enumeration of Mortality and Morbidity

The Physiological and Operative Severity Score for the Enumeration of Mortality and Morbidity (POSSUM) score has been validated in subsets of surgical patients, including those undergoing emergency surgery.[15] It includes 12 factors, a four-grade physiological score, and a six-factor operative physiological score. The parameters used to calculate the POSSUM score are enumerated in **Table 5**. The aforementioned study had a small sample size of 100 patients. A systematic review found that the predictability was low to moderate in patients undergoing emergency surgeries.[16] The POSSUM scoring system underestimates morbidity rates.[17]

### Portsmouth-Physiological and Operative Severity Score for the Enumeration of Mortality and Morbidity (P-POSSUM)

The P-POSSUM score **(Table 6)** is a modification of the POSSUM score, including the mode of surgery in the operative parameters.[18] Like the POSSUM score for emergency surgeries,[17] the P-POSSUM score also had low to moderate predictability of morbidity and mortality.

Similar scoring systems, such as modified P-POSSUM (mP-POSSUM) and the Simplified Acute Physiology Score (SAPS II), all have low or moderate predictability.[17]

### Acute Physiology and Chronic Health Evaluation II

The Acute Physiology and Chronic Health Evaluation II (APACHE II) score predicted mortality moderately and admission to the intensive care unit (ICU) poorly.[19]

## SCORING SYSTEMS DEVELOPED FOR EMERGENCY SURGERIES

Some scoring systems have been specifically developed to predict mortality and morbidity in patients undergoing surgery. Some of these are listed here.

**TABLE 4:** American Society of Anesthesiologists Physical Status (ASA PS) classification.

| ASA PS classification | Definition | Adult examples, including but not limited to | Pediatric examples, including but not limited to | Obstetric examples, including but not limited to |
|---|---|---|---|---|
| ASA I | A normal healthy patient | Healthy, nonsmoking, no or minimal alcohol use | Healthy (no acute or chronic disease), normal BMI percentile for age | |
| ASA II | A patient with mild systemic disease | Mild diseases only without substantive functional limitations. Current smoker, social alcohol drinker, pregnancy, obesity (30 < BMI <40), well-controlled DM/HTN, mild lung disease | Asymptomatic congenital cardiac disease, well-controlled dysrhythmias, asthma without exacerbation, well-controlled epilepsy, noninsulin-dependent diabetes mellitus, abnormal BMI percentile for age, mild/moderate OSA, oncologic state in remission, autism with mild limitations | Normal pregnancy*, well-controlled gestational HTN, controlled preeclampsia without severe features, diet-controlled gestational DM |
| ASA III | A patient with severe systemic disease | Substantive functional limitations; one or more moderate to severe diseases. Poorly controlled DM or HTN, COPD, morbid obesity (BMI ≥40 kg/m²), active hepatitis, alcohol dependence or abuse, implanted pacemaker, moderate reduction of ejection fraction, ESRD undergoing regularly scheduled dialysis, history (>3 months) of MI, CVA, TIA, or CAD/stents | Uncorrected stable congenital cardiac abnormality, asthma with exacerbation, poorly controlled epilepsy, insulin-dependent DM, morbid obesity, malnutrition, severe OSA, oncologic state, renal failure, muscular dystrophy, cystic fibrosis, history of organ transplantation, brain/spinal cord malformation, symptomatic hydrocephalus, premature infant PCA <60 weeks, autism with severe limitations, metabolic disease, difficult airway, long term parenteral nutrition. Full-term infants <6 weeks of age | Preeclampsia with severe features, gestational DM with complications or high insulin requirements, a thrombophilic disease requiring anticoagulation |
| ASA IV | A patient with severe systemic disease that is a | Recent (<3 months) MI, CVA, TIA or CAD/stents, ongoing cardiac ischemia or severe | Symptomatic congenital cardiac abnormality, congestive heart failure, active sequelae of prematurity, acute hypoxic-ischemic | Preeclampsia with severe features complicated by HELLP or other adverse event, |

*Contd...*

Contd...

| ASA PS classification | Definition | Adult examples, including but not limited to | Pediatric examples, including but not limited to | Obstetric examples, including but not limited to |
|---|---|---|---|---|
| | constant threat to life | valve dysfunction, severe reduction of ejection fraction, shock, sepsis, DIC, ARD or ESRD not undergoing regularly scheduled dialysis | encephalopathy, shock, sepsis, disseminated intravascular coagulation, automatic implantable cardioverter-defibrillator, ventilator dependence, endocrinopathy, severe trauma, severe respiratory distress, advanced oncologic state | peripartum cardiomyopathy with EF <40, uncorrected/ decompensated heart disease, acquired or congenital |
| ASA V | A moribund patient who is not expected to survive without the operation | Ruptured abdominal/thoracic aneurysm, massive trauma, intracranial bleed with mass effect, ischemic bowel in the face of significant cardiac pathology or multiple organ/system dysfunction | Massive trauma, intracranial hemorrhage with mass effect, patient requiring ECMO, respiratory failure or arrest, malignant HTN, decompensated congestive heart failure, hepatic encephalopathy, ischemic bowel or multiple organ/system dysfunction | Uterine rupture |
| ASA VI | A declared brain-dead patient whose organs are being removed for donor purposes | | | |

*Although pregnancy is not a disease, the parturient's physiologic state is significantly altered from when the woman is not pregnant, hence the assignment of ASA 2 for a woman with uncomplicated pregnancy.
**The addition of "E" denotes Emergency surgery: (An emergency is defined as existing when a delay in treatment of the patient would lead to a significant increase in the threat to life or body part).
(ARD: acute renal disease; BMI: body mass index; CAD: coronary artery disease; COPD: chronic obstructive pulmonary disease; CVA: cerebrovascular accident; DIC: disseminated intravascular coagulation; DM: diabetes mellitus; ECMO: extracorporeal membrane oxygenation; EF: ejection fraction; ESRD: end-stage renal disease; HTN: hypertension; MI: myocardial infarction; OSA: obstructive sleep apnea; PCA: postconceptional age; TIA: transient ischemic attack)
Source: American Society of Anesthesiologists.[14]

**TABLE 5:** The Physiological and Operative Severity Score for the Enumeration of Mortality and Morbidity (POSSUM) score parameters.

| Physiological parameters | Operative parameters |
|---|---|
| • Age | • Operative severity |
| • Cardiac signs | • Operative urgency |
| • Respiratory history | • Multiple procedures |
| • Systolic blood pressure | • Total blood loss |
| • Pulse | • Peritoneal soiling |
| • Glasgow Coma Scale | • Presence of malignancy |
| • Hemoglobin | • Mode of surgery |
| • White cell count | |
| • Urea | |
| • Sodium | |
| • Potassium | |
| • Electrogram | |

*Surgical APGAR score:* The surgical Apgar score is a predictive system developed by Gawande et al. It is a 10-point system proposed based on three factors: Estimated blood loss, lowest mean arterial pressure, and lowest heart rate.[20] The score has been evaluated for various emergency surgeries, such as spine surgeries and general surgeries. However, it seems to perform poorly in orthopedic surgeries.[21]

*ACS-NSQIP Universal Surgical Risk Calculator:* The American College of Surgeons National Quality Improvement program database validated for the emergency general surgical (EGS) population. This predicts the chance of an unfavorable outcome, such as complication or death. Hyder et al. showed that ACS NSQIP slightly underestimated the risk of emergency general surgery compared to the risk of elective surgery.[22] For calculating postoperative death and complications in the EGS population, ACS-NSQIP is reasonably accurate. This uses 20 patient characteristics (age, sex, type of surgery, etc.) that can be quickly entered online.[23] The advantages are that it can be used in the early phases of care for auditing purposes and helps inform patients about the risks of surgery.[24]

*Physiological Emergency Surgery Acuity Score (PESAS):* The physiological emergency surgery acuity score was created to assess the operative risk of mortality using objective data. It is derived from sequential analysis of ACS-NSQIP data and subsequently validated on ACS-NSQIP data from 2012. This score comprises 10 physiological points linked to advanced clinical acuity and postoperative mortality.[25] This score can be applied to early patient care and used for auditing. The disadvantage is that PESAS does not assess morbidity.

*Charlson Comorbidity Index (CCI) and Charlson Age-comorbidity Index (CACI):* The CCI has been approved for medical, critically ill, trauma patients, and elective surgical settings. 19 comorbid conditions were classified, and a weighted index was developed that accounted for the number and seriousness of comorbid diseases.[26] Charlson later modified this to add age to the comorbidity index (CACI).[26] CACI combines 19 medical conditions weighted 1-6, with age weighted 1 for every decade past 40 years.[26] Literature suggests CCI and CACI may accurately estimate morbidity and mortality in

**TABLE 6:** The Portsmouth-Physiological and Operative Severity Score for the enumeration of Mortality and Morbidity (P-POSSUM) scoring parameters.

| Physiologic variable | Points | | | | | | | |
|---|---|---|---|---|---|---|---|---|
| | 4 | 3 | 2 | 1 | 0 | 1 | 3 | 4 |
| Temperature (°C) | >41 | 39–40.9 | | 38.5–38.9 | 36–38.4 | 34–35.9 | 30–31.9 | <29.9 |
| Mean arterial pressure (mm Hg) | >160 | 130–159 | 110–129 | | 70–109 | | 50–69 | <49 |
| Heart rate (beats/min) | >180 | 140–179 | 110–139 | | 70–109 | | 55–69 | 40–54 | <39 |
| Respiratory rate (breaths/min) | >50 | 35–49 | | 25–34 | 12–24 | 10–11 | 6–9 | <5 |
| Oxygenation<br>• $FiO_2$ >0.5 (use A-a$DO_2$)<br>• $FiO_2$ <0.5 (use $PaO_2$) | >500 | 350–499 | 200–349 | | • <200<br>• >70 | 61–70 | 55–60 | <55 |
| Arterial pH | >7.7 | 7.6–7.69 | | 7.5–7.59 | 7.33–7.49 | | 7.25–7.32 | 7.15–7.24 | <7.15 |
| Serum sodium (mMol/L) | >180 | 160–179 | 155–159 | 150–154 | 130–149 | | 120–129 | 111–119 | <110 |
| Serum potassium (mMol/L) | >7 | 6–6.9 | | 5.5–5.9 | 3.5–5.4 | 3–3.4 | 2.5–2.9 | <2.5 |
| Serum creatinine (mg/dL): double point score for acute renal failure | >3.5 | 2–3.4 | 1.5–1.9 | | 0.6–1.4 | | 0.6 | |
| Hct (%) | >60 | | 50–59.9 | 46–49.9 | 30–45.9 | | 20–29.9 | <20 |
| WBC (1,000s) | >40 | 20–39.9 | | 15–19.9 | 3–14.9 | | 1–2.9 | <1 |
| Glasgow Coma Scale (GCS) | Score = 15 minus actual GCS | | | | | | | |

(A-a $DO_2$: alveolar-arterial oxygen gradient; $FiO_2$: fractional inspired oxygen; Hct: hematocrit; WBC: white blood cell) the EGS population. The limitation of the use is that it is a cumbersome calculation in EGS, which estimates mortality and morbidity in the EGS population. The role of CCI and CACI in the emergency setting is less. The literature suggests that CCI and CACI may accurately predict mortality and morbidity in the EGS population.

*Emergency surgery acuity score:* The emergency surgery acuity score estimates perioperative mortality in emergency surgery patients.[25] The preoperative risk stratification system considers patient comorbidities and acute physiology at presentation. The ESAS includes three demographic variables, 10 comorbidities, and nine laboratory variables. It is based entirely on objective factors that can be easily identified preoperatively. This risk score could be used in nonoperative patients.[27] The advantage is that this score is easy to apply clinically and can be used for auditing.

*Surgical Outcome Risk Tool (SORT):* Surgical Outcome Risk Tool scores can be used in preoperative settings. The tool has six variables. An app and web-based calculators are available to help with calculations.[28] Compared to ASA-PS and the SRS, SORT is more accurate. Its ability to accurately predict mortality and morbidity risk in the EGS patient population is unknown. It is a preoperative risk prediction tool for death within 30 days of surgery in adult noncardiac, non-neurologic patients and can be used for auditing.[28]

*Surgical Risk Scale:* The surgical risk score consists of three components: Confidential Enquiry into Perioperative Deaths grade (elective, scheduled, urgent, and emergency), the ASA-PS grade, and the British United Provident Association (BUPA) operative grade.[29] This tool has yet to be studied for risk prediction in the EGS population. The score can be applied early in patient care and may be clinically helpful. It cannot be used in nonoperative patients. This score can be applied in early patient care trajectory. This score is not suitable for auditing.

## ■ LIMITATIONS OF SCORING SYSTEMS

Acute injury requires comprehensive care for all general surgical emergencies. In this setting, the trauma scoring system does not evaluate inclusively the comorbid conditions of the EGS population. ACS-NSQIP surgical calculator has shown broad statistical reliability but does not apply to nonoperative patients. The CCI includes the comorbid conditions but does not consider the acute physiologic changes that may contribute to postoperative outcomes. It does not assess risk from a procedural standpoint. SRS, POSSUM, and P-POSSUM contain comprehensive information but have shown significant limitations in EGS. ESAS is the ideal scoring system, but it does not apply to nonoperative patients and has yet to be available as a consumer application.

## ■ ROLE OF ARTIFICIAL INTELLIGENCE IN RISK PREDICTION

The artificial intelligence (AI) risk prediction algorithms, such as the smartphone-available Predictive Optimal Trees in Emergency Surgery Risk (POTTER) for emergency general surgery, are superior to traditional risk calculators, because they account for complex nonlinear interactions between variables. It is a clinical decision support tool to aid medical providers in predicting emergency surgery mortality and morbidity likelihood. POTTER is a highly accurate and user-friendly emergency surgery risk calculator. This tool could prove helpful as a bedside adjunct to surgeons when preoperatively counseling patients.[30]

## ■ CONCLUSION

An operative or nonoperative strategy can manage emergency general surgery conditions. Whether to adopt an operative or nonoperative management strategy is guided by a graphic representation of the relationship between risk prediction and patient management. Ultimately, the patient has to decide whether or not to undergo surgery. Objective risk assessment may help the surgeon guide the patient in decision-making, give informed consent, and provide realistic expectations. In surgical management, predicting perioperative morbidity and mortality is thus essential. Risk prediction may be used to indicate the need for monitoring in high dependency unit (HDU) before or after surgery. Risk assessment highlights the need for quality improvement efforts in the emergency patient population.

## ■ REFERENCES

1. Shaydakov ME, Tuma F. Operative Risk. (2023). In: StatPearls [Internet]. Treasure Island (FL): StatPearls Publishing; 2024. Available from: https://www.ncbi.nlm.nih.gov/books/NBK532240/. [Last accessed July, 2024].
2. Bould MD, Hunter D, Haxby EJ. Clinical risk management in anaesthesia. BJA Educ. 2006;6:240-43.
3. O'Connell PR, McCaskie AW, Williams NS (Eds). Bailey & Love's Short Practice of Surgery, 28th edition. New Delhi: CBS; 2023.
4. De Simone B, Kluger Y, Moore EE, Sartelli M, Abu-Zidan FM, Coccolini F, et al. The new timing in acute care surgery (new TACS) classification: a WSES Delphi consensus study. World J Emerg Surg. 2023;18:1-10.
5. Stewart B, Khanduri P, McCord C, Ohene-Yeboah M, Uranues S, Vega Rivera F, et al. Global disease burden of conditions requiring emergency surgery. Br J Surg. 2014;101(1):9-22.
6. Mullen MG, Michaels AD, Mehaffey HJ, Guidry CA, Turrentine FE, Hedrick TL, et al. Risk associated with complications and mortality after urgent surgery vs elective and emergency surgery: Implications for defining "quality" and reporting outcomes for urgent surgery. JAMA Surg. 2017;152(8):768-774.
7. Gray LD, Morris CG. Organisation and planning of anaesthesia for emergency surgery. Anaesthesia. 2013;68(Suppl. 1):3-13.
8. Lake C. Assessment of the emergency surgical patient. Anaesth Intensive Care Med. 2015;16(9):431-4.
9. Mutschler M, Paffrath T, Wölfl C, Probst C, Nienaber U, Schipper IB, et al. The ATLS® classification of hypovolaemic shock: a well established teaching tool on the edge? Injury. 2014;45:S35-S38.
10. Bonanno FG. The need for a physiological classification of hemorrhagic shock. J Emerg Trauma Shock. 2020;13(3):177-82.
11. Mutschler M, Nienaber U, Brockamp T, Wafaisade A, Wyen H, Peiniger S, et al. A critical reappraisal of the ATLS classification of hypovolaemic shock: does it really reflect clinical reality? Resuscitation. 2013;84(3):309-13.
12. Gardner-Thorpe J, Love N, Wrightson J, Walsh S, Keeling N. The value of Modified Early Warning Score (MEWS) in surgical in-patients: A prospective observational study. Ann R Coll Surg Engl. 2006;88:571-5.
13. Doyle DJ, Hendrix JM, Garmon EH. American Society of Anesthesiologists Classification. (2023). In: StatPearls [Internet]. Treasure Island (FL): StatPearls Publishing. Available from: https://www.ncbi.nlm.nih.gov/books/NBK441940/ [Last accessed July, 2024].
14. American Society of Anesthesiologists. Statement on ASA Physical Status Classification System. (2020). Available from: https://www.asahq.org/standards-and-practice-

parameters/statement-on-asa-physical-status-classification-system [Last accessed July, 2024].
15. Markus PM, Martell J, Leister I, Horstmann O, Brinker J, Becker H. Predicting postoperative morbidity by clinical assessment. Br J Surg. 2005;92:101-6.
16. Sreeharsha H, Sp R, Sreekar H, Reddy R. Efficacy of POSSUM score in predicting the outcome in patients undergoing emergency laparotomy. Pol Przegl Chir. 2014;86:159-65.
17. Oliver CM, Walker E, Giannaris S, Grocott MP, Moonesinghe SR. Risk assessment tools validated for patients undergoing emergency laparotomy: a systematic review. Br J Anaesth. 2015;115(6):849-60.
18. Igari K, Ochiai T, Yamazaki S. POSSUM and P-POSSUM for risk assessment in general surgery in the elderly. Hepatogastroenterology. 2013;60(126):1320-7.
19. Hansted AK, Møller MH, Møller AM, Vester-Andersen M. APACHE II score validation in emergency abdominal surgery. A post hoc analysis of the InCare trial. Acta Anaesthesiol Scand. 2020;64(2):180-7.
20. Gawande AA, Kwaan MR, Regenbogen SE, Lipsitz SA, Zinner MJ. An Apgar score for surgery. J Am Coll Surg. 2007;204(2):201-8.
21. Nair A, Bharuka A, Rayani BK. The Reliability of Surgical Apgar Score in Predicting Immediate and Late Postoperative Morbidity and Mortality: A Narrative Review. Rambam Maimonides Med J. 2018;9(1):e0004.
22. Havens JM, Columbus AB, Seshadri AJ, Brown CVR, Tominaga GT, Mowery NT, et al. Risk stratification tools in emergency general surgery. Trauma Surg Acute Care Open. 2018;3(1):e000160.
23. Parkin CJ, Moritz P, Kirkland O, Doane M, Glover, A. Utility of the American College of Surgeons National Surgical Quality Improvement Program surgical risk calculator in predicting mortality in an Australian acute surgical unit. ANZ J Surg. 2020;90:746-51.
24. van der Hulst HC, Dekker JWT, Bastiaannet E, van der Bol JM, van den Bos F, Hamaker ME, et al. Validation of the ACS NSQIP surgical risk calculator in older patients with colorectal cancer undergoing elective surgery. J Geriatr Oncol. 2022;13(6):788-95.
25. Sangji NF, Bohnen JD, Ramly EP, Yeh DD, King DR, DeMoya M, et al. Derivation and validation of a novel Emergency Surgery Acuity Score (ESAS). J Trauma Acute Care Surg. 2016;81(2):213-20.
26. Charlson M, Szatrowski TP, Peterson J, Gold J. Validation of a combined comorbidity index. J Clin Epidemiol. 1994;47:1245-51.
27. Wang H, Luu V, Jiang E, Kirkland O, Kabir S, Davis SS, et al. Evaluation of a modified emergency surgical acuity score in predicting operative and non-operative mortality and morbidity in an acute surgical unit. ANZ J Surg. 2023;93(10):2297-302.
28. Protopapa KL, Simpson JC, Smith NC, Moonesinghe SR. Development and validation of the Surgical Outcome Risk Tool (SORT). Br J Surg. 2014;101:1774-83.
29. Sutton R, Bann S, Brooks M, Sarin S. The Surgical Risk Scale as an improved tool for risk-adjusted analysis in comparative surgical audit. Br J Surg. 2002;89:763-8.
30. El Moheb M, Gebran A, Maurer LR, Naar L, El Hechi M, Breen K, et al. Artificial intelligence versus surgeon gestalt in predicting risk of emergency general surgery. J Trauma Acute Care Surg. 2023;95(4):565-72.

# CHAPTER 4

# Upcoming Role of Artificial Intelligence in Airway Management

*Reeta Singh, Susheela Taxak*

## ABSTRACT

Airway management is critical in anesthesia, resuscitation, and critical care medicine. Predicting airway difficulties remains challenging due to the inaccurate diagnostic accuracies of the existing prediction methods. Artificial intelligence (AI) can replicate and amplify human knowledge and recent research into AI applications in difficult airway management. Benefits can be seen in accurate prediction of difficult airways, enhanced decision-making in selecting the appropriate airway device, real-time feedback, and guidance during airway management and in providing improved training and education opportunities in simulating difficult airway scenarios, allowing clinicians to practice and improve their skills in a safe and controlled environment. Investing in high-quality research, gaining a comprehensive understanding of AI systems, and stepping up with improvements in AI technology are essential for present anesthesiologists to improve clinical outcomes.

**Keywords:** Airway management; Difficult airway; Difficult mask ventilation; Intubation; Artificial intelligence; Machine learning

## KEY POINTS

- Failure to identify difficult intubation is the leading cause of anesthesia-related death and morbidity.
- Closed claims analysis related to managing airway difficulties indicates that inadequate planning, inability to predict and anticipate difficult airways, and judgment failures are the core issues leading to mishaps.
- Artificial intelligence (AI)-based algorithms with machine learning models using clinical, imaging, and facial analysis techniques have recently been developed and validated to predict difficult airways, potentially improving safety and clinical outcomes in contrast to the low sensitivity and specificity of the presently used prediction algorithms.
- This chapter deals with the present state of research on using AI-based techniques in airway management and the near-futuristic application of the intelligent models in clinical practice by anesthesiologists.

## ■ INTRODUCTION

The revised definition of difficult airway (DA) is: "the clinical situation in which anticipated or unanticipated difficulty or failure is experienced by a physician trained in anesthesia care, including but not limited to one or more of the following: facemask ventilation, laryngoscopy, ventilation using a supraglottic airway, tracheal intubation, extubation, or invasive airway". Prediction and anticipation of DAs in the preoperative period remain challenging, as the diagnostic accuracies of the existing prediction methods are still relatively low.[1]

Artificial intelligence (AI) is a multidisciplinary branch of computer science that researches and develops technology, principles, techniques, algorithms, and application systems for replicating and amplifying human knowledge, and can have potential benefits in airway management. It can be utilized for improved accuracy in predicting DAs, enhanced decision-making in selecting the appropriate airway device based on patient characteristics and other factors, real-time assistance (feedback and guidance) during airway management, and providing improved training and education opportunities in simulating DA scenarios, allowing healthcare providers to practice and improve their skills in a safe and controlled environment.[2]

We aim to review recent advances and research in developing and applying AI models, with the possible clinical impact on airway management.

## ■ WHAT IS ARTIFICIAL INTELLIGENCE?

Artificial intelligence encompasses various concepts, such as machine learning (ML) and deep learning (DL), which involve neural networks, natural language processing, computer vision, robotics, expert systems, and more. It is about creating systems that can perform tasks that require human intelligence, such as reasoning, problem-solving, perception, and learning. DL is a subset of machine learning that utilizes neural networks with multiple layers (hence "deep") to learn representations of data. DL involves:

- "Data representation", where data is represented in layers, with each layer transforming the data into a more abstract and meaningful form.
- "Learning features", wherein DL models automatically learn hierarchical features from the input data through backpropagation.
- "Complex models" can learn complex patterns and relationships in data, making them well-suited for tasks such as image recognition, natural language processing, and speech recognition.
- "Scalability", so the DL models can scale effectively with large amounts of data and computational resources, allowing them to handle increasingly complex tasks and datasets.

The AI diagnostic applications are being used in multiple fields of medicine and are presently gaining approvals for therapeutic and interventional use.[3] Anesthesiology as a field is well positioned to benefit from advances in AI, as anesthesiologists are familiar with AI applications already in use in multiple clinical areas of their practice. Failure to identify a DA and inability to oxygenate/intubate is the leading cause of anesthesia-related death and morbidity, where AI can better the decision-making process and improve outcomes. Presently, physical airway examination remains an essential tool to identify DAs. Still, a multidimensional analysis using ML models can be a game changer in predicting and guiding the management of DAs.

## ■ USE OF AI IN AIRWAY ASSESSMENT AND MANAGEMENT

Airway-related severe complications occur in one in every 22,000 anesthetics. Death or brain injury occurs in one in 180,000, with statistical analysis suggesting only 25% of relevant incidents may have been reported.[4] Despite preoperative airway assessment, 75–93% of difficult intubations (DIs) are unanticipated, and airway examination methods underperform, with sensitivities of 20–62% and specificities of 82–97%.[5] The catastrophic complications that ensue with failure of oxygenation or maintenance of a patent airway serve to justify the numerous developments, research, guidelines, and algorithms developed in this area.

The use of AI in airway management can provide several benefits, including:
- *Prediction models:* AI algorithms can analyze patient data and identify patterns based on anatomy, medical history, and previous airway management experiences, thus improving accuracy in predicting DAs. This can help healthcare providers prepare and plan the correct approach for managing difficulties in airway management, therefore reducing incidents and complications.
- *Image analysis:* Computer vision algorithms can analyze medical images, such as X-rays and CT/MRI scans, to help identify anatomical features that may contribute to airway difficulty.
- *Decision support systems:* AI systems can enhance decision-making and provide real-time guidance and feedback during airway management by suggesting appropriate techniques, selecting the proper airway device, and making interventions based on the specific patient's characteristics, condition, and procedure context.
- *Simulation and improved training and education:* AI-powered platforms can simulate DA scenarios, allowing providers to practice and improve their skills in a safe and controlled environment.
- *Remote consultation:* AI-enabled telemedicine and augmented reality platforms can provide real-time views of the patient in OT to airway management experts, allowing them to virtually participate, remotely monitor, and advise colleagues in remote locations in challenging cases.

## ■ USE OF AI IN PREDICTING A DIFFICULT AIRWAY

Ever-expanding innovations in using advanced diagnostic modalities to refine airway assessment, assist in the prediction of DA, and formulate safer, precise airway management strategies significantly reduce human error and improve patient safety. The use of these innovations like X-rays to assess airway structures, ultrasonography (USG) to identify cricothyroid membrane in emergency cricothyrotomy and DA prediction, computed tomography (CT) scan for a finer characterization of pathology and image reconstruction,[6,7] magnetic resonance imaging (MRI) to define soft tissue airway lesions, nasal endoscopy for bedside visualization of glottis and subglottic areas, virtual endoscopic evaluation of airway, and three-dimensional (3D) printing to provide a simulated airway model to enable planning, practice, and education are proving helpful in guiding complex treatment decisions.[8-11]

In recent years, AI technology and image analysis systems have continued to develop and evolve. AI has been explored to predict difficult mask ventilation (DMV) and DI to outperform conventional airway examinations by integrating subjective factors, such as facial appearance, speech features, habitus, and other poorly known features, along with the above innovative diagnostic modalities.[12] Compared with conventional prediction tools and regression approaches, modern ML approaches have several advantages, such as incorporating high-order, nonlinear interactions between predictors and mitigating overfitting.

## PREDICTIVE MACHINE LEARNING MODEL USING CLINICAL ASSESSMENT FOR DIFFICULT AIRWAYS

Zhou et al.[13] examined whether ML and DL can predict DA intubation in patients undergoing thyroid surgery. They used 10 ML and DL algorithms to establish a corresponding model through a training group and then verified the results in a test group. In the training group, the area under curve (AUC) values and accuracy and the gradient boosting precision were 0.932, 0.929, and 100%, respectively. In this analysis of 500 patients, 48 of whom showed difficult laryngoscopy, they concluded that gradient boosting performed best overall, with an AUC >0.8, an accuracy >90%, and a precision of 100%. Besides, the top five weighting factors identified by the ML algorithm for DAs were age, sex, weight, height, and body mass index (BMI).

Multiple other ML studies have shown a correlation of DA with increased neck circumference (NC >33.5 cm), age (40–59), male sex, high BMI (especially in patients with obstructive sleep apnea syndrome), increased neck circumference to thyromental distance (NC/TMD) ratio and Mallampati score. Individually, these were not good predictors, but in the AI models and ML algorithm, they can advise anesthesiologists on DAs with excellent sensitivity and specificity. Langeron et al., in a cohort study with a 6.1% incidence of DI, demonstrated conventional methods using BMI, age, Mallampati grade, TMD, mouth opening, macroglossia, gender, receding chin, and snoring parameters had a low predictive value but computer-assisted models using complex interaction between variables enable an accurate prediction of difficult tracheal intubation with a low proportion of patients in the inconclusive zone.[14]

Kim et al. used age, Mallampati grade, BMI, sternomental distance, and NC to predict difficult laryngoscopy. Preanesthesia and anesthesia data of 616 patients who had undergone anesthesia at a single center were included. The dataset was divided into a base training set (n = 492) and a base test set (n = 124), with equal distribution of difficult laryngoscopy. Training data sets were trained with six algorithms (multilayer perception, logistic regression, supportive vector machine, random forest, extreme gradient boosting, and light gradient boosting machine) and cross-validated. The model with the highest area under the receiver operating characteristic (AUROC) was chosen as the final and validated with the test set. The predicted AUROC for the challenging laryngoscopy class was 0.71 (95% confidence interval (CI), 0.59–0.83; p = 0.014), and the recall (sensitivity) was 0.85.[15]

## AI USED IN ANALYSIS OF RADIOLOGICAL IMAGES, FACE SCANS, AND SPEECH FOR AIRWAY ASSESSMENT

### AI in X-ray Identification of Difficult Airways

Several X-ray-based ML and DL have recently been developed and validated to predict DAs and first-pass success compared to conventional approaches. X-rays are commonly used to verify the placement of endotracheal tubes (ETTs) and tracheostomy tubes (TTs), to determine the appropriate size of ETT/TT, and to identify complications arising from complex airway management. X-rays can also serve as a valuable tool for assessing bony and soft tissues of the airway, enabling the identification of tumors, masses, trauma, abscesses, epiglottitis, tracheal compression, degenerative diseases, or stenosis, etc.[4] AI models using X-ray for DA assessment incorporate objective distance parameters. In 90 patients with acromegaly undergoing pituitary tumor surgery, Lee et al.[7] found that the difficult laryngoscopy group had longer alveolar line to hyoid bone (ALH) and mandible to hyoid bone (MPH) distance. However, although the X-ray makes up for the lack of subjective evaluation and provides a good tool for measuring bone markers, they still cannot be used clinically as a necessary tool for the assessment of DAs, considering its adverse hazards such as radiation and the problems of sensitivity and specificity of diagnosis.

Harris et al.[16] used a box-based ML model to localize the ETT and carina, measuring the distance in centimeters. This strategy offered information about malpositioning and distance measurement, allowing quantitative details on how many centimeters the tube should be moved to achieve the correct positioning. Chen et al.[17] developed an automatic tool for detecting ETT and carina using portable chest X-rays using an AI model [Mask region-based convolutional neural network (Mask R-CNN)]. DL models demonstrated high interobserver agreement compared to radiologists. However, pixel segmentation-based tube and carina identification models did not produce accurate findings (as the Carina Net model). This suggests the need for implementing a novel segmentation-based model for more precise localization of the tube tip.[18]

## AI in CT Identification of Difficult Airways

The CT scans are often used for 3D reconstruction of airway anatomy. Han et al.[19] made an airway model using CT 3D reconstruction technology for DAs. This allowed a tailored individualized management algorithm by first practicing on the 3D reconstructed model. Grimes et al.[20] found that CT scans had a predictive value and positive predictive value (PPV) of 90.7% and 71.4%, respectively, to predict difficulties in nasal intubation. The authors found that a nasal diameter of ≤6.3 mm can indicate nasal intubation difficulty. Lee et al.[7] reported that CT measurement of the tongue area can predict difficult laryngoscopy, with 2,600 mm$^2$ as the best-predicted cutoff point. A CT scan can also help detect complications of endotracheal intubation, such as selective intubation of the right bronchus.

However, 3D CT use as an auxiliary tool to evaluate DAs is limited due to radiation risk, the requirement of extra workforce, CT equipment, and additional costs. Therefore, CT is neither simple nor convenient as a tool for DA assessment. In conclusion, preoperatively, CT may only be recommended to identify potentially DAs in high-risk head, neck, and maxillofacial surgery patients.

## AI in MRI Identification of Difficult Airways

The MRI has the advantage of not using harmful ionizing radiation. AI image recognition algorithms to analyze MRI scans of the neck and airway can be trained to identify anatomical airway features that may make intubation challenging, such as a high-arched palate, a narrow oropharynx, or a short neck. Münster et al.[21] reported in 142 patients a correlation between difficult laryngoscopy and the anatomical position of the vocal cords with the cervical vertebrae as assessed by MRI. However, there is very little research evidence to support the effectiveness of MRI in evaluating DAs, and studies are limited due to MRI being time-consuming and expensive.

## Ultrasound in Predicting Difficult Airway

Ultrasound is readily available, portable, inexpensive, with no radiation, and can scan airway structures in the form of images in real-time, making it a promising tool for airway assessment. Ultrasound can assist in measuring the thickness of the anterior cervical soft tissue, anterior epiglottis, anterior hyoid bone, anterior vocal cord, the lateral pharyngeal wall, and the distance from the base of the tongue to the skin. Other indicators of a DA include tongue thickness and volume, oral exposure ratio, range of temporomandibular joint movement, distance from the epiglottis to the midpoint of the vocal cords, hyomental distance (HMD), and its derivative ratio.[22,23] In the future, AI may arrive at a comprehensive evaluation model to predict difficulty in intubation using USG and patient clinical parameters; however, as of date, more extensive studies are needed.

## AI-based Facial Analysis Techniques

AI-based facial analysis techniques have been used to predict DMV, videolaryngoscopy (VL), and DIs. Langeron O et al.[10] in a prospective study of 1,502 patients, defined DMV as the inability of an unassisted anesthesiologist to maintain the measured oxygen saturation as measured by pulse oximetry >92% or to prevent or reverse signs of inadequate ventilation during positive-pressure mask ventilation under general anesthesia (GA). A univariate analysis was performed to identify potential factors predicting DMV, followed by a multivariate analysis, and the odds ratio and 95% CI were calculated. DMV was reported in 75 patients (5%; 95% CI, 3.9-6.1%), with one case of impossible ventilation. The anesthesiologist anticipated DMV in only 13 patients (17% of the DMV cases). BMI, age, macroglossia, beard, lack of teeth, history of snoring, increased Mallampati grade, and lower TMD were identified in the univariate analysis as potential DMV risk factors. Using a multivariate analysis, five criteria were recognized as independent factors for a DMV (age older than 55 years, BMI >26 kg/m$^2$, beard, lack of teeth, history of snoring), the presence of two indicating a high likelihood of DMV (sensitivity, 0.72; specificity, 0.73).

However, the diagnostic accuracy of DMV prediction based on these factors has been proven to be poor, with up to 94% of DMV patients ultimately failing to be predicted. For this reason, the difficult facemask (DIFFMASK) score (which incorporated age, sex, BMI, history of DI, history of snoring, TMD, modified Mallampati test, beard, sleep apnea, and history of neck radiation) ranging from 0 to 18 points was developed and validated in a large cohort of 46,804 patients.[24] Patients with a sum score ≥5 were deemed to be at risk for DMV. DL techniques in facial image analysis are gaining momentum in medical research with better detection of medical conditions.[12]

Bei Pei et al. used a prediction model for DMV with morphometric data and ML algorithms. In this study, 669 patients undergoing elective GA were enrolled, including 634 patients with easy mask ventilation (MV) and 35 patients with DMV, and the 3D facial scan was designed to predict DMV. This model demonstrated better predictive performance than the DIFFMASK score, which obtained an AUC of 0.785 and a sensitivity of 0.686. Their study exemplified the application of 3D scans for DMV prediction and found that using multiple principal components (PCs) as inputs, with the linear regression (LR) algorithm, allowed for effective DMV prediction, achieving an AUC of 0.825 (95% CI, 0.765-0.885), which outperformed the DIFFMASK score. This proposed that 3D geometric morphometric analysis of facial scans combined with ML algorithms could be an alternative tool to predict DMV in patients scheduled for GA.[25]

AI-based facial analysis is a feasible technique for predicting difficulty during videolaryngoscopy, and the model developed using neural networks has higher predictive performance than traditional methods and better overall success rates of tracheal intubation. In their study, Xia M et al.[26] aimed to create an AI model to identify difficult videolaryngoscopy using a neural network. Baseline characteristics, medical history, bedside examination, and seven facial images were included as predictor variables. ResNet-18 was introduced to recognize images and extract features. Different ML algorithms were utilized to develop predictive models. A videolaryngoscopy view of Cormack–Lehane grade of 1 or 2 was classified as "nondifficult", while grade 3 or 4 was classified as "difficult". A total of 5,849 patients were included, of whom 5,335 had nondifficult, and 514 had difficult video. The facial model (only including facial images) using the light gradient boosting machine algorithm showed the highest AUC (95% CI) of 0.779 (0.733–0.825) with a sensitivity (95% CI) of 0.757 (0.650–0.845) and specificity (95% CI) of 0.721 (0.626–0.794) in the test set.

Cuendet et al.[27] proposed the first noninvasive automatic face-analysis system to detect morphological traits related to DI and improve its prediction. He collected a database of 970 patients using the importance ranking specified by the random forest algorithm. With an AUC of 0.779, this algorithmic AI model based on face scanning reported a precision level comparable to the standard methods for predicting DAs. Hayasaka et al.[28] created an AI model to classify intubation difficulties from the patient's facial image using a CNN, which links the facial image with the actual intubation difficulty. This model had an AUC of 0.864 and was helpful in tracheal intubation performed by inexperienced medical staff in emergencies or under GA. The accuracy was 80.5%, sensitivity 81.8%, and specificity 83.3%.

Recently, Wang et al.[29] used 1,000 patients scheduled for elective surgery under GA, using a multichannel information fusion method to fuse images captured from nine specific and different viewpoints. The fused information used the patient's maximum mouth opening, Mallampati score, neck length, NC, neck movements, TMD, and other vital indicators. Using a semisupervised learning method, compared with an existing supervised learning algorithm, they achieved similar classification accuracy and improved efficiency, with only a small amount of labeled data, thus predicting a reduced demand for human and material resources. Tavolara et al.[30] developed a DL model to identify difficult-to-intubate patients using an extensive database of frontal facial images to train CNNs on 11 corresponding facial portions to improve the model's overall performance, significantly surpassing conventional bedside tests.

Overall, these studies demonstrate the potential of facial analysis techniques in AI in predicting DI. With smartphones with cameras readily available, these predictive models could easily optimize usability during preoperative evaluation. They can also lay a foundation for rationalizing the collection of preoperative images and creating accessible registries.

## Airway Management and Speech Features Analysis by AI

Multiple studies in recent times have reflected the potential value of voice parameters and acoustics produced during speech as novel predictors of a DA in patients scheduled for GA. Xia M[31] in a study including 225 adult patients using univariate and multivariate logistic regression analysis, analyzed the association between acoustic features and difficult laryngoscopy in patients scheduled to undergo orthognathic surgery. Clinical airway evaluation was performed preoperatively, and the acoustic data were collected. Twelve phonemes were recorded, and their formants (f1–f4) and bandwidths (bw1–bw4) were extracted. Difficult laryngoscopy was defined as direct laryngoscopy with a Cormack–Lehane grade of 3 or 4. Difficult laryngoscopy was reported in 59/225 (26.2%) patients. The AUC attained a value of 0.761 in the training set but a value of 0.709 in the testing set. The sensitivity and specificity of the model in the testing set are 86.7% and 63.0%, respectively, leading them to conclude that acoustic features may be considered valuable predictors of difficult laryngoscopy during orthognathic surgery.

De Carvalho CC et al.[32] examined the potential for voice sounds to predict a DA as compared with the prediction by the modified Mallampati test. A total of 453 patients scheduled for elective surgery under GA with tracheal intubation were studied. Five phonemes were recorded, and their formants were analyzed. Among the five regression models evaluated, voice presented a significant association with difficult laryngoscopy (Cormack–Lehane grade 3 or 4) during GA, and the model combining both modified Mallampati score (MMS) and voice performed an even better probability of correctly classifying a randomly selected patient. Cao et al.[33] conducted a similar study including 1,160 patients and collected the clinical variables usually reported as predictors of DMV before surgery for comparison with similar results.

In the future, AI-based acoustic systems have the potential to identify patients with DAs based on speech from remote locations. However, multicentric studies involving diverse populations are necessary to confirm the promising role of voice technology in predicting DAs.

## ROLE OF AI IN FIBEROPTIC VISUALIZING DEVICES USED IN INTUBATION

Artificial intelligence technology has achieved significant progress in image classification, segmentation, and object detection, and its applications in intelligent devices such as fiberoptic bronchoscopy (FOB), Vivasight, and videolaryngoscopy, with automatic airway image recognition, are now achieving success. Videolaryngoscopes have helped to improve the view of the glottic opening and shortened the tracheal intubation time. They are often preferred for airway management due to their highest first-pass success rate across clinical settings. The Vivasight is a recently introduced disposable polyvinylchloride (PVC) ETT with an embedded video camera and light source at its distal end for continuous airway visualization on a connected monitor. This device can improve the intubation success rate without a direct laryngoscope or FOB and may be faster than the latter.[34] AI algorithms can automatically identify the pharynx and trachea based on video laryngoscope and FOB, thus assisting the anesthetist in intubation and positioning. Patrini et al.[35] developed a DL-based strategy to automatically select information-rich laryngoscope video frames, thereby reducing the amount of data to be processed for diagnosis.

Choi et al.[36] tried to develop an AI model for segmenting structures in the oral cavity using VL images acquired while performing emergency intubations, having excellent precision and specificity for vocal cords, epiglottis, and cricoid cartilage. However, this study needed to be improved by adequate model validation. Carlson and colleagues evaluated the efficacy of augmented reality videolaryngoscopy by video recording the intubation attempts performed on mannequins.[37]

With the development of technology, the level of tracheal intubation visualization continues to advance. It reduces the surgical damage to the patients, reduces the physician's stress and improves the first-attempt success. Future innovation and research focus on improving the design of video devices and refining blades for 3D visualization of airway structures with a real-time feedback system using an AI interface.

## ROBOTICS IN AIRWAY MANAGEMENT

Tighe and colleagues[38] performed the first robotic-aided endotracheal intubation in a mannequin using the Da Vinci system, an expensive and bulky device. Diagrammatic representation in **Figure 1** shows how AI and ML work in predicting airway difficulty and assisting in decision-making and treatment planning. The robot used took 75 seconds to advance the bronchoscope tip from the oropharynx to carinal visualization and 67 seconds to advance the tip from nasal entry to carinal visualization.

Hemmerling designed a Kepler intubation robot system (KIS) for intubation in mannequins,[39] consisting of a remote-control center (joystick and intubation cockpit) linked to a standard VL via a robotic arm. A single operator performed 90 intubations using a direct view, an indirect view where the operator could not see the mannequin, and a semiautomated view (30 each). All intubations were successful at the first attempt. The mean intubation times were 46 seconds, 51 seconds, and 41 seconds for the direct, indirect, and semiautomated groups, respectively. Each successive trial required less time, and automated intubations were highly reproducible. He followed up with the first human studies using the KIS.[40] They conducted a pilot study with 12 patients (11 men and one woman) requiring tracheal intubation for elective surgical procedures. Tracheal intubation was successful in 11 out of 12 patients, and the meantime taken was 93 seconds, with no complications observed. It was a small study which cannot be generalized. However, the KIS is currently a prototype, and future efforts can be directed toward enhancing its technical aspects by making it smaller, portable, and more semiautomatic. Other robots in the development stage are the IntuBot developed by Cheng et al.,[41] The portable remote robot-assisted intubation system (RRAIS) developed by Wang X et al.,[42] and the recent REALITI (robotic endoscope-automated via laryngeal imaging for tracheal intubation) system by Biro and colleagues.[43]

## CHALLENGES, LIMITATIONS, AND THE FUTURE OF AI IN AIRWAY MANAGEMENT

The healthcare industry is at a turning point, with multiple opportunities and formidable challenges as the practice, medicine, and application of technology converge in the real world to implement large-scale innovations.[44] AI-based airway management research and breakthroughs are at an investigative and development stage. It is critical to understand that AI is a tool that must be deployed in the right situation to answer an appropriate question or solve an applicable problem. AI without ethical considerations can lead to harm and wasteful research if clinicians, patients, and regulators do not oversee the correct implementation of AI technology into healthcare, especially in critical lifesaving techniques such as managing DAs.

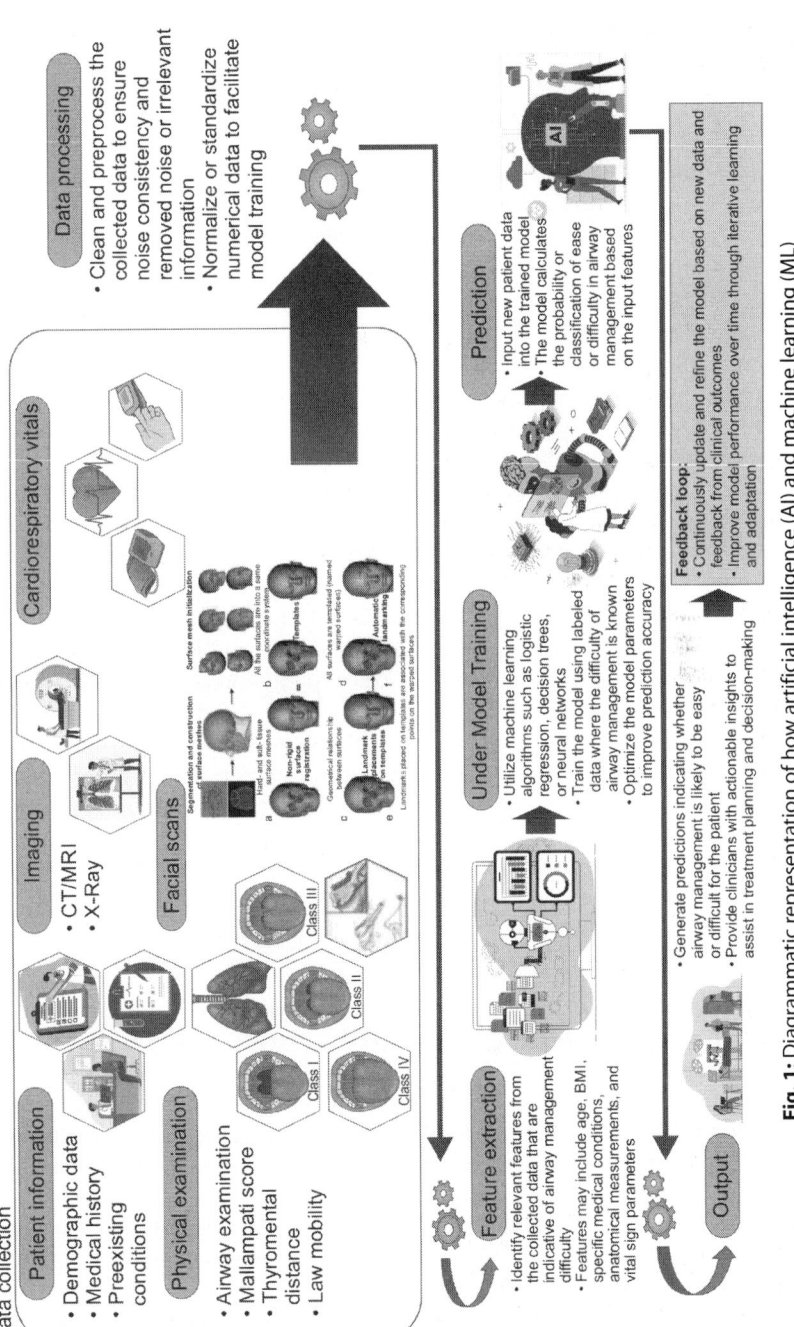

**Fig. 1:** Diagrammatic representation of how artificial intelligence (AI) and machine learning (ML) work in predicting airway difficulty and assist in decision making and treatment planning.

The AI is based on data, and data ethics should not be ignored. AI systems can exacerbate the bias if the selected data are inaccurate. There is a potential threat to data privacy and security; hence, robust policies and regulations for data management need to be implemented. AI systems can cause ethical and legal liabilities in a faulty clinical application. When we apply data such as patients' facial images, there is a need to comply with relevant laws and regulations strictly, and data confidentiality and authorization should make data leakage and misuse difficult, if not impossible. In addition, the actual use of AI in clinical settings requires regulatory approval, and the need for AI to be interpretable can make it challenging to pass regulations.

The ML-based models are challenging to interpret, as they can result in black box results, which are notified to the clinician but do not elaborate on why the prediction was made. The interpretability and transparency make a model relevant to medical decision-making. Another challenge of using AI/ML models is ensuring ethics and eliminating operator bias and prejudice during their application. Some DA prediction models are overfitted to improve accuracy, resulting in poor extrapolation. In contrast, many models are built from small single-center data, and these single-center data may also be biased. Extending the training dataset, establishing comprehensive quality control and standardization tools, and using multi-institutional data sharing and validation are essential to improve the generalization and robustness of model algorithms.[3,45,46]

The AI can quickly and efficiently analyze data and bring to focus essential patterns and correlations that may be difficult to notice by the human brain. It does not surpass the clinicians' ability to apply the findings to clinical use, and it cannot take over human performance, mainly when critical thinking and skills acquired from experience and practice are needed. Even with all the unprecedented AI advancements, the medical and surgical field practice is still a uniquely human endeavor, both a science and an art. Integration and data analysis by models do not mean the models understand the implications of that data for specific patients.[47] Anesthesiologists should continue to partner with data scientists and engineers to provide their valuable clinical insight into the development of AI in airway management.

## ■ CONCLUSION

Airway management is a critical step in anesthesia safety. AI is a transformative evolving technology that can use multivariate models to better predict airway management difficulties. AI, when ethically implemented, minimizes data and user bias and can achieve performance that is close to or exceeds that of humans. The recent research into AI applications in DA management is full of promise. This chapter has reviewed the present state of the use of AI in airway management. Further studies are required to validate this novel tool's generalizability and clinical utility on a larger scale. Regardless of risks and challenges, adopting improvements in AI technology and investing in high-quality research is essential to embrace the benefits of AI in improving clinical outcomes in airway management. This obligates anesthesiologists to understand the need to contribute and strengthen data size, quality, and validation by reporting experiences and establishing robust regulations and guidelines in our day-to-day practice to resolve ethical and legal obligations.

# REFERENCES

1. Apfelbaum JL, Hagberg CA, Connis RT, Abdelmalak BB, Agarkar M, Dutton RP, et al. 2022 American Society of Anesthesiologists Practice Guidelines for Management of the Difficult Airway. Anaesthesiology. 2022;136(1):31-81.
2. Tolsgaard MG, Pusic MV, Sebok-Syer SS, Gin B, Svendsen MB, Syer MD, et al. The fundamentals of Artificial Intelligence in medical education research: AMEE Guide No. 156. Med Teach. 2023;45(6):565-73.
3. Hashimoto DA, Witkowski E, Gao L, Meireles O, Rosman G. Artificial intelligence in anesthesiology: Current techniques, clinical applications, and limitations. Anesthesiology. 2020;132(2):379-94.
4. Ravindran B. Innovations in the management of the difficult airway: a narrative review. Cureus. 2023;15(2):e35117.
5. Yentis SM. Predicting difficult intubation–worthwhile exercise or pointless ritual? Anaesthesia. 2002;57(2):105-9.
6. Zhou CM, Wang Y, Xue Q, Yang JJ, Zhu Y. Predicting difficult airway intubation in thyroid surgery using multiple machine learning and deep learning algorithms. Front Public Health. 2022;10:937471.
7. Lee HC, Kim MK, Kim YH, Park HP. Radiographic predictors of difficult laryngoscopy in acromegaly patients. J Neurosurg Anesthesiol. 2019;31(1):50-6.
8. Senthilnathan M, Kundra P. Predictive machine learning algorithms in anticipating problems with airway management airway. 2023;6(1):4-9.
9. Jain K, Gupta N, Yadav M, Thulkar S, Bhatnagar S. Radiological evaluation of airway-what an anaesthesiologist needs to know! Indian J Anaesth. 2019;63(4):257-64.
10. Ahmad I, Millhoff B, John M, Andi K, Oakley R. Virtual endoscopy—a new assessment tool in difficult airway management. J Clin Anesth. 2015;27(6):508-13.
11. Chao I, Young J, Coles-Black J, Chuen J, Weinberg L, Rachbuch C. The application of three-dimensional printing technology in anaesthesia: a systematic review. Anaesthesia. 2017;72(5):641-50.
12. Su Z, Liang B, Shi F, Gelfond J, Šegalo S, Wang J, et al. Deep learning-based facial image analysis in medical research: a systematic review protocol. BMJ Open. 2021;11(11):e047549.
13. Zhou C-M, Xue Q, Ye H-T, Wang Y, Tong J, Ji MH, et al. Constructing a prediction model for difficult intubation of obese patients based on machine learning. J Clin Anesth. 2021;72:110278.
14. Langeron O, Masso, E, Huraux C, Guggiari M, Bianchi A, Coriat P, et al. Prediction of difficult mask ventilation. Anesthesiology. 2000;92(5):1229-36.
15. Ho Kim, Kim JH, Jang JS, Hwang SM, Lim SY, Lee JJ, et al. Development and validation of a difficult laryngoscopy prediction model using machine learning of neck circumference and thyromental height. BMC Anesthesiol. 2021;21(1):125.
16. Harris RJ, Baginski SG, Bronstein Y, Kim S, Lohr J, Towey J, et al. Measurement of endotracheal tube positioning on chest X-ray using object detection. J Digit Imaging. 2021;34(4):846-52.
17. Chen C, Huang M, Sun Y, Lai C. Development of automatic endotracheal tube and carina detection on portable supine chest radiographs using artificial intelligence. Comput Vision Pattern Recog. 2022.
18. Oliver M, Renou A, Allou N, Moscatelli L, Ferdynus C, Allyn J. Image augmentation and automated measurement of endotracheal-tube-to-carina distance on chest radiographs in intensive care unit using a deep learning model with external validation. Crit Care. 2023;27(1):40.
19. Han B, Liu Y, Zhang X, Wang J. Three-dimensional printing as an aid to airway evaluation after tracheotomy in a patient with laryngeal carcinoma. BMC Anesthesiol. 2016;16:6.

20. Grimes D, MacLeod I, Taylor T, O'Connor M, Sidebottom A. Computed tomography as an aid to planning intubation in the difficult airway. Br J Oral Maxillofac Surg. 2016;54(1):80-2.
21. Münster T, Hoffmann M, Schlaffer S, Ihmsen H, Schmitt H, Tzabazis A. Anatomical location of the vocal cords in relation to cervical vertebrae: a new predictor of difficult laryngoscopy? Eur J Anaesthesiol. 2016;33(4):257-62.
22. Yao W, Zhou Y, Wang B, Yu T, Shen Z, Wu H, et al. Can mandibular condylar mobility sonography measurements predict difficult laryngoscopy? Anesth Analg. 2017;124(3):800-6.
23. Gupta D, Srirajakalidindi A, Ittiara B, Apple L, Toshniwal G, Haber H. Ultrasonographic modification of Cormack Lehane classification for pre-anesthetic airway assessment. Middle East J Anaesthesiol. 2012;21(6):835-42.
24. Lundstrøm LH, Rosenstock CV, Wetterslev J, Nørskov AK. The DIFFMASK score for predicting difficult facemask ventilation: a cohort study of 46,804 patients. Anaesthesia. 2019;74(10):1267-76.
25. Pei B, Jin C, Cao S, Ji N, Xia M, Jiang H. Geometric morphometrics and machine learning from three-dimensional facial scans for difficult mask ventilation prediction. Front Med (Lausanne) 2023;10:1203023.
26. M Xia, C Jin, Y Zheng, J Wang, M Zhao, S Cao, et al. Jian Deep learning-based facial analysis for predicting difficult videolaryngoscopy: a feasibility study. Anaesthesia. 2024;79(4):399-409.
27. Cuendet GL, Schoettker P, Yüce A, Sorci M, Gao H, Perruchoud C, et al. Facial image analysis for fully automatic prediction of difficult endotracheal intubation. IEEE Trans Biomed Eng. 2016;63(2):328-39.
28. Hayasaka T, Kawano K, Kurihara K, Suzuki H, Nakane M, Kawamae K, et al. Creation of an artificial intelligence model for intubation difficulty classification by deep learning (convolutional neural network) using face images: an observational study. J Intensive Care. 2021;9(1):38.
29. Wang G, Li C, Tang F, Wang Y, Wu S, Zhi H, et al. A fully-automatic semi-supervised deep learning model for difficult airway assessment. Heliyon. 2023;9(5):e15629.
30. Tavolara TE, Gurcan MN, Segal S, Niazi MKK. Identification of difficult to intubate patients from frontal face images using an ensemble of deep learning models. Comput Biol Med. 2021;136:104737.
31. Xia M, Cao S, Zhou R, Wang JY, Xu TY, Zhou ZK, et al. Acoustic features as novel predictors of difficult laryngoscopy in orthognathic surgery: an observational study. Ann Transl Med. 2021;9(18):1466.
32. de Carvalho CC, da Silva DM, de Carvalho Junior AD, Santos Neto JM, Rio BR, Neto CN, et al. Pre-operative voice evaluation as a hypothetical predictor of difficult laryngoscopy. Anaesthesia. 2019;74(9):1147-52.
33. Cao S, Xia M, Zhou R, Wang J, Jin CY, Pei B, et al. Voice parameters for difficult mask ventilation evaluation: an observational study. Ann Transl Med. 2021;9(23):1740.
34. Huitink JM, Koopman EM, Bouwman RA, Craenen A, Verwoert M, Krage R, et al. Tracheal intubation with a camera embedded in the tube tip (Vivasight™). Anaesthesia. 2013;68(1):74-8.
35. Patrini I, Ruperti M, Moccia S, Mattos LS, Frontoni E, De Momi E. Transfer learning for informative-frame selection in laryngoscopic videos through learned features. Med Biol Eng Comput. 2020;58(6):1225-38.
36. Choi SJ, Kim DK, Kim BS, Cho M, Jeong JM, Jo YH, et al. Mask R-CNN based multiclass segmentation model for endotracheal intubation using video laryngoscope. Digit Health. 2023;9:2055-76.
37. Carlson JN, Das S, De la Torre F, Frisch A, Guyette FX, Hodgins JK, et al. A Novel artificial intelligence system for endotracheal intubation. Prehosp Emerg Care. 2016;20(5):667-71.

38. Tighe PJ, Badiyan SJ, Luria I, Lampotang S, Parekattil S. Robot-assisted airway support: a simulated case. Anesth Analg. 2010;111(4):929-31.
39. Hemmerling TM, Wehbe M, Zaouter C, Taddei R, Morse J. The Kepler intubation system. Anesth Analg. 2012;114(3):590-4.
40. Hemmerling TM, Taddei R, Wehbe M, Zaouter C, Cyr S, Morse J. First robotic tracheal intubations in humans using the Kepler intubation system J. Br J Anaesth. 2012;108(6):1011-6.
41. Cheng X, Jiang G, Lee K, Yheoshua LN. IntuBot: Design and prototyping of a robotic intubation device. 2018 IEEE International Conference on Robotics and Automation (ICRA) 2018:1482-7.
42. Wang X, Tao Y, Tao X, Chen J, Jin Y, Shan Z, et al. An original design of remote robot-assisted intubation system. Sci Rep. 2018;8(1):13403.
43. Biro P, Hofmann P, Gage D, Boehler Q, Chautems C, Braun J, et al. Automated tracheal intubation in an airway manikin using a robotic endoscope: a proof of concept study. Anaesthesia. 2020;75(7):881-6.
44. Naik NB, Mathew PJ, Kundra P. Scope of artificial intelligence in airway management. Indian J Anaesth. 2024;68(1):105-10.
45. Buch VH, Ahmed I, Maruthappu M. Artificial intelligence in medicine: current trends and future possibilities. Br J Gen Pract. 2018;68(668):143-4.
46. Collins GS, Reitsma JB, Altman DG, Moons KG. Transparent reporting of a multivariable prediction model for individual prognosis or diagnosis (TRIPOD): the TRIPOD statement. BMJ. 2015;350:g7594.
47. Chen H, Zheng Y, Fu Q, Peng Li. A review of the current status and progress in difficult airway assessment research. Eur J Med Res. 2024;29:172.

# CHAPTER 5

# Maternal Cardiac Arrest

*Michael J Furdyna, Michaela K Farber*

## ABSTRACT

Maternal mortality rates are increasing in developed countries due to increased maternal age and comorbidities. Maternal cardiac arrest (MCA) represents the culmination of physiologic deterioration and a final opportunity for life-saving intervention. Obstetric anesthesiologists must establish MCA preparedness, expertise, rapid management, and team leadership to optimize maternal and newborn survival. Identifying risk factors, recognizing signs of deterioration, and establishing a rapid differential diagnosis when MCA occurs are vital components of care. Facilitating resuscitative hysterotomy within 5 minutes of arrest promotes the return of spontaneous circulation. Leading etiologies of MCA—maternal hemorrhage, amniotic fluid or pulmonary embolism, anesthesia complications, and cardiovascular complications—are discussed. Updates in basic and advanced management strategies for the obstetric anesthesiologist are reviewed. Crisis management, team training, and identification of unit deficiencies can best be done with simulation training for such rare events. Mastery of these aspects will ensure preparedness when MCA occurs.

**Keywords:** Maternal cardiac arrest; ACLS; Resuscitative hysterotomy; POCUS; Postpartum hemorrhage; Amniotic fluid embolism; High spinal; Local anesthetic systemic toxicity

## KEY POINTS

- Cardiopulmonary resuscitation during maternal cardiac arrest (MCA utilizes the same chest compression location, frequency, and quality as in nonpregnant patients. Manual left uterine displacement should be performed to relieve aortocaval compression without compromising cardiopulmonary resuscitation (CPR) quality. Medications that would be used in the management of cardiac arrest should not be withheld due to pregnancy status.
- A resuscitative hysterotomy, or perimortem cesarean delivery, should be performed within 5 minutes in all cases at 20-week gestation or more for best maternal survival.
- Understanding the causes of arrest that are more common in, or unique to, pregnancy and the peripartum period can expedite diagnosis and targeted treatment. Anesthesiologists should be familiar with the manifestations and management of such etiologies, including postpartum hemorrhage, amniotic fluid embolism, high spinal, and peripartum cardiomyopathy.
- Anesthetic complications are significant contributors to MCA. An anesthesiologist must recognize and understand both direct and indirect anesthesia-related causes of MCA so that vigilance can be maintained at all times.

# INTRODUCTION

The global burden of maternal mortality is alarmingly high, with approximately 800 maternal deaths occurring in the world every day.[1] Maternal cardiac arrest (MCA) represents the culmination of physiologic deterioration and a final opportunity for life-saving intervention. Obstetric anesthesiologists play a critical role in leading resuscitation when MCA occurs in a hospital. Preparedness for the best maternal chance of survival requires that anesthesiologists recognize both general and obstetric-specific risk factors for MCA, adhere to established best practices for cardiopulmonary resuscitation (CPR) and advanced cardiovascular life support (ACLS), establish crisis response systems for emergencies tailored to their local practice, and adopt procedural safeguards to eliminate iatrogenic causes of arrest. This chapter reviews MCA's epidemiology and critical management principles, highlighting specific clinical scenarios and anesthesia strategies for successful resuscitation.

# EPIDEMIOLOGY

The pooled incidence of MCA in a 2023 systematic review of 63,859,400 maternities worldwide was 5.83 per 100,000 maternities.[2] In this series, 42% of women survived till hospital discharge. Population-based studies from the United Kingdom (UK), United States (US), and Canada extrapolate national incidences of MCA to be 1 in 12,000 to 1 in 36,000 (2.8–8.3 per 100,000), with inhospital survival rates as high as 59%.[3-5] Higher overall inhospital survival after MCA may reflect reversible causes of arrest such as hemorrhage and respiratory failure from high spinal.[6] The global maternal mortality rate is declining, according to the World Health Organization, yet in the US, maternal death has worsened from 7.2 per 100,000 live births in 1987 to 19 per 100,000 live births in 2023.[7] Trends of increased mortality have also been noted in other developed countries such as the UK[8] and likely reflect increasing maternal age, comorbidity burden, and worsening racial disparities in care. Recognizing drivers of MCA, including patient risk factors, signs of deterioration, etiology, and outcomes, is a task that must be undertaken by anesthesia care providers at the local clinic or hospital level, given the heterogeneity of this vulnerable patient population and accessibility to care.

# MANAGEMENT OF MATERNAL CARDIAC ARREST

The general principles of MCA management are the same as those for cardiac arrest in nonpregnant patients **(Table 1)**.[9-14] Critical general management features and considerations specific to obstetric patients are reviewed here. At the time of MCA, it is essential to stop all medications that have potential validator or negative inotropic effects, including general anesthetic agents, oxytocin, magnesium, local anesthetics, and other agents.[15]

## Uterine Displacement

In nonpregnant cardiac arrest patients, optimized chest compressions yield a cardiac output of approximately 30%.[16] At approximately 20 weeks of gestational age, the uterus size may compress the abdomen's aorta and inferior vena cava (aortocaval compression). Relief of aortocaval compression is recommended during CPR, as this improves venous return and improves cardiac output.[9] Previously, this was sometimes accomplished by tilting the patient. However, it has been demonstrated that tilting

**TABLE 1:** General principles of MCA management.

Core similarities between obstetric and nonobstetric advanced cardiovascular life support (ACLS)

| | |
|---|---|
| Chest Compressions[9] | • Hand over hand, lower half of sternum (avoid xiphoid process)<br>• Compress to 5–6 cm and allow full recoil<br>  Compress at a rate of 100–120 compressions per minute |
| Epinephrine*[10] | 1 mg IV or IO every 3–5 minutes |
| Amiodarone[9] | • 300 mg IV or IO after 3rd defibrillation<br>  150 mg IV or IO after the 4th defibrillation |
| Lidocaine†[10] | • It can be used in place of amiodarone<br>• 1–1.5 mg/kg IV or IO after 3rd defibrillation<br>• 0.5–0.75mg/kg IV or IO after 4th defibrillation |
| Defibrillation‡[9,11-14] | • Every 2 minutes, if a shockable rhythm<br>• Pads placed anterior/lateral or anterior/posterior<br>• 200 J biphasic or 360 J monophasic |

*When local anesthetic systemic toxicity is suspected, doses of less than 1 mcg/kg are recommended.
†Lidocaine should not be used if local anesthetic toxicity is suspected.
‡If possible, remove fetal monitors before defibrillation, given the theoretical risk of electrical arcing, but do not delay defibrillation for this.

patients in this fashion during CPR results in lower-quality chest compressions.[17] Instead, lateral uterine displacement should be performed manually with the patient placed supine.

## Airway Management

Prompt airway management is vital in cases of MCA and should be a priority when hypoxemia is suspected as the etiology. Due to the increased metabolic demand and diminished pregnancy reserve, bag-mask ventilation should be performed with 100% oxygen. Chest compressions should alternate with rescue breaths in a 30:2 ratio until an advanced airway is secured.[13] Early intubation should be prioritized due to the elevated aspiration risk in late pregnancy. However, intubation attempts should not interfere with high-quality CPR, nor should they delay a resuscitative hysterotomy.[13] Once an advanced airway is in place, standard ACLS guidelines recommend a rate of 10-12 breaths per minute to avoid lung overdistension and its potential hemodynamic effects.[9] Once the return of spontaneous circulation (ROSC) is achieved, ventilation should be titrated appropriately for pregnant physiology.

## Vascular Access

Vascular access is critical in MCA, with some considerations specific to pregnancy. Due to aortocaval compression, the inferior vena cava may have impaired or variable venous return. Therefore, vascular access should be obtained above the diaphragm to ensure reliable delivery of medications, and preexisting upper extremity vascular access should be used preferentially over femoral access for resuscitation. If intravenous access cannot be quickly secured, intraosseous access should be obtained via humeral or sternal sites.[13]

## Resuscitative Hysterotomy

One of the most notable differences in the management of cardiac arrest in pregnant versus nonpregnant patients is the concept of resuscitative hysterotomy or performing a cesarean delivery during ongoing resuscitation. Historically referred to as a perimortem cesarean delivery (PMCD), the term resuscitative hysterotomy better reflects its intent to benefit both maternal and fetal survival.[18] Instrumental delivery may be attempted when the fetal position is favorable.

### Hemodynamic Principles and Benefit

Aortocaval compression by the gravid uterus impairs venous return and cardiac output. Similar to lateral uterine displacement, delivery of the fetus relieves this impairment and promotes improved cardiac output. Eliminating the fetoplacental circulation and contraction of the uterus following delivery redirects cardiac output to other vital organs.[18] Additionally, delivery of the fetus removes it from a hypoperfused environment for resuscitation and optimal survival. Multiple studies have shown that resuscitative hysterotomies can improve both maternal and fetal outcomes, and their use is widely endorsed.[13,18-21]

### Eligibility

Resuscitative hysterotomy should be considered in all patients at 20 week gestation or more, in which delivery of the gravid uterus may improve maternal hemodynamics (20 weeks onward) or improve fetal survival (23-24 weeks onward). If gestational age is unknown, a palpable or visible uterus above the umbilicus suggests a size large enough to cause aortocaval compression.[18-20] Point-of-care obstetric ultrasound can be used if it is immediately available and if large body habitus impedes the ability to verify pregnancy by direct visualization or palpation; fetal biparietal diameter ≥45 mm or fetal femur length over ≥30 mm indicates sufficient size.[22]

### Timing

Evidence suggests that prompt resuscitative hysterotomy performance improves maternal and fetal outcomes.[20] The guideline consensus is that it should be performed if there is no maternal ROSC by 4 minutes, with the goal of delivery by 5 minutes.[13,18] Resuscitative hysterotomy can be considered before 5 minutes in specific circumstances, such as an unknown duration of arrest or a nonshockable rhythm.[21] It is technically challenging to achieve a resuscitative hysterotomy within 5 minutes of a witnessed MCA. Failure to achieve the goal should not lead to deprioritization by the team; maternal and fetal patients can still achieve favorable outcomes with emergent delivery that extends far beyond the goal of 5 minutes postarrest, mainly if high-quality CPR is administered from the time of arrest to the time delivery can be achieved.

## Advanced Management

### Point-of-Care Ultrasound

Obstetric anesthesiologists and critical care specialists increasingly utilize point-of-care ultrasound (POCUS) (**Fig. 1**). While the full extent of ultrasonographic techniques

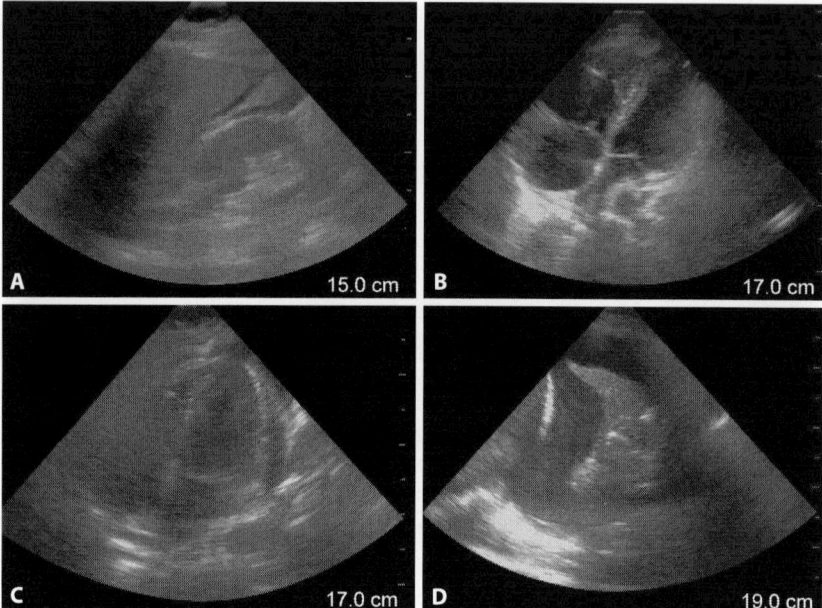

**Figs. 1A to D:** (A) Abdominal POCUS with free fluid in the abdomen between the liver and kidney, as can be seen with uterine rupture or other intraperitoneal hemorrhage; (B) Dilated right ventricle on cardiac POCUS, as can be seen with pulmonary embolism; (C) Pericardial effusion on cardiac POCUS, causing tamponade; and (D) Pleural effusion on lung POCUS, as can be seen in heart failure. (POCUS: point-of-care ultrasound)

and their applications are outside the scope of this chapter, POCUS holds promise for the prevention, differential diagnosis, and management of MCA. A brief overview of standard POCUS techniques and potential uses is described here.

*Cardiac POCUS* can be one of the most valuable forms of ultrasound in MCA or peri-arrest periods and is increasingly considered a vital skill to care for critically ill pregnant patients.[23-25] Several protocols for rapid, qualitative assessments of cardiac pathology exist, such as the Focus Assessed Transthoracic Echocardiography (FATE) protocol and others. Such tools can be used to identify cardiac pathology, including cardiac tamponade, acute right ventricular failure, and hypovolemic shock.[23,25,26] For those with training, protocols such as the Rapid Obstetric Screening Echocardiography (ROSE) protocol can be used to make advanced measurements to diagnose hypotension or periarrest.[27] Additional experience with critical care echocardiography allows for more detailed quantitative assessments to guide management.[23] In cardiac arrest, the subxiphoid view can often be obtained without interfering with chest compressions. It can identify potential pathologies, assess compression quality, and assess cardiac activity during pulse checks.

*Lung POCUS* has several uses in peri-arrest or cardiac arrest. Examining the lung fields and bases can suggest pathologies such as interstitial edema, consolidation (i.e., pneumonia), and pleural effusions. Additionally, examination of lung movement can be used to identify or rule out a pneumothorax, which in the setting of arrest may be a tension pneumothorax, or identify esophageal or unilateral intubation.[25]

*Abdominal POCUS* has several potential applications. It is a component of the Focused Assessment with Sonography (FAST) exam, designed to investigate hypotension and possible bleeding in trauma patients. Still, its techniques can be applied to the obstetric population as well. Hemorrhagic etiologies of hypotension or arrest can be suggested by the presence of free fluid in the abdomen, including uterine rupture, a bleeding placenta percreta, postoperative bleeding, and subcapsular hematoma.[25] Abdominal POCUS can be used to rapidly assess uterine and fetal status and guide decision-making, such as identification of retained products of conception or confirmation of pregnancy when an examination is unclear.[22,25]

*Gastric POCUS* is a growing subcategory of abdominal ultrasound focused on measuring stomach contents and quantity to assess aspiration risk. While it is unlikely to be directly helpful in cardiac arrest, identifying a full or empty stomach can help clinicians make better informed anesthetic decisions, potentially avoiding catastrophic events such as aspiration.[28]

*Vascular POCUS* is one of the modalities most familiar to anesthesiologists and can help obtain rapid access to invasive blood pressure monitoring. Additionally, multiple protocols exist using ultrasonography to rapidly evaluate for the presence of deep venous thromboses (DVTs), for which pregnant patients are at higher risk. In a patient with unexplained MCA, the presence of DVTs should raise suspicion for pulmonary embolism and prompt consideration for thrombolysis or thrombectomy.[25,29,30]

### Transesophageal Echocardiography

Transesophageal echocardiography (TEE) is an advanced cardiac imaging modality that can be beneficial in managing MCA. Advanced training and TEE availability are limiting factors. Still, if available, its use should be considered, mainly when the etiology of arrest is uncertain or when guiding prolonged resuscitation in an intubated patient. TEE allows a more detailed evaluation of cardiac structures and function without tissue or air obstruction and does not interfere with chest compressions.

### Extracorporeal Membrane Oxygenation

The usage of extracorporeal membrane oxygenation (ECMO) in pregnancy is increasing for cardiac and respiratory arrest.[31] As per a recent systematic review, most ECMO cannulations for MCA occurred in the immediate postpartum period. The overall survival rate among MCA cases utilizing ECMO was 87.7%.[31] If available, the use of ECMO or E-CPR may be considered in MCA. ECMO should not be used in place of or to delay resuscitative hysterotomy, but rather in situations where a resuscitative hysterotomy has failed to achieve ROSC or does not apply.[21]

## CAUSES OF MATERNAL CARDIAC ARREST AND SPECIFIC MANAGEMENT

It is important to remember that women who are pregnant or postpartum can suffer cardiac arrest for all the reasons that nonpregnant patients can, including septic or hypovolemic shock. A firm grasp of the differential for cardiac arrest unrelated to pregnancy, as well as the significant forms of shock, is essential. However, focusing on causes of arrest that are more common in, or unique to, pregnancy and the peripartum period, whether due to physiologic changes, specific intrapartum events, or commonly used anesthetics, can expedite diagnosis and targeted treatment.

## Postpartum Hemorrhage

Hemorrhage is a leading cause of MCA in the peripartum period; antepartum, intrapartum, or postpartum hemorrhage is a potential contributing factor in over 50% of MCAs in high-resource countries.[4] In the perianesthetic period, hemorrhage has been implicated in 25.0–40.2% of arrests.[32,33] Most instances of hemorrhagic shock and cardiac arrest that occur during or in temporal proximity to anesthesia are due to postpartum hemorrhage. However, antepartum hemorrhage, trauma, aortic dissection, and other etiologies also contribute. It is essential to recognize and treat the various etiologies of postpartum hemorrhage, including uterine atony, abnormal placentation (e.g., placenta accreta), retained products of conception, vascular or tissue damage (e.g., vaginal laceration or hysterotomy extension), and coagulopathy.

Targeted management of bleeding based on etiology requires vigilance and engagement on the part of the anesthesiologist to address uncontrolled bleeding, correct coagulopathy, and prevent hemorrhagic shock and cardiac arrest, which itself has a mortality rate as dismal as cardiac arrest from amniotic fluid embolism in a recent database study.[5,34] Delayed recognition and treatment of hemorrhage remains a common and avoidable cause of arrest; in one series, inadequate early resuscitation contributed to 6 out of 7 hemorrhagic arrests.[32,35] Anesthesiologists should be vigilant for warning signs of impending hypovolemic shock, such as a shock index (heart rate divided by systolic blood pressure) of 1.0 or higher; a heart rate consistently above systolic blood pressure should prompt a reevaluation of the scope of blood loss and escalation of care.[35] As described earlier, cardiac POCUS can also help determine volume status. Anesthesiologists must promptly administer the appropriate uterotonics and other hemorrhage medications, including oxytocin or carbetocin, secondary uterotonics, calcium, tranexamic acid, and fibrinogen concentrate.[36,37]

There are no universally accepted guidelines on blood product ratios for major transfusion during obstetric hemorrhage. Still, most societies have historically recommended some variation of balanced ratio (e.g., 1:1:1) to avoid worsening coagulopathy.[37] Growing evidence shows that fibrinogen is critical in maternal hemostasis and that fixed-ratio transfusions may dilute intrinsic maternal serum fibrinogen. Likewise, evidence suggests that goal-directed, as opposed to fixed-ratio, transfusions lead to improved outcomes.[37-39] In particular, viscoelastic testing (thromboelastography and rotational thromboelastometry) may allow for more targeted transfusions.[37-39] Obstetric hemorrhage that is acute and unstable may preclude the ability to assess for coagulopathy and provide goal-directed therapy. The critical role of the anesthesiologist is to recognize such situations and provide aggressive volume resuscitation, continuously evaluating the surgical condition and patient status. Once a patient stabilizes, avoiding overtransfusion can lower the risks of transfusion-associated circulatory overload and transfusion-related acute lung injury.

## Amniotic Fluid Embolism

Amniotic fluid embolism (AFE) is among the most unpredictable and feared causes of MCA, accounting for an estimated 12.6–16.7% of arrests during delivery hospitalization and up to 14.3–31.0% of arrests in the perianesthetic period.[4,5,32,33,40]

The pathophysiology of AFE is not fully understood. Still, it is believed to stem from disruption of the maternal–fetal interface, the introduction of fetal material into maternal circulation, and abnormal immunologic response. The presentation of AFE is variable but classically begins with profound pulmonary vasoconstriction, leading to hypoxemia; right ventricular failure; and cardiovascular collapse. Patients may also experience altered mental status and seizures. Left ventricular failure, including ongoing hypotension and pulmonary edema, is usually a delayed manifestation.[41] Disseminated intravascular coagulation (DIC) is a common finding and may be present in over 80% of AFEs; while classically seen as a delayed manifestation, it can also occur in the early phase. DIC can lead to ongoing hemorrhage, further patient instability, as well as subsequent multiorgan failure.[41] Given its severe consequences, AFE should be suspected when a woman experiences cardiorespiratory collapse either during labor or shortly after vaginal or cesarean delivery so that aggressive supportive measures can be initiated promptly.[41]

Management of cardiac arrest or peri-arrest due to AFE should include the core concepts discussed in this chapter, such as the ACLS algorithm, preparation for possible resuscitative hysterotomy, and consideration of ECMO. The clinical challenge of AFE is its variable manifestation of cardiac arrest, which can range from transient to refractory. Reversible causes of cardiac arrest—hemorrhage, local anesthetic systemic toxicity (LAST), magnesium toxicity, and hypoxemia—must be ruled out early. For such patients with refractory cardiac arrest and suspected AFE, urgent consideration for ECMO or cardiopulmonary bypass can be a life-saving maneuver.

Once ROSC has been achieved in suspected AFE, no single treatment or therapy exists; additional supportive care should be tailored to the condition's unique features. As acute right ventricular dysfunction is often an early manifestation, anesthesiologists should be mindful of both under and overresuscitation when treating a suspected AFE. Agents with inotropic properties (e.g., epinephrine, norepinephrine, and milrinone) should be used to support the right heart, and pure vasoconstrictors that increase right heart afterload (e.g., phenylephrine) should be used judiciously. Inhaled or intravenous pulmonary vasodilators (e.g., nitric oxide) can also be beneficial if available.[41] Cardiac POCUS can be helpful throughout this period to evaluate volume status and the quality of right heart function and monitor for the delayed onset of left ventricular dysfunction. If left-sided dysfunction and systemic vasodilation develop, continued inotrope and vasopressor usage will likely be required.

Preparations should be made for massive bleeding and blood product transfusion as soon as an AFE is suspected, including massive transfusion protocol activation, large-bore intravenous access, and invasive blood pressure monitoring. Multiple factors may cause hemorrhage, even if it was not present initially. Uterine atony after delivery is often seen during an AFE, and if identified, it should be treated aggressively with uterotonics.[41] Additionally, it is recommended to begin serially assessing for coagulopathy when an AFE is suspected, as its time course is variable.[41] Clinically, this may manifest as increased bleeding from surgical or venipuncture sites, vaginal bleeding, hematuria, or bleeding from other locations. A goal-directed approach to blood replacement and coagulation management using laboratory testing, including fibrinogen measurement, is recommended to avoid overtransfusion or worsening coagulopathy.[41] Serial viscoelastic testing can help further tailor the response usage of antifibrinolytic agents such as tranexamic acid.[41]

## Anesthetic Complications

Anesthetic complications significantly contribute to MCA, and they are involved in up to 67.9% of cases. In high-resource settings, anesthetic factors are a leading cause of MCA.[3,5,32,33,40] Direct anesthetic complications that can lead to MCA include high spinal or failed intubation, both of which manifest as a hypoxemic arrest.[3,32,33] Such cardiac arrests from anesthesia complications have a higher rate of ROSC and lower mortality than other causes. Indirect anesthetic factors can include failure to recognize or treat other etiologies, such as inadequate resuscitation in an ongoing postpartum hemorrhage, as discussed earlier. They can also include anesthetic decisions or techniques that compound other factors, such as induction of anesthesia in tenuous patients. An anesthesiologist must recognize and understand both direct and indirect anesthesia-related causes of MCA so that vigilance can be maintained at all times.

### High Spinal Block

Total spinal anesthesia is a direct anesthetic cause of hypoxemic cardiac arrest when local anesthetic ascends to cause paralysis of the diaphragm at C3, 4, and 5 (respiratory weakness/failure) to the midbrain, including the recurrent pharyngeal innervation (loss of phonation). This complication can occur after de novo spinal; a commonly described clinical scenario is spinal administration after an epidural failed to provide adequate anesthesia for cesarean delivery.[3,32,35] In such cases, thecal sac compression from epidural volume may lead to unpredictable and high spinal blocks. A high spinal can also occur from epidural dosing of unrecognized intrathecal catheters, most commonly when converting to cesarean anesthesia.[3,32,33] This can occur due to a catheter placed intrathecally and not tested or not recognized or due to a catheter that previously behaved like an epidural but migrated to the intrathecal space. True catheter migration is considered unlikely with flexible, wire-reinforced catheters. However, subdural catheters can potentially rupture the subarachnoid membrane, particularly when large volumes are administered quickly, with unpredictable effects.[35] While there is no test for a subdural catheter, unpredictable behavior or unusual sensorimotor blockade should prompt its consideration.

Fractionating larger boluses into smaller doses may reduce the risk of subarachnoid membrane rupture or identify it before administration of a full dose.[35] Overall, safe anesthesia practices such as catheter aspiration before any epidural injection and considering every dose to be a test dose can lower the risk of an unrecognized intrathecal catheter in an obstetric patient. Bag valve masks and airway equipment must be immediately available for airway support of patients who develop a high spinal with respiratory failure. Labor and delivery units should be equipped with safety monitors such as call buttons within reach of the patient, policies to encourage spouse or support person's presence during labor, and safe supervision ratios of patients to nurses, midwives, and physicians.

### Bradyarrhythmia

Bradyarrhythmias progressing to cardiac arrest are a factor in 2.3–21.4% of arrests overall, in high-resource countries.[32,33] In most of these cases, cardiac arrest occurred in the setting of spinal anesthesia, ranging from less than 10–30 minutes after medication administration.[32] The Bezold-Jarisch reflex, or reflexive slowing of the heart rate in response to decreased venous return, is believed to be the primary mechanism, compounded by the blockade of cardiac accelerator fibers in the high thoracic sympathetic chain.[32,35] Additionally, alpha-adrenergic vasopressors such as phenylephrine are frequently used as first-line infusions or boluses in cesarean deliveries and can worsen bradycardia as well.

While the degree of bradycardia after spinal anesthesia cannot be predicted, specific strategies may mitigate the risk of deterioration to cardiac arrest. Fluid coloading during neuraxial administration can reduce the decrease in venous return from vasodilation. Vasopressors with beta-adrenergic agonism, such as norepinephrine, are being reexamined as potential alternatives to pure alpha-adrenergic agents.[35] Ondansetron, an antiemetic with 5-HT3 receptor antagonism, is frequently used in cesarean deliveries; evidence suggests that administering ondansetron before spinal medications may likewise blunt the Bezold–Jarisch reflex.

## Difficult Airway

Physiologic changes during pregnancy and labor lead to changes in the maternal airway that can make intubation challenging, including increased airway edema and tissue friability.[10] In one study of general anesthesia for cesarean delivery in a high-resource country, the risk of difficult intubation was 1 in 49 patients, and the risk of failed intubation was 1 in 808 patients.[42] Difficult or failed intubations can contribute directly to cardiac arrest from hypoxemia.[3,32,33] Additionally, a challenging maternal airway can complicate resuscitation after cardiac arrest has occurred, regardless of the cause of the arrest.

Providers should be familiar with locally available airway equipment and societal difficult airway algorithms to address airway issues quickly. When a pregnant patient is being induced for general anesthesia in a controlled setting, adequate preoxygenation is critical, given increased oxygen demand and decreased reserve.[13] A rapid sequence induction should be performed for patients who are not adequately NPO or are beyond 20 weeks gestation, given the elevated aspiration risk.[10] The total number of attempts should be minimized given the potential for airway trauma and worsening view; repeated attempts should be limited to experienced providers.[10] Videolaryngoscopy can increase the likelihood of successful intubation; however, while it is increasingly available, its usage remains limited in the obstetric setting, even in high-utilization environments.[35,42] In the event of an inability to intubate, laryngeal mask airways can establish ventilation with some reduction in aspiration risk.[10] Other means of establishing ventilation may also be attempted. Still, providers should be prepared for a "cannot intubate, cannot ventilate" situation and its contingencies, including emergence from anesthesia or establishing a surgical airway.[10]

While general anesthesia cannot be avoided altogether in obstetrics, the use of neuraxial analgesia significantly lowers the risk of emergency general anesthetics. Functional labor epidurals can be converted for anesthesia within minutes, and anesthesiologists can anticipate such need by monitoring fetal heart tracings in labor in conjunction with the obstetric and nursing teams. Personalized patient care, considering factors such as body habitus, airway, anticipated difficulty of neuraxial, and anticipated need for surgery, is essential to planning labor analgesia or neuraxial anesthesia and minimizing the need for intubation.[35]

## Local Anesthetic Systemic Toxicity

Local anesthetic systemic toxicity is a rare but life-threatening condition caused when local anesthetics reach a toxic blood concentration, which can occur via direct vascular injection or tissue absorption.[43,44] Effects are primarily neurologic and cardiovascular. Neurologic manifestations typically begin as excitatory symptoms, including paresthesia, tinnitus, agitation, altered mental status, and seizure, followed by central nervous system depression.[44] The estimated incidence of LAST in the general population is less than 11 per 10,000 epidurals; the described incidence among peripheral nerve blocks varies between similar rates up to 1 in 500 epidurals.[43,44] Pregnant patients are at elevated risk of developing LAST due to increased neuronal sensitivity to local anesthetics, increased propensity for arrhythmias, increased local anesthetic absorption from extravascular tissues, and increased unbound fraction of plasma local anesthetics.[43,44]

Despite a higher risk in obstetrics, LAST as a cause of MCA is exceedingly rare, accounting for less than 0.5% of cases.[4,5,32] A 2024 scoping review identified 22 instances of reported LAST in peripartum patients, three of which had cardiac arrest; of these, two died. However, nine more had severe symptoms, including seizures, arrhythmias, and respiratory arrest, with the potential to progress to cardiac arrest without intervention.[43] Half of these occurred in the setting of a transversus abdominis plane (TAP) block after cesarean delivery. Of the cardiac arrests, two were attributed to accidental intravascular infusions of bupivacaine and one due to an overdose of ropivacaine after a TAP block.[43]

Suppose LAST is suspected as the cause of cardiac arrest; in that case, any local anesthetic administration should be stopped, and a 20% lipid emulsion should be administered intravenously, in addition to care, as outlined earlier in this chapter. Intralipid should be stocked, and immediately available on any patient unit where neuraxial and peripheral local anesthetics are administered due to the risk of LAST, and labor and delivery units are no exception. An initial bolus of 1.5 mL/kg intralipid should be given over 1 minute, followed by an infusion at 15 mL/kg/h, using ideal body weight. This bolus can be repeated twice with 5 minutes in between if there is cardiovascular instability. After the first 5 minutes, the infusion can be doubled to 30 mL/kg/h if needed; this should be continued until clinical stability or a maximum of 12 mL/kg is reached.[44] In the event of a shockable arrhythmia during arrest, Lidocaine should *not* be used in place of amiodarone. A smaller bolus of epinephrine should be considered (starting with ≤1 μg/kg) in place of the standard 1 mg dose, escalating if need be. Vasopressin should be avoided.[45]

## Pulmonary Embolism

Pregnant and postpartum patients are at elevated risk of pulmonary embolism. Pregnancy is an inherently hypercoagulable state. Additionally, multiple iatrogenic factors promote clots in obstetric patients, including prolonged bed rest as well as inflammatory changes after cesarean delivery. Up to 14.1% of MCAs are related to venous thromboembolic events, with up to 3.5% occurring during the immediate perianesthetic period.[3,33]

Pulmonary embolism should be suspected in pregnant patients experiencing acute tachycardia, hypotension, or hypoxemia. While D-dimer tests are elevated and thereby less diagnostic for pulmonary embolism in pregnancy, levels <500 ng/mL with low clinical suspicion can help rule out the diagnosis.[46] In many cases, imaging and clinical judgment are required for diagnosis. In the context of cardiac arrest, ultrasonography can be used to support or refute pulmonary embolism in real time. A pulmonary embolism large enough to cause hemodynamic collapse will likely cause acute right heart failure as well, which can be detected with cardiac POCUS.

Treatment options for pulmonary embolism vary with severity, with options for massive emboli including thrombolytics and mechanical or open thrombectomies. As with other interventions in MCA, appropriate care should not be withheld for pregnancy status. Furthermore, thrombolytics, such as the tissue plasminogen activator, do not cross the placenta due to their large molecular size.[47] However, bleeding risk should be carefully considered, particularly following recent delivery.

## Peripartum Cardiomyopathy, Preeclampsia, and other Cardiovascular Pathologies

Cardiovascular pathologies such as heart failure and myocardial infarction can precipitate cardiac arrest in pregnant patients, as with nonobstetric patients. However, a few points worthy of discussion pertain to obstetric patients. First, the presence of underlying cardiovascular disease increases the risk of MCA occurring, both during the delivery hospitalization and specifically in the perianesthetic period; pulmonary hypertension and chronic ischemic heart disease were among the comorbidities most strongly associated.[25,32] Second, there are cardiovascular diseases that can precipitate MCA that are either unique to or more likely to be seen in obstetric patients. Peripartum cardiomyopathy (PPCM) is a form of heart failure with reduced ejection fraction that occurs in the final months of pregnancy up to several months postpartum. While the symptoms of heart failure can be insidious in onset and challenging to differentiate from the symptoms of pregnancy itself, PPCM can also develop rapidly and result in cardiogenic shock or lethal arrhythmia.[41] Treatment is supportive.

Spontaneous coronary artery dissection (SCAD) is a rare condition in which a tear or bleed in a coronary wall leads to an occlusive myocardial infarction; it primarily affects younger women in whom acute coronary syndrome might otherwise not be suspected. Pregnancy-associated SCAD, possibly related to hormonal or other physiologic changes, has been implicated in roughly 40–50% of acute coronary syndromes in pregnancy and the postpartum period.[42] Therefore, even if a pregnant or recently pregnant patient does not fit the risk profile for myocardial infarction, physicians should be aware that acute coronary events are possible.

Preeclampsia is a disorder of pregnancy that is commonly associated with hypertension as well as the risk of seizures or eclampsia. Eclamptic seizures and cerebral edema can lead to cardiac arrest, whether due to hypoxia, hemorrhagic stroke, or other mechanisms. In addition, the cardiopulmonary manifestations of preeclampsia are of high morbidity. Preeclampsia with severe features can be associated with heart failure with preserved or reduced ejection fraction, manifesting as diastolic dysfunction with pulmonary edema. Respiratory distress from flash pulmonary edema can occur. Applying POCUS to appreciate such manifestations and manage such high-risk patients is helpful. Anesthesiologists should be aware of the multiple potential mechanisms of decompensation when caring for patients with preeclampsia.

## Magnesium Toxicity

Magnesium toxicity is a rare cause of MCA, accounting for 1.4% or fewer cases.[10] It can occur in the context of magnesium administration for seizure prophylaxis in patients with preeclampsia or for fetal neuroprotection in patients with preterm labor and imminent delivery, in which, conditions for supranormal magnesium levels are targeted. Potential toxicity from magnesium varies by serum concentration, ranging from milder symptoms, such as loss of deep tendon reflexes, to more severe manifestations, including respiratory depression, heart block, and cardiac arrest.

If magnesium toxicity is suspected, the magnesium infusion should immediately be stopped, and calcium should be administered to counteract the magnesium at neuronal junctions. At least 10 mL of a 10% calcium chloride solution should be given. If only calcium gluconate is available, three times as much should be administered to achieve the same dose of calcium.[10,15]

## ■ POSTARREST CARE

After ROSC is achieved, it is critically important to continue supportive care postarrest to minimize mortality and improve outcomes.[33,48-50] In addition to the original insult, sedation, and mechanical ventilation, clinicians may need to manage a host of sequelae of cardiac arrest, known as postcardiac arrest syndrome (PCAS).[50] PCAS develops due to whole-body ischemia-reperfusion injury during cardiac arrest and is characterized by systemic inflammation and multiorgan dysfunction.[50] A complete discussion of postarrest care is outside the scope of this chapter, but careful multidisciplinary care is required, frequently in an intensive care unit. Most maternal postcardiac arrest patients will have been delivered and benefit from typical postpartum considerations as well. For example, if the mother wishes to breastfeed, the use of breast pumps for a critical patient may preserve lactation and enable breastfeeding later in recovery. In the less common scenario where the patient is still pregnant, additional aspects of pregnancy physiology and fetal care must be a focus of care. Left uterine displacement should be maintained if the gestational age is appropriate. A multidisciplinary team of critical care, obstetric, and anesthesiology physicians can facilitate delivery planning. Fetal monitoring may be warranted in general and with specific interventions such as postarrest cooling.[49]

## ■ PREVENTION AND PREPARATION

A recurrent theme in the field of MCA is the importance of preventing events before they happen, whether through safe anesthetic practices to avoid error or vigilance to recognize impending collapse. When MCA *does* occur, a prompt and coordinated multidisciplinary response can make the difference between a good and poor outcome. However, studies have found that deviations from routine ACLS guidelines happen with some frequency, whether in the operating room or general healthcare setting. Common examples of deviation include alterations in medication dosing and delayed time to resuscitative hysterotomy.[3,33] Simulation exercises suggest that even clinicians trained in ACLS are prone to neglecting aspects of maternal resuscitation covered in this chapter, such as left uterine displacement.[51,52]

Fortunately, while simulation training has uncovered knowledge gaps, it also effectively bridges them. Multiple studies have found that simulation improves knowledge and responsiveness to obstetric emergencies, including MCA.[52-54]

In addition to enhancing human factors, simulation training can potentially uncover systems-level issues that can be addressed, such as equipment availability or prompt notification of teams.[54]

## ■ CONCLUSION

Maternal cardiac arrest is a rare emergency, with more than one life at stake. Whether in the operating room, labor ward, or elsewhere, anesthesiologists offer a skillset crucial to improving chances of survival and must be prepared to encounter these crises. Proper training, including understanding the unique aspects of maternal resuscitation, knowledge of common etiologies of MCA, and multidisciplinary simulation, is critical. Mastery of these aspects will ensure that the anesthesiologist, as well as the healthcare system at large, is best prepared to meet this challenge.

## ■ REFERENCES

1. World Health Organization. (2023). Trends in maternal mortality 2000 to 2020: Estimates by WHO, UNICEF, UNFPA, World Bank Group and UNDESA/Population Division. Available from: https://iris.who.int/bitstream/handle/10665/366225/9789240068759-eng.pdf?sequence=1 [Last accessed July, 2024].
2. Nagraj S, Safiriyu I, Kokkinidis D, Kharawala A, Seo J, Varrias D, et al. Abstract 13677: Incidence and survival to hospital discharge after maternal cardiac arrest: A systematic review and meta-analysis. Circulation. 2023;148(Suppl 1):A13677.
3. Beckett VA, Knight M, Sharpe P. The CAPS Study: Incidence, management and outcomes of cardiac arrest in pregnancy in the UK: a prospective, descriptive study. BJOG. 2017;124(9):1374-81.
4. Balki M, Liu S, León JA, Baghirzada L. Epidemiology of cardiac arrest during hospitalization for delivery in Canada: a nationwide study. Anesth Analg. 2017; 124(3):890-7.
5. Mhyre JM, Tsen LC, Einav S, Kuklina EV, Leffert LR, Bateman BT. Cardiac arrest during hospitalization for delivery in the United States, 1998–2011. Anesthesiology. 2014;120(4):810-8.
6. Nagraj S, Kong S. (2024). Maternal cardiac arrest: The present and the future. Future Cardiology. Available from: https://www.tandfonline.com/doi/full/10.1080/14796678.2024.2341535 [Last accessed July, 2024].
7. National Center for Health Statistics. (2024). Maternal Mortality Surveillance. Available from: https://www.cdc.gov/nchs/nvss/vsrr/provisional-maternal-deaths-rates.htm. [Last accessed July, 2024].
8. Rimmer A. Maternal death rate in UK rises to highest level in 20 years. BMJ. 2024;384:q62.
9. Pacheco LD, Shepherd MC, Saade GS. Septic shock and cardiac arrest in obstetrics. Obstet Gynecol Clin North Am. 2022;49(3):461-71.
10. Fardelmann KL, Alian AA. Anesthesia for obstetric disasters. Anesthesiol Clin. 2020;38(1):85-105.
11. Zelop CM, Einav S, Mhyre JM, Lipman SS, Arafeh J, Shaw RE, et al. Characteristics and outcomes of maternal cardiac arrest: a descriptive analysis of Get with the guidelines data. Resuscitation. 2018;132:17-20.
12. Bircher NG, Chan PS, Xu Y; American Heart Association's Get With The Guidelines-Resuscitation Investigators. Delays in cardiopulmonary resuscitation, defibrillation, and epinephrine administration all decrease survival in in-hospital cardiac arrest. Anesthesiology. 2019;130(3):414-22.
13. American College of Obstetricians and Gynecologists' Presidential Task Force on Pregnancy and Heart Disease and Committee on Practice Bulletins—Obstetrics. ACOG Practice Bulletin No. 212: Pregnancy and heart disease. Obstet Gynecol. 2019;133(5): e320-56.

14. Sumer RW, Woods WA. Cardiac arrest in special populations. Cardiol Clin. 2024;42(2):289-306.
15. Knapp C, Bhatia K. Maternal collapse in pregnancy. Br J Hosp Med (Lond). 2022;83(12):1-12.
16. Sanders AB, Meislin HW, Ewy GA. The physiology of cardiopulmonary resuscitation. An update. JAMA. 1984;252(23):3283-6.
17. Enomoto N, Yamashita T, Furuta M, Tanaka H, Ng ESW, Matsunaga S, et al. Japan Resuscitation Council Maternal task force. Effect of maternal positioning during cardiopulmonary resuscitation: a systematic review and meta-analyses. BMC Pregnancy Childbirth. 2022;22(1):159.
18. Rose CH, Faksh A, Traynor KD, Cabrera D, Arendt KW, Brost BC. Challenging the 4- to 5-minute rule: From perimortem cesarean to resuscitative hysterotomy. AJOG. 2015;213(5):653.
19. Downing J, Sjeklocha L. Trauma in Pregnancy. Emerg Med Clin North Am. 2023;41(2):223-45.
20. Liggett MR, Amro A, Son M, Schwulst S. Management of the pregnant trauma patient: a systematic literature review. J Surg Res. 2023;285:187-96.
21. American Red Cross. Management of cardiac arrest in pregnancy. In: Focused Updates and Guidelines 2020. Available from: https://www.redcross.org/content/dam/redcross/training-services/course-fact-sheets/American-Red-Cross-Focused-Updates-and-Guidelines-2020.pdf [Last accessed July, 2024].
22. de Assis V, Shields AD, Johansson A, Shumbusho DI, York BM. Resuscitation of traumatic maternal cardiac arrest: a case report and summary of recommendations from Obstetric Life Support™. Trauma Case Rep. 2023;44:100800.
23. Padilla C, Ortner C, Dennis A, Zieleskiewicz L. The need for maternal critical care education, point-of-care ultrasound and critical care echocardiography in obstetric anesthesiologists training. Int J Obstet Anesth. 2023;55:103880.
24. Ortner CM, Padilla C, Carvalho B. Cardiac ultrasonography in obstetrics: a necessary skill for the present and future anesthesiologist. Int J Obstet Anesth. 2022;50:103545.
25. Easter SR, Hameed AB, Shamshirsaz A, Fox K, Zelop CM. Point of care maternal ultrasound in obstetrics. Am J Obstet Gynecol. 2022;228(5):509:e1-509.e13.
26. Zieleskiewicz L, Bouvet L, Einav S, Duclos G, Leone M. Diagnostic point-of-care ultrasound: Applications in obstetric anaesthetic management. Anaesthesia. 2018;73(10):1265-79.
27. Dennis A, Stenson A. The use of transthoracic echocardiography in postpartum hypotension. Anesth Analg. 2012;115(5):1033-7.
28. Perlas A, Van De Putte P, Van Houwe P, Chan VWS. I-AIM framework for point-of-care gastric ultrasound. Br J Anaesth. 2016;116(1):7-11.
29. Lee JH, Lee SH, Yun SJ. Comparison of 2-point and 3-point point-of-care ultrasound techniques for deep vein thrombosis at the emergency department: a meta-analysis. Medicine (Baltimore). 2019;98(22):e15791.
30. Devis P, Knuttinen MG. Deep venous thrombosis in pregnancy: Incidence, pathogenesis, and endovascular management. Cardiovasc Diagn Ther. 2017;7(Suppl 3):S309-19.
31. Naoum EE, Chalupka A, Haft J, MacEachern M, Vandeven CJM, Easter SR, et al. Extracorporeal life support in pregnancy: a systematic review. J Am Heart Assoc. 2020;9(13):e016072.
32. Lucas DN, Kursumovic E, Cook TM, Kane AD, Armstrong RA, Plaat F, et al. Cardiac arrest in obstetric patients receiving anaesthetic care: Results from the 7th National Audit Project of the Royal College of Anaesthetists. Anaesthesia. 2024;79(5):514-23.
33. Furdyna, Michael. Etiologies and management of maternal cardiac arrest during peripartum anesthetic care: a study from the Multicenter Perioperative Outcomes Group Consortium. Orally presented at SOAP 56th Annual Meeting, Denver, Colorado; 2024.

34. Patek K, Friedman P. Postpartum hemorrhage—Epidemiology, risk factors, and causes. Clin Obstet Gynecol. 2023;66(2):344-56.
35. Monks DT, Singh PM, Palanisamy A. Preventing maternal cardiac arrest: How do we reach the next level of safety in obstetric anaesthesia? Anaesthesia. 2024;79(5):461-4.
36. Liu LY, Nathan L, Sheen JJ, Goffman D. Review of current insights and therapeutic approaches for the treatment of refractory postpartum hemorrhage. Int J Womens Health. 2023;15:905-26.
37. Kumaraswami S, Butwick A. Latest advances in postpartum hemorrhage management. Best Pract Res Clin Anaesthesiol. 2022;36(1):123-34.
38. Waters JH, Bonnet MP. When and how should I transfuse during obstetric hemorrhage? Int J Obstet Anesth. 2021;46:102973.
39. Massoth C, Wenk M, Meybohm P, Kranke P. Coagulation management and transfusion in massive postpartum hemorrhage. Curr Opin Anaesthesiol. 2023;36(3):281-7.
40. Ford ND, DeSisto CL, Galang RR, Kuklina EV, Sperling LS, Ko JY. Cardiac arrest during delivery hospitalization: A cohort study. Ann Intern Med. 2023;176(4):472-9.
41. Pacheco LD, Saade G, Hankins GDV, Clark SL. Amniotic fluid embolism: Diagnosis and management. Am J Obstet Gynecol. 2016;215(2):B16-24.
42. Reale SC, Bauer ME, Klumpner TT, Aziz MF, Fields KG, Hurwitz R, et al. Frequency and risk factors for difficult intubation in women undergoing general anesthesia for cesarean delivery: a multicenter retrospective cohort analysis. Anesthesiology. 2022;136(5):697-708.
43. Tsuji M, Nii M, Furuta M, Baba S, Maenaka T, Matsunaga S, et al. Intravenous lipid emulsion for local anaesthetic systemic toxicity in pregnant women: a scoping review. BMC Pregnancy Childbirth. 2024;24(1):138.
44. Christie LE, Picard J, Weinberg GL. Local anaesthetic systemic toxicity. BJA Education. 2015;15(3):136-42.
45. Neal JM, Neal EJ, Weinberg GL. American Society of Regional Anesthesia and Pain Medicine Local Anesthetic Systemic Toxicity checklist: 2020 version. Reg Anesth Pain Med. 2021;46(1):81-2.
46. van der Pol LM, Tromeur C, Bistervels IM, Ni Ainle F, van Bemmel T, Bertoletti L, et al. Pregnancy-Adapted YEARS Algorithm for diagnosis of suspected pulmonary embolism. N Engl J Med. 2019;380(12):1139-49.
47. Gartman EJ. The use of thrombolytic therapy in pregnancy. Obstet Med. 2013;6(3):105-11.
48. Hirsch KG, Abella BS, Amorim E, Bader MK, Barletta JF, Berg K, et al. Critical care management of patients after cardiac arrest: a scientific statement from the American Heart Association and Neurocritical Care Society. Circulation. 2023;149(2).
49. Lipman S, Cohen S, Einav S, Jeejeebhoy F, Mhyre JM, Morrison LJ, et al. The Society for Obstetric Anesthesia and Perinatology Consensus Statement on the Management of Cardiac Arrest in Pregnancy. Anesth Analg. 2014;118(5):1003-16.
50. Lazzarin T, Tonon CR, Martins D, Fávero EL, Baumgratz TD, Pereira FWL, et al. Post-cardiac arrest: Mechanisms, management, and future perspectives. J Clin Med. 2022;12(1):259.
51. Lipman SS, Daniels KI, Carvalho B, Arafeh J, Harney K, Puck A, et al. Deficits in the provision of cardiopulmonary resuscitation during simulated obstetric crises. Am J Obstet and Gynecol. 2010;203(2):179.e1-5.
52. Boucetta N, El Alaoui M. Clinical simulation training for the adequate management of obstetrics emergencies: a narrative review. Medwave. 2023;23(10):e2712.
53. Fisher N, Eisen LA, Bayya JV, Dulu A, Bernstein PS, Merkatz IR, et al. Improved performance of maternal-fetal medicine staff after maternal cardiac arrest simulation-based training. Am J Obstet Gynecol. 2011;205(3):239.e1-5.
54. Lee A, Sheen JJ, Richards S. Intrapartum maternal cardiac arrest: a simulation case for multidisciplinary providers. MedEdPORTAL. 2018;14:10768.

# CHAPTER 6

# Anesthetic Management of Tracheoesophageal Fistula

*Anju Gupta, Manjula Sarkar, Nishkarsh Gupta*

## ABSTRACT

Tracheoesophageal fistula (TEF) is one of the most common congenital anomalies. Recent advancements in the field of surgery, anesthesia, and neonatal critical care have improved the survival of neonates with complex congenital anomalies, including TEF. Airway management in the case of TEF is challenging and requires the bypassing of the fistula to be effective. The technique of choice for securing the airway should consider the type and location of the fistula, the preoperative chest condition, pulmonary compliance, and other associated comorbid conditions. One-lung ventilation is generally not required for open surgery but may be a prerequisite for thoracoscopic surgery.

**Keywords:** Tracheoesophageal fistula; Neonate; Anesthesia; Minimally invasive surgery

## KEY POINTS

- The most common form of esophageal atresia/tracheoesophageal fistula (Gross type C) represents 90% of all cases of this anomaly.
- Anticipating potential perioperative problems and communicating with the surgeon are essential for optimal outcomes.
- Neonatal intensive and surgical care improvements have improved these infants' survival rates.
- Airway management in the case of esophageal atresia with tracheoesophageal fistula is challenging, but bronchoscopy dramatically aids in this process.
- The technique of choice for securing the airway must consider the type and location of the fistula, the preoperative chest condition, pulmonary compliance, and other associated comorbid conditions.
- The traditional technique of endobronchial intubation followed by gradual withdrawal into the trachea remains the most popular among anesthesiologists.
- The long-term sequelae following repair, such as gastroesophageal reflux, tracheomalacia, obstructive and restrictive ventilatory defects, airway reactivity, and recurrent pneumonia, should be suspected in patients with a history of tracheoesophageal fistula repair.
- Minimally invasive surgery is being increasingly used for younger age groups with comorbidities, including preterm patients with complex congenital heart disease.
- The application of the thoracoscopic technique is challenging in the neonatal population due to the requirement of lung isolation and the induction of capnothorax, which has several ramifications on the physiology of this tender age group.

## INTRODUCTION

Esophageal atresia (EA) is a congenital discontinuance of the esophageal lumen. EA is the most common congenital anomaly of the esophagus. It is associated with a tracheoesophageal fistula (TEF) in >90% of affected patients.[1-3] TEF results from a congenital fistulous communication between the esophagus and trachea or one of its main branches. The anomaly was first described in 1703, but it was not until 1939 that its first successful repair could be performed.[4] Congenital EA/TEF has an incidence of 1:2,500–1:4,500 live births.[2,3] Most cases of TEF are sporadic, and the recurrence rate is 1% in siblings.

### Classification of Tracheoesophageal Fistula/Esophageal Atresia

Anatomical classifications of TEF are based on the location of the fistula. The Gross and Vogt classifications are commonly used and are described in **Table 1**. A diagrammatic depiction of the same is shown in **Figure 1**. There are six types of TEF according to the classic Gross classification **(Figs. 1A to E)**.[2,5] Gross type "F" refers to esophageal stenosis without fistula. Vogt classification describes TEF/EA into five types: I, II, IIa, III, IIIa.[2] Vogt type I refers to esophageal agenesis. It does not include the "H" type. The Gross classification and corresponding Vogt classification are described in **Table 1**.

The most common form of EA/TEF (Gross type C), representing 90% of all cases of this anomaly, manifests as a blind upper esophageal pouch and a distal esophagus that forms a fistula with the trachea on the posterior aspect near the carina or less commonly to one of the bronchi.[1,2,4,5]

### Classification According to Prognosis

In 1962, Waterston developed the first classification of the prognosis of TEF, as described in **Table 2**.[7]

The survival of TEF babies has improved over the years because of advancements in intensive care unit care, anesthesia, and surgical technique and a better understanding of pathophysiology.

In contemporary practice, the survival in Waterston groups A and B approach 100%, and birth weight >1.5 kg no longer independently predicts mortality.[8] New classification systems have been developed to provide more meaningful information.[8,9] Of these, perhaps the most useful is the Spitz classification **(Table 3)**, which is based

**TABLE 1:** Esophageal atresia (EA)/tracheoesophageal fistula (TEF) classification (Gross and corresponding Vogt classification).[2,5,6]

| Gross classification | Vogt classification | Incidence | Type of fistula |
|---|---|---|---|
| – | Vogt I | Rare | Esophageal agenesis |
| Gross A | Vogt II | 8% | Isolated EA |
| Gross B | Vogt III | <1% | EA with proximal TEF |
| Gross C | Vogt IIb | 75–80% | EA with distal TEF |
| Gross D | Vogt IIIa | 2% | EA with proximal and distal TEF |
| Gross E (H-Type) | – | 4% | TEF without EA |
| Gross F | – | Rare | Esophageal stenosis |

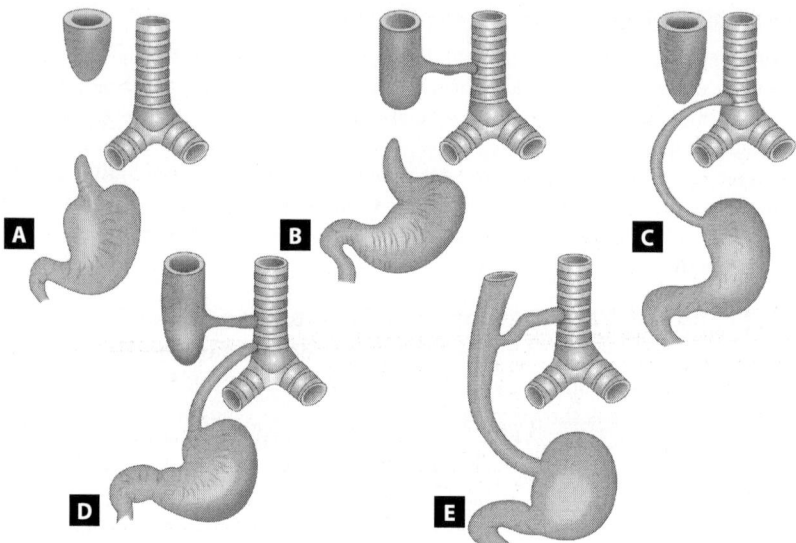

**Figs. 1A to E:** Types of esophageal atresia (EA)/tracheoesophageal fistula (TEF) (Gross classification A to E).
(*Source:* Redrawn from Ravitch MM, et al. eds. Pediatric Surgery, Vol. 1, 3rd edition. Chicago: Yearbook Medical Publishers; 1979.)

| TABLE 2: Waterston classification.[7] | | |
|---|---|---|
| **Group** | **Description** | **Survival** |
| Group A | Birth weight >2.5 kg, healthy | 95% |
| Group B | Birth weight 1.8–2.5 kg and healthy, or >2.5 kg with moderate pneumonia, or other anomalies | 68% |
| Group C | Birth weight <1.8 kg or >1.8 kg with severe pneumonia or severe congenital anomaly | 6% |

| TABLE 3: Spitz classification. | | |
|---|---|---|
| **Group** | **Description** | **Survival** |
| Group I | Birth weight >1.5 kg, no major cardiac disease | 97% |
| Group II | Birth weight <1.5 kg, or major cardiac disease | 59% |
| Group III | Birth weight <1.5 kg and major cardiac disease | 22% |

on the data from a review of 372 infants from 1980 to 1992.[9] It was shown that cardiac disease remains the leading risk factor for mortality in the TEF group.

Further and ongoing improvements in neonatal intensive and surgical care have led to even better survival rates in these infants, as shown in a more recent review of 188 cases from 1993 to 2004 where Spitz group I survival was 99%, group II 82%, and group III 50%.[10,11]

## ■ DIAGNOSIS AND PATHOPHYSIOLOGY

*Antenatal diagnosis:* The diagnosis of TEF is suspected prenatally by the presence of polyhydramnios, which is secondary to the failure of the fetus to swallow amniotic fluid due to EA. However, polyhydramnios and most other signs on prenatal imaging are not pathognomic of TEF. Other defects, including duodenal atresia, anencephaly, congenital diaphragmatic hernia, and Trisomy 18 may also cause "Polyhydramnios".[12] On prenatal ultrasound, there will be no fluid-filled stomach bubble and a dilated blind-ending upper pouch of the esophagus (upper pouch sign).[12] MRI imaging may help as the intrathoracic portion of the esophagus would not be visible in the case of TEF.

*Postnatal diagnosis:* In the most typical form of this anomaly, the distal trachea is connected to the lower esophagus through a fistula. This causes three problems. First, inhaled air enters the stomach and distends it. In extreme cases, diaphragmatic splinting will impede ventilation and cause atelectasis. Second, acidic stomach contents can leak back into the trachea and damage lung tissue. Third, oral secretions tend to pool in the proximal esophageal pouch, resulting in intermittent aspiration, swallowing problems, coughing, and cyanosis. A neonate with TEF will, therefore, present with copious drooling, coughing, and cyanosis when attempting to feed the baby. Usually, in the delivery room itself, diagnosis can be confirmed when an orogastric tube (OGT) cannot be passed >9–10 cm from the alveolar ridge and will coil up in the upper esophageal pouch rather than pass into the stomach.[6] On chest X-ray, a radio-opaque OGT will be coiled in the proximal esophageal pouch, which would be dilated, whereas an abdominal X-ray may show air in the bowels entering through the fistula **(Fig. 2)**. Nonetheless, H-type (Gross type "E") fistula patients usually present later in life with recurrent pneumonia.[13]

## ■ EMBRYOLOGY

The trachea originates as a ventral diverticulum from the primitive foregut during embryologic development's 4th and 5th weeks. The foregut differentiates into a separate esophagus and trachea. An abnormality in the physical separation process of

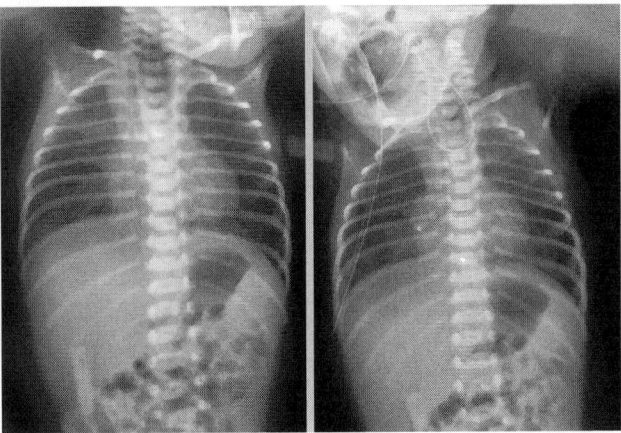

**Fig. 2:** Chest X-ray of a neonate without and with coiled oral gastric tube in situ.

the two structures has been recognized as the crucial event leading to the development of the EA/TEF.[14]

Multiple theories have been proposed in this relation.[15-17] The most commonly accepted theory states that a mesenchymal tracheoesophageal septum develops at the site where the longitudinal tracheoesophageal folds fuse. This septum divides the foregut into a ventral laryngotracheal tube and a dorsal esophagus. EA results if the tracheoesophageal septum is deviated posteriorly, causing an incomplete separation of the esophagus from the laryngotracheal tube and causing a TEF. Isolated EA is attributable to failure of the recanalization of the esophagus during the 8th week of development and is not associated with TEF. However, multiple genetic and environmental factors are said to contribute to the development of TEF, and the specific genetic syndrome is found in only 6–10% of these patients.[14,18]

## Associated Congenital Anomalies

Multisystem involvement or the presence of a chromosomal disorder along with TEF/EA not only has significant implications for mortality and morbidity but also influences decision-making about therapeutic options and surgical/anesthetic management. Nearly 50% of patients with EA/TEF possess one or more additional congenital malformations, and 30% are born prematurely **(Table 4)**.[1,2,5,6]

The Gross A group (isolated EA) has the highest incidence of associated congenital disabilities (50–70%). In comparison, they are least common (10%) in infants with the H-type fistula (Type E).[2,13] EA/TEF occurs as a subset of VATER/VACTERL [Vertebral, Atresia (duodenal and anorectal), Cardiac, Tracheoesophageal, Renal, and Limb] associations in 10–20% of cases.[2,5,18] A patient is considered to have VACTERL association with three or more of these lesions.[18] TEF/EA is also associated with chromosomal anomalies such as trisomy 18, 14, and 21 and syndromes such as Potter's and DiGeorge's syndrome.[2,5,8,18]

**TABLE 4:** Associated anomalies in patients with tracheoesophageal fistula (TEF)/esophageal atresia (EA)[1,2,5,6,8,18]

| Organ system | Incidence | Examples |
| --- | --- | --- |
| Cardiovascular | 29% | VSD, TOF, PDA, ASD, HLHS, right-sided aortic arch |
| Gastrointestinal | 14% | Imperforate anus, duodenal atresia, pyloric stenosis, malrotation, and omphalocele |
| Genitourinary | 14% | Renal agenesis, horseshoe kidneys, hypospadias, and ureteric abnormalities |
| Musculoskeletal | 10% | Radial limb abnormalities, hemivertebrae, rib defects, scoliosis, and micrognathia |
| Respiratory | 6% | Trachea-bronchomalacia, pulmonary hypoplasia, tracheal agenesis/stenosis |
| Chromosomal abnormalities | 5.5% | 13q deletion; Trisomy 14, 18, and 21 |
| Central nervous system | 10% | Hydrocephaly and cerebellar hypoplasia |

(ASD: atrial septal defect; HLHS: hypoplastic left heart syndrome; PDA: patent ductus arteriosus; TOF: Tetralogy of Fallot; VSD: ventricular septal defect)

Cardiac defects are the most typical associated anomaly and may be a subset of VACTERL or may have CHARGE group of anomalies (Coloboma, Heart, Atresia choanal, Retarded growth, Genital hypoplasia, and Ear deformities).[2,5,18,19]

## ■ PREOPERATIVE EVALUATION

Preoperative evaluation should focus on assessing the presence and severity of pulmonary disease and identifying significant anomalies (i.e., cardiac and renal). Assessment of the patient's pulmonary status allows the team to predict if single-lung ventilation would be tolerated intraoperatively and whether a ventilator other than that associated with the anesthesia machine should be made available. Clinical examination and chest X-ray would rule out aspiration pneumonia. A plain chest X-ray would show infiltrates in case of aspiration pneumonia. In premature infants, there may be additional respiratory distress due to immature lungs. In addition, children with significant cardiac anomalies may be dyspneic because of congestive heart failure. Contrast dye to delineate the fistula should be used with caution because of the risk of aspiration and, if indicated, should preferably be given under fluoroscopy so that any aspiration can be immediately detected. Second, an echocardiogram is mandatory as major cardiac defects strongly influence survival and may have an impact on anesthetic management.[6,19] In addition, one wants to look for the presence of a right-sided aortic arch (2.5-5%) because this will require positioning the infant with the opposite side down from usual.[5,18,19] X-ray spine and/or sacral ultrasound should be done to exclude vertebral anomalies, especially if a sacral dimple is present and neuraxial catheterization is planned as an analgesic modality.[5] Renal ultrasound should be done to rule out abnormalities, especially single kidney/hydronephrosis. In addition, complete blood count, arterial blood gas analysis, and serum electrolytes should be determined, and packed red blood cells should be typed and cross-matched.

## ■ PREOPERATIVE PREPARATION AND OPTIMIZATION

Primary TEF repair is considered a standard of care in contemporary practice. Usually, the procedure is done as an urgent one, but anesthesiologists can buy sufficient time to optimize the preoperative condition of the child. Aspiration pneumonitis is directly implicated as a cause of perioperative morbidity and mortality in the majority of these patients.[20] As soon as the diagnosis of TEF is made, the following measures are undertaken to prevent and treat aspiration pneumonia:

- Keeping the baby "nil per oral (NPO)".
- Baby placed in a warmed isolete with the head elevated at least 30°, semi-prone to minimize reflux through the fistula.
- Nasogastric tube (NGT) is placed in the upper pouch with intermittent suctioning to prevent aspiration of oral secretions.
- Administration of antibiotics to treat aspiration pneumonia and/or sepsis.

Infective endocarditis prophylaxis should be given to those infants having significant congenital heart disease. In case features of congestive heart failure are present, the condition should be optimized using diuretics. If the child has severe tetralogy of Fallot, he may require placement of a temporary shunt between the systemic arterial and pulmonary circulation before repair of the TEF.[19,20] Some critically ill infants may need mechanical ventilation preoperatively for 24-72 hours while their general condition is stabilized, hemodynamic parameters are improved, other anomalies are defined, and the surgical plan is formulated.

## Neonate with Severe Respiratory Disease

In severe respiratory compromise requiring ventilatory support (severe pneumonia or respiratory distress syndrome), especially in premature infants, stomach dilation due to air leak from the fistula may worsen pulmonary compliance by elevating the diaphragm.[6,11] The poor lung compliance coupled with loss of ventilation through the fistula may prevent delivery of adequate tidal volumes. One technique to optimize ventilation while minimizing gastric distention is to employ high-frequency oscillatory ventilation to reduce the peak inspiratory pressure.[11,21] Alternatively, a simple gastrostomy performed under local anesthesia allows the drainage of gastric fluid (to minimize further aspiration). It prevents or relieves gastric distention that can occur with positive pressure ventilation. However, in the case of poorly compliant lungs, gastrostomy placement allows the gases to follow the path of least resistance and escape through the stomach.[20,22] This can make it difficult or impossible to ventilate the baby adequately. This problem can be partially alleviated if the gastrostomy tube is placed underneath a water seal, allowing gas to escape only when the pressure exceeds a predetermined threshold.[6,22] Another technique successfully entailed retrograde occlusion of the fistula through a gastrostomy using a Fogarty catheter advanced through a gastrostomy to a position just above the gastroesophageal junction using fluoroscopy.[23] The balloon was inflated, and the catheter was clamped or placed under a water seal. In this way, gastric distention or inadequate ventilation due to bypass of the lungs is avoided. Nonetheless, there is a potential risk of esophageal rupture and fatal pneumothorax if the catheter is not placed correctly.[23,24] Mortality remains higher in the premature infant (14%) compared to the term infant (<5%).[8,18]

## ■ SURGICAL TECHNIQUE

In most Type C cases, TEF repair is done as a single-stage procedure, where the fistula is ligated, and the esophagus is primarily anastomosed. Unless the aortic arch is right-sided, the surgical approach for open repair involves a right thoracotomy using a posterolateral incision and a retropleural approach. Following ligation of the fistula, the anesthesiologist inserts an orogastric catheter into the blind upper pouch to help to identify the upper esophagus. The upper esophagus is mobilized, then the distal esophagus. The catheter is threaded into the lower part of the esophagus, and the anastomosis is completed over the catheter. After the anastomosis, the catheter is withdrawn to rest just above the suture line, and the proximal end of the orogastric tube is marked at the mouth. This distance is noted to guide suctioning postoperatively.

Sometimes, the gap between the upper and lower esophageal pouch is too long to permit a primary anastomosis. If the gap is more than two vertebral bodies, it is referred to as a long gap EA (also considered a gap >3 cm), and primary anastomosis may not be feasible.[25] Type A (pure EA) is usually associated with such wide interruption, and delayed anastomosis might be needed.[6] In such cases, limited thoracotomy is done where the fistula is ligated, and a gastrostomy is inserted in the newborn. The baby is posted for definitive repair between 3 and 6 months of age. In such cases, techniques based on inducing the growth of innate esophageal tissue are preferred over the interposition techniques using gastric/bowel segments as they provide superior function.[26]

In neonates where primary repair of TEF is associated with unacceptable risk (significant associated congenital anomalies, bilateral pneumonia, or sepsis), limited thoracotomy may focus on ligation of the TEF followed by placement of a gastrostomy.

## ■ ANESTHETIC MANAGEMENT

### Monitoring

Standard monitoring should include an electrocardiogram, noninvasive blood pressure, end-tidal carbon dioxide ($EtCO_2$), oxygen saturation, and rectal/oropharyngeal temperature. Upper- and lower-extremity pulse oximeter monitoring preductal and postductal oxygen saturation, especially in those with right-to-left shunting, provides valuable information on shunting and pulmonary hypertension. Peak airway pressures and tidal volumes should be carefully monitored. Precordial stethoscopes positioned in the left axilla can provide continuous monitoring to ensure ventilation to the dependent lung. A second precordial stethoscope placed over the stomach may be helpful to assess whether the fistula is being ventilated. In infants with unstable cardiorespiratory status, congenital heart disease, or significant lung disease preoperatively, an arterial catheter (umbilical or radial) should be secured.[19] Another school of thought is that since lung retraction is required for surgery and intermittent compression of the trachea and great vessels are possibilities, an arterial line is mandatory for all cases of TEF repair for beat-to-beat blood pressure monitoring and arterial blood gas analysis.[5,20] The gradient between arterial partial pressure of $CO_2$ and $EtCO_2$ provides valuable information on shunt fraction. A qualified neonatologist can conveniently place an umbilical arterial line in the neonatal intensive care unit (NICU).

### Role of Bronchoscopy

Preoperative rigid or fiberoptic bronchoscopy can aid in detecting the number and location of the fistulae, help to guide the surgical technique (cervical fistula can be approached through the neck), assess other airway anomalies (e.g., tracheomalacia), and precisely place an endotracheal tube to bypass the fistula or a Fogarty catheter to block the fistula.[6,23,24,27] The routine preoperative bronchoscopy had modified the surgical management of 24% of patients in a study.[27] Previous investigators have described using a rigid bronchoscope to guide the placement of a Fogarty arterial embolectomy catheter/other devices into the TEF to achieve its occlusion to counter ventilatory problems in large TEFs.[23,24,27] Additionally, a catheter placed in the fistula during bronchoscopy may help its subsequent identification by the surgeon. Recurrent TEF may be approached bronchoscopically by placing fibrin glue directly into the fistula, precluding the need for a second thoracotomy.[6]

Bronchoscopy is usually performed before surgical repair. Glycopyrrolate intravenously administered and topicalized over the vocal cords and trachea with lidocaine and inhalational anesthetics to provide suitable conditions for bronchoscopy under spontaneous respiration.

### Airway Management

The goal of intubation and subsequent ventilation is to allow adequate gas exchange with the lowest possible inspiratory pressure needed to inflate the lungs, avoid stomach distention, and avoid atelectasis. Positive pressure mask ventilation should be avoided during induction of anesthesia and intubation.[20,22,23] In all cases, the surgeon should be present during induction of anesthesia for urgent percutaneous/ultrasound-guided needle decompression of the distended stomach whenever required.[28]

There are several options for induction of anesthesia to achieve this goal:
- "Awake intubation" was traditionally considered the safest way of securing the airway in an infant with TEF as theoretically it eliminates the risk for gastric distention from positive pressure ventilation.[29,30] However, awake intubation can be pretty stressful in vigorous infants and carries the risk of intracranial hemorrhage, especially in preterm neonates. Therefore, in most cases where it is practiced, awake sedated intubation is preferred using small-titrated doses of sedatives [e.g., fentanyl (0.5–1 µg/kg) or midazolam (0.01–0.05 mg/kg)].[30]
- Intubation can be performed after inhalation induction.[6,29] Good intubating conditions can be achieved with a deep volatile agent, but ensuing apnea may require gentle respiration assistance.
- Rapid sequence of intravenous (IV) induction and intubation while avoiding IPPV or providing controlled ventilation with low inspiratory pressure (10–12 mm Hg) is currently favored.[20,29]
- Maintain spontaneous ventilation until the fistula is ligated.[29,30] Maintaining adequate ventilation and surgical conditions during a thoracotomy without a relaxant may be challenging. This technique requires deep inhalation with gentle assistance of each breath to minimize atelectasis.

Further, correctly positioning the ETT tip to ensure that the tip is distal to the fistula yet proximal to the carina is a fundamental goal in preventing gastric distention and worsening lung compliance during surgery. Gastric rupture has been reported in cases with failure to achieve fistula isolation.[28] A previous bronchoscopic study on 113 patients of TEF/EA noted that the fistula was infracarinal in up to 11% of patients. In contrast, in 22% of the patients, the fistula was close (within 1 cm) to the carina.[31] If the tube is in a favorable position, the child can be paralyzed, and normal IPPV is maintained. Several methods have been described in the literature to achieve this goal:
- Endotracheal tube (ETT) is deliberately inserted endobronchial (usually into the right bronchus when inserted blindly), then gradually pulled back until breath sounds appear on the left. At this point, the ETT would have bypassed the fistula in most cases.[6,29,30]
- Salem and colleagues had mentioned that the ETT, with its bevel facing anteriorly, should be positioned as distal as possible so that its posterior wall occludes the fistula.[32]
- If the patient has a gastrostomy in situ, it should be placed under a water seal, and the ETT should be pulled back almost until gas begins to bubble from the end of the gastric tube and then re-advanced until the bubbling stops.[20]
- Inserting a 2/3 Fr (balloon diameter 4 and 5 mm) Fogarty catheter (or another balloon-tipped device) via the side port of a rigid bronchoscope into the TEF or retrograde via the gastrostomy can effectively occlude the fistula.[23,24] However, precise positioning of the catheter is difficult to achieve, and even if the positioning is perfect initially, displacement of the balloon can happen later. It will be disastrous if it impedes the trachea.[33,34] The high-pressure balloon may

- encroach on small pulmonary vessels or airways and compromise pulmonary blood flow or ventilation.[33]
- Using a cuffed tube (preferably microcuff ETT with a distal cuff) with its tip just above the carina and inflation of the cuff at the level of the fistula will isolate any underlying or proximal fistula.[35]
- If the fistula is present below the carina, then left mainstream intubation will help to isolate the fistula and right lung simultaneously and may be tolerated by a child with well-preserved pulmonary function. After fistula ligation, the ETT is withdrawn back into the trachea.[36]

## Intraoperative Management

The various choices for induction and airway management are described in the previous section. Awake intubation is losing favor among anesthetists due to the reasons previously mentioned. Inhalational or IV induction with/without muscle relaxants is used by the majority in contemporary practice.[6,29] In a series on TEF repair, muscle relaxants were employed in 93% of cases before intubation.[20] After initial careful positioning of the ETT, the difficulty lies in maintaining the correct position during subsequent repositioning for surgery, positive pressure ventilation, and surgical manipulation. The neonate is positioned in left lateral decubitus for right thoracotomy (after the right aortic arch has been ruled out) using gel blocks under the head and left thorax using tapes to secure the position. Establish IV access (at least one peripheral IV before induction and a second one after the patient is anesthetized). Avoid placing lines in the right arm, as this arm is elevated above the head during right thoracotomy, and access will be limited. The selection of an anesthetic technique during surgical correction of EA/TEF depends on the physiologic status of the neonate. Low-dose volatile agents in conjunction with air, oxygen, and an opioid are usually well tolerated if the neonate is adequately hydrated. It is advocated to maintain spontaneous ventilation till ligation of the fistula, following which neuromuscular blockers can be administered. However, maintaining adequate ventilation and depth for thoracotomy can be difficult without muscle paralysis, and a nondepolarizing muscle relaxant can be administered after the airway is secured optimally and ventilation is deemed satisfactory.[6] Intraoperative analgesia can be opioid-based, especially when postoperative ventilation is planned. In some cases, epidural analgesia (caudal catheter threaded to thoracic levels or thoracic epidural) may be provided if expertise and proper equipment are available.[6,20,24,29] Caudal insertion of epidural catheter avoids the risk of direct spinal cord trauma compared to more proximal approaches. If a gastrostomy tube is present, the end may be placed underneath a water seal during induction and maintenance of anesthesia.[20] Bubbling will indicate that the fistula is being ventilated, thereby indicating that the tip of the ETT is proximal to the opening of the fistula. Alternatively, a capnograph attached to the gastrostomy tube will indicate the same thing.[30]

Hypoxia and inadequate ventilation have many possible causes, as mentioned in **Box 1**, and these should be ruled out whenever such an event happens.[5,6,11,19,20,22,25] Lung retraction (or isolation) leads to atelectasis and may interfere with oxygenation and ventilation, especially in premature infants with respiratory distress syndrome, aspiration pneumonia, or congenital heart disease. It is crucial to maintain close communication with the surgeon. Volume-controlled and intermittent manual

**BOX 1:** Main reasons for hypoxemia during TEF repair.[5,6,11,19,20,22,25]

*Causes of desaturation in TEF surgery*
- Preexisting pulmonary dysfunction
- Stomach distention resulting in diaphragmatic splint
- Intubation of fistula
- Dislodgment of Fogarty catheter resulting in tracheal obstruction
- Retraction of lung for surgery
- Kinking of trachea or main bronchi
- Endobronchial intubation
- ETT obstruction by blood/secretions
- Kinking and compression of heart and great vessels
- Accidental ligation of bronchi instead of fistula during surgery

(ETT: endotracheal tube; TEF: tracheoesophageal fistula)

ventilation is usually employed to counter poor lung compliance and achieve desired ventilatory parameters. Increasing the inspired oxygen concentration and intermittent pressure release by the surgeon to allow reinflation of the lungs is sufficient to improve oxygenation and ventilation in the majority. The risk of oxygen toxicity and barotrauma should be kept in mind.

In some cases, precarious preoperative ventilatory status, large fistula and very high peak airway pressures, hypercarbia, and unacceptably low tidal volumes indicate the need for advanced ventilatory modes like high-frequency oscillatory ventilation may be required. One case report described the successful ventilatory management of two preterm infants who were refractory to conventional ventilation due to a large fistula leading to loss of tidal volumes.[21] An advanced NICU ventilator may be more suitable in such cases, and a ventilatory strategy should be devised in coordination with the NICU team.[21] Frequent endotracheal suctioning to clear blood clots or secretions may be required. After the completion of the procedure, the thoracic cavity is filled with saline, and positive pressure is applied to exclude any leak from the anastomosis. The lung should be carefully re-expanded to eliminate atelectasis before closure.

## Fluid and Temperature Management

Careful attention to fluid and temperature management is of utmost importance. Neonates (especially premature infants) are prone to develop hypothermia due to multiple causes, including limited subcutaneous fat.[29,30] Moreover, nonshivering thermogenesis, which is the prime mechanism of temperature regulation in neonates, is up to 70% inhibited by inhaled anesthetics.[30] The child should be transported to the operation theater (OT) in a prone/propped-up position in a warmed incubator. The OT should be prewarmed to at least 27–29°C. Surgical irrigation, IV fluids, and blood products should be warmed before transfusion. A forced-air warming system is most effective.[29,30] Using a warmed mattress, overhead radiating warmer, keeping the head and extremities wrapped in plastic, and placing a heat and moisture exchanger in the airway can be very useful. Since the majority of these patients belong to the early neonatal age group and have kept NPO since birth, it is essential to include a glucose-containing solution in IV fluid therapy intraoperatively. 10% dextrose solution administered IV at a maintenance rate using an infusion pump is a common technique to avoid hypoglycemia. Third-space losses should be replaced with isotonic solution (Ringer lactate/Plasmalyte) at 2–4 mL/kg/hour. Blood loss may be replaced with 5% albumin and packed red cells to maintain a >35% hematocrit.[29,30] In the neonatal population during anesthesia, hypotension is usually defined using mean arterial pressures (MAP). In preterm neonates, the minimum acceptable blood pressure in terms of MAP is approximately equivalent to the gestational age in weeks, with 30 mm Hg as the lowest limit.[37] Urine output should be maintained at 0.5–2 mL/kg/hour.

## Common Intraoperative Problems

Interference with ventilation and desaturation is the most common problem and can have many causes (**Box 1**). Lung retraction, which results in atelectasis, leads to frequent desaturation. The retracted lung may need to be intermittently reexpanded to avoid severe hypoxia. Sometimes, barotrauma and pneumothorax are possible due to very high peak airway pressures.[38] The $PCO_2$ may rise to 70–80 mm Hg despite all attempts to optimize ventilation. If the patient has a Fogarty catheter in the fistula, it may be displaced into the trachea, causing total airway obstruction.[23,33] Surgical manipulation of the soft trachea makes it vulnerable to kinking or displacement of ETT distal (into the right mainstem) or proximally (above the fistula). Frequent compression of vital structures in the mediastinum can lead to profound hemodynamic compromise. Blood and secretions are a constant problem during surgery, which risks obstructing the small bore ETT of the neonate. The ETT should be suctioned frequently, more so if blood is seen. Severe gastric distention before ligation of the TEF may require emergent gastric needle decompression.[6,29,30] Diaz and colleagues described the incidence of intraoperative critical events in open TEF repair in patients with and without associated cardiac anomalies in a recent series of cases.[19] This report found the highest incidence of clinically significant events in the group with complex ductus-dependent lesions who were mechanically ventilated preoperatively when compared to infants with no/minor heart disease. The primary critical events included intubation difficulties, desaturation during lung retraction, hypotension, and ETT obstruction.[19] Perioperative mortality in the highest-risk group was 23%, consistent with the survival rates reported by Lopez and associates for similar patients.[10]

## Timing of Extubation

Many of the full-term infants with significant anomalies and uneventful intraoperative courses may be extubated on the OT table. Many surgeons prefer early extubation as an ETT, and positive pressure ventilation is a source of constant pressure over the anastomosis.[12,30] Thoracoscopic procedures result in faster extubation times (37.6 vs. 54 hours) and discharge from the NICU (2.75 vs. 3.4 days) than open thoracotomies, with comparable postoperative complication rates.[39,40] Neck extension must be carefully avoided to minimize stress on the anastomosis. However, the presence of copious secretions and tracheomalacia at the site of the fistula, which predisposes to airway collapse, mandates reintubation in many infants who have been extubated. Neonates with underlying cardiopulmonary comorbidities, prematurity, low birth weight, or patients with a complicated intraoperative course (e.g., trachea perforation, pneumothorax, need for vasopressors, etc.) are electively ventilated during early postoperative course until stable.[3,4,19,25] Finally, after repair of "long-gap" of EA, any stretch on the esophageal repair may predispose to anastomotic leaks, and most surgeons would request elective postoperative ventilatory support for up to 1 week to maintain anastomotic integrity.[3,4,30] Patients must be sedated well to eliminate brisk neck movements and negative intrapleural pressure due to spontaneous respiration to affect the anastomosis.

## ■ POSTOPERATIVE ANALGESIA

Multimodal analgesia, including regional anesthesia, would be the preferred technique. An epidural catheter (caudal/thoracic) may be used for postoperative analgesia using intermittent boluses or continuous infusions of low-concentration of local anesthetics (LA) (0.1% bupivacaine/0.2% ropivacaine/0.1% levobupivacaine) along with opioids.[41,42] The test dose should be administered before a full LA dose.[42] Doses should be appropriately reduced for the neonatal age group given pharmacological differences (reduced protein binding and immature metabolic pathways).[42,43] The correct catheter placement should ideally be confirmed using fluoroscopy/ultrasonography before use.[44,45] Other regional anesthetic techniques that can provide helpful analgesia include intercostal blocks (percutaneous/under direct vision), intrapleural analgesia (LA infusion using a catheter in the pleural cavity), single shot or continuous paravertebral block (percutaneous/LA infiltrated by the surgeon under direct vision) and wound infiltration.[24,29,41,42] Paracetamol suppository inserted before the start of a procedure or intravenously at the end will provide supplemental analgesia in the early postoperative period. If the patient is going to be electively ventilated postoperatively, then a high dose of narcotic is used intraoperatively (fentanyl 10–20 µg/kg) and continued postoperatively as required will provide good hemodynamic stability and postoperative analgesia.[11,12,19]

## ■ POSTOPERATIVE COMPLICATIONS

Anastomosis leakage is the most typical early complication (up to 7–25% after open repair and 17–36% after thoracoscopic repair).[46] It responds to conservative treatment in the majority, but significant persistent leaks with pneumothorax, mediastinitis, or sepsis mandate re-exploration. Tracheomalacia may become evident postoperatively, and vocal cord paresis due to vagal nerve injury has been reported.[19,47,48] Respiratory complications and gastroesophageal reflux are common among premature infants.[25] Delayed complications include esophageal dysmotility, recurrent fistula, esophageal stricture, and thoracic wall deformities.[25,49]

A posterolateral incision for thoracotomy in infancy has been associated with musculoskeletal deformities, including fused ribs, scoliosis, shoulder girdle weakness, and chest wall deformity later in life.[25,49] With thoracoscopy, these complications are reduced in incidence and severity.[46]

## ■ ANESTHESIA FOR THORACOSCOPIC TRACHEOESOPHAGEAL FISTULA/ESOPHAGEAL ATRESIA REPAIR

Lobe and Rothenberg reported the first thoracoscopic EA/TEF repair in 1999.[50,51] Thoracoscopic approaches have many advantages and have been widely adopted as a preferred surgical approach. Advancements in surgical and anesthetic techniques and equipment have made complex thoracoscopic procedures feasible and safe even in infants with complex heart diseases (hypoplastic left heart syndrome and single ventricle physiology).[52,53] The problem of excessive insufflation pressures in neonates has been resolved because of the development of suitable equipment (neonatal insufflator with low flow and valved trocars).[30] This approach is generally contraindicated in children weighing <2 kg, long-gap EA, severe pulmonary parenchymal disease, pulmonary arterial hypertension, and hemodynamic instability.[30,46,50,51]

Traditional repair through a right posterolateral thoracotomy has many disadvantages, including increased postoperative pain, larger scar, and increased chances of scoliosis and winged scapula later in life.[46,49] Minimally invasive surgery offers the benefit of magnified visualization of the fistula and the surrounding anatomy, including the vagus nerve, to the surgeon, less traction on the trachea and surrounding structures with possible decreased risk of postoperative stridor and hoarseness.[6,50,51]

Anesthetic implications of neonatal thoracoscopic surgery include managing the patient's underlying comorbid conditions, need for lung isolation, ventilatory management, and physiologic alterations induced by thoracoscopy and capnothorax.[50,51] Physiologic changes during endoscopic approach can be aggravated in those with coexisting significant cardiac abnormalities. Single-lung ventilation increases pulmonary vascular resistance (PVR) through hypoxic pulmonary vasoconstriction.[52,53] Increases in PVR can lead to a transition back to fetal circulation with the reopening of foramen ovale or ductus arteriosus, even in neonates without congenital heart disease. Right-sided thoracoscopy reduces venous return, cardiac index, and mean arterial blood pressure even at low insufflation pressures due to direct compression of the vena cava and right atrium.[19,52] Carbon dioxide ($CO_2$) absorption from pleura produces hypercarbia and acidosis.

## Lung Isolation

The surgeon and anesthesiologist must discuss the need for one-lung ventilation (OLV) and whether the patient can tolerate the technique. Given the few options for lung isolation in the neonatal population, lung isolation is challenging. Also, true lung isolation may not be achieved in infants with poor lung compliance and high peak pressures.

Some surgeons may prefer to achieve lung collapse with the use of $CO_2$ insufflation of right hemithorax up to 4-6 mm Hg pressures in the semiprone position.[30,50,51] When it is indicated, single-lung ventilation in newborn infants implies selective endobronchial intubation of the contralateral lung or insertion of bronchial blockers (BB) (Fogarty embolectomy catheter, atrial septostomy catheters, and pulmonary artery catheters) on the ipsilateral surgical side.[51,54-56] Mainstem intubation may be beneficial if the fistula is close to the carina. The ETT should be selected in one-half to one size smaller than calculated based on age. With selective mainstem intubation, providing intermittent two-lung ventilation would not be possible as that would require intermittently pulling back the ETT from its position in the bronchus into the trachea.[54] Also, left endobronchial intubation can result in bronchial edema and postoperative left upper lobe collapse.[11]

The use of BBs is another option for OLV in young infants. BBs can be placed through or along the ETT's side into the operative side's mainstem bronchus.[55,56] However, in neonates, these devices can significantly reduce the cross-sectional area and increase resistance when placed within the lumen. Therefore, placing the bronchial blocker alongside the ETT in these patients may be preferable. Also, there is a risk of dislodgment during the surgical procedure or a change in position, which may result in airway obstruction.[33,54] Monitoring breath sounds continuously using a precordial stethoscope in the left axilla and monitoring airway pressures and respiratory compliance should help to identify this problem rapidly.

One report described the management of lung isolation for a neonate with a type C TEF at the level of the carina, using two BBs, one to occlude the fistula and the other for lung isolation alongside the conventional ETT.[57] This prevented the loss of ventilation to the large TEF and provided effective OLV. Fiberoptic bronchoscopy facilitated the precise placement of the blockers in this case.

Though OLV facilitates the surgical procedure, it may not be tolerated in those having baseline pulmonary dysfunction. Close communication with the surgeon should be maintained. Oxygen insufflation or the application of continuous positive airway pressure (CPAP) to the operative lung prevents dangerous hypoxemia or hypercarbia.[54,55] If desaturation still occurs, intermittent release of insufflation pressure and institution of two-lung ventilation may be required.

## Intraoperative Complications and Challenges

Thoracoscopic procedures impose their unique challenges due to the operative requirements, including semi-prone positioning, $CO_2$ insufflation, prolonged capnothorax leading to hypercarbia, and long duration of procedures.[50,51,55] These conditions can lead to complications, including distal migration of ETT, hypoxia, and hypercarbia. Intrathoracic pressures during gas insufflation into the thorax should not exceed 10 mm Hg and preferably below 6 mm Hg.[6,55] It is common for neonates to desaturate after capnothorax to achieve lung collapse.[11,50,51] This usually responds to increasing the inspired oxygen concentration and gentle hand ventilation. Arterial oxygen saturation of >85% should be considered acceptable.[55,56] Ventilation can be challenging to monitor due to frequently inaccurate or absent $EtCO_2$ during ongoing procedures.[6,55] Arterial lines should be in place, and frequent blood gas monitoring should be done. With $CO_2$ insufflation, hypercarbia and acidosis are frequently present in blood gas analysis. Gastric distention and consequent diaphragmatic splinting can occur if the ETT position is not optimal, the fistula is large/near the carina, or due to ventilation with high peak airway pressures. Carbon dioxide embolism is a rare complication.

## ■ CONCLUSION

The neonate who presents to repair EA and TEF can be incredibly challenging for the anesthesiologist. Pediatric anesthesiologists must keep up-to-date with the latest developments in the surgical field and its anesthetic implications to provide the best outcome for every patient. Minimally invasive surgery is being increasingly used for younger age groups with comorbidities. The application of this surgical technique is challenging in the neonatal population due to the requirement of lung isolation and induction of capnothorax, which has several ramifications on the physiology of this tender age group.

*Conflicts of interest:* None.

*Funding:* None.

*Acknowledgments:* None.

## REFERENCES

1. Sparey C, Jawaheer G, Barrett AM, Robson SC. Esophageal atresia in the Northern Region Congenital Anomaly Survey, 1985-1997: prenatal diagnosis and outcome. Am J Obstet Gynecol 2000;182:427-31.
2. Spitz L. Oesophageal atresia. Orphanet J Rare Dis. 2007;11:24.
3. Holland AJ, Fitzgerald DA. Oesophageal atresia and tracheo-oesophageal fistula: current management strategies and complications. Paediatr Respir Rev. 2010;11:100-6.
4. Spitz L. Esophageal atresia: lessons I have learned in a 40-year experience. J Pediatr Surg. 2006;41:1635-40.
5. Pinheiro PF, Simões e Silva AC, Pereira RM. Current knowledge on esophageal atresia. World J Gastroenterol. 2012;18:3662-72.
6. Broemling N, Campbell F. Anesthetic management of congenital tracheoesophageal fistula. Pediatr Anesth. 2011;21:1092-9.
7. Waterston DJ, Carter RE, Aberdeen E. Oesophageal atresia: tracheo-oesophageal fistula. A study of survival in 218 infants. Lancet. 1962;1:819-22.
8. Okamoto T, Takamizawa S, Arai H, Bitoh Y, Nakao M, Yokoi A, et al. Esophageal atresia: prognostic classification revisited. Surgery. 2009;145:675-81.
9. Spitz L, Kiely EM, Morecroft JA, Drake DP.. Oesophageal atresia: at-risk groups for the 1990s. J Pediatr Surg. 1994;29:723-5.
10. Lopez PJ, Keys C, Pierro A, Drake DP, Kiely EM, Curry JI, et al. Oesophageal atresia: improved outcome in high-risk groups? J Pediatr Surg. 2006;41:331-4.
11. Krosnar S, Baxter A. Thoracoscopic repair of esophageal atresia with tracheoesophageal fistula: anesthetic and intensive care management of a series of eight neonates. Pediatr Anesth. 2005;15:541-6.
12. Houben CH, Curry JI. Current status of prenatal diagnosis, operative management and outcome of esophageal atresia/tracheoesophageal fistula. Prenat Diagn. 2008;28:667-75.
13. Crabbe DC. Isolated tracheo-oesophageal fistula. Paediatr Respir Rev. 2003;4:74-8.
14. Merei J, Huston J. Embryogenesis of tracheoesophageal anomalies. Saudi Med J. 2003;24:39-40.
15. Ioannides AS, Chaudhry B, Henderson DJ, Spitz L, Copp AJ. Dorsoventral patterning in oesophageal atresia with tracheo-oesophageal fistula: evidence from a new mouse model. J Pediatr Surg. 2002;37:185-91.
16. Crisera CA, Connelly PR, Marmureanu AR, Colen KL, Rose MI, Li M, et al. Esophageal atresia with tracheoesophageal fistula: suggested mechanism in faulty organogenesis. J Pediatr Surg. 1999;34:204-8.
17. Crisera CA, Connelly PR, Marmureanu AR, Li M, Rose MI, Longaker MT, et al. TTF-1 and HNF-3b in the developing tracheoesophageal fistula: further evidence for the respiratory origin of the "distal esophagus". J Pediatr Surg. 1999;34:1322-6.
18. Shaw-Smith C. Oesophageal atresia, tracheo-oesophageal fistula, and the VACTERL association: review of genetics and epidemiology. J Med Genet. 2006;43:545-54.
19. Diaz LK, Akpek EA, Dinavahi R, Andropoulos DB. Tracheoesophageal fistula and associated congenital heart disease: implications for anesthetic management and survival. Pediatr Anesth 2005;15:862-9.
20. Andropoulos DB, Rowe RW, Betts JM. Anaesthetic and surgical airway management during tracheo-oesophageal fistula repair. Pediatr Anesth. 1998;8:313-9.
21. Donn SM, Zak LK, Bozynski ME, Coran AG, Oldham KT. Use of high-frequency jet ventilation in the management of congenital tracheoesophageal fistula associated with respiratory distress syndrome. J Pediatr Surg. 1990;25:1219-21.
22. Richenbacher WE, Ballantine TV. Esophageal atresia, distal tracheoesophageal fistula, and an air shunt that compromised mechanical ventilation. J Pediatr Surg. 1990;25:1216-8.

23. Reeves ST, Burt N, Smith CD. Is it time to reevaluate the airway management of tracheoesophageal fistula? Anesth Analg. 1995;81:866-9.
24. Gayle JA, Gomez SA, Baluch A, Fox C, Lock S, Kaye A. Anaesthetic considerations for the neonate with tracheoesophageal fistula. Middle East J Anesth. 2008;19:1241-54.
25. Castilloux J, Noble AJ, Faure C. Risk factors for short- and long-term morbidity in children with esophageal atresia. J Pediatr. 2010;156:755-60.
26. Foker JE, Kendall TC, Catton K, Khan KM. A flexible approach to achieve a true primary repair for all infants with esophageal atresia. Semin Pediatr Surg. 2005;14:8-15.
27. Atzori P, Iacobellia BD, Bottero S, Spirydakis J, Laviani R, Trucchi A, et al. Preoperative tracheobronchoscopy in newborns with esophageal atresia: does it matter? J Pediatr Surg. 2006;41:1054-7.
28. Maoate K, Myers NA, Beasley SW. Gastric perforation in infants with oesophageal atresia and distal tracheo-oesophageal fistula. Pediatr Surg Int. 1999;15:24-7.
29. Pani N, Panda C. Anesthetic considerations for neonatal surgical emergencies. Indian J Anaesth. 2012;56:463-9.
30. Davis PJ, Cladis FP, Motoyama EK. Smith's anesthesia for infants and children, 8th edition. Philadelphia: Mosby, Elsevier Science; 2011. p. 577.
31. Holzki J. Bronchoscopic findings and treatment in congenital tracheo-oesophageal fistula. Paediatr Anaesth. 1992;2:297-303.
32. Salem MR, Wong AY, Lin HV, Firor HV, Bennett EJ. Prevention of gastric distention during anesthesia for newborns with tracheoesophageal fistulas. Anesthesiol. 1973;38:82-3.
33. Cooper MG. Bronchial blocker placement in infants: A technique and some considerations. Paed Anaesth. 1994;4:73-4.
34. Kaplan R, Guzzi L. An aid in the placement of right-sided lung ventilation during video-assisted thoracoscopic surgical bronchial blocker in small children. Paed Anaesth. 1993;3263.
35. Greenberg M, Cheng G, Lassasso B, Collins D, Vanderwall K. Endotracheal tube positioning using a flexible fiberoptic bronchoscope during tracheoesophageal fistula repair. Internet J Anesthesiol. 2006;12:1.
36. Tercan E, Sungun MB, Boyaci A, Kucukaydin M. One lung ventilation of a preterm newborn during esophageal atresia and tracheoesophageal fistula repair. Acta Anaesthesiol Scand. 2002;46:332-3.
37. Park MK, Lee DH. Normative arm and calf blood pressure values in the newborn. Pediatrics. 1989;83:240-3.
38. Park S, Lee H. Tension pneumothorax during tracheoesophageal fistula repair: a case report. Anesth Pain Med. 2015;10:134-7.
39. Al Tokhais T, Zamakhshary M, Aldekhayel S, Mandora H, Sayed S, AlHarbi K, et al. Thoracoscopic repair of tracheoesophageal fistulas: a case-control matched study. J Pediatr Surg. 2008;43:805-9.
40. Holcomb GW 3rd, Rothenberg SS, Bax KM, Martinez-Ferro M, Albanese CT, Ostlie DJ, et al. Thoracoscopic repair of esophageal atresia and tracheoesophageal fistula: a multi-institutional analysis. Ann Surg. 2005;242:422-8; discussion 428-30.
41. Walker A, Stokes M, Moriarty A. Anesthesia for major general surgery in neonates with complex cardiac defects. Pediatr Anesth. 2009;19:119-25.
42. Tobias JD, Lowe S, O'Dell N, Holcomb GW 3rd. Thoracic epidural anaesthesia in infants and children. Can J Anesth. 1993;40:879-82.
43. Skinner A. Neonatal Pharmacology. Anaesth Intensive Care Med. 2008;9:99-103.
44. Tsui BC, Suresh S. Ultrasound imaging for regional anesthesia in infants, children, and adolescents: a review of current literature and its application in the practice of neuraxial blocks. Anesthesiology. 2010;112:719-28.
45. Valairucha S, Seefelder C, Houck CS. Thoracic epidural catheters placed by the caudal route in infants: the importance of radiographic confirmation. Pediatr Anesth. 2002;12:424-8.

46. Davenport M, Rothenberg SS, Crabbe DC, Wulkan ML. The great debate: open or thoracoscopic repair for oesophageal atresia or diaphragmatic hernia. J Pediatr Surg. 2015;50:240-6.
47. Oestreicher-Kedem Y, DeRowe A, Nagar H, Fishman G, Ben-Ari J. Vocal fold paralysis in infants with tracheoesophageal fistula. Ann Otol Rhinol Laryngol. 2008;117:896-901.
48. Cozzi DA, Zani A, Conforti A, Colarizi P, Moretti C, Cozzi F. Pathogenesis of apparent life-threatening events in infants with esophageal atresia. Pediatr Pulmonol. 2006;41:488-93.
49. Kovesi T, Rubin S. Long-term complications of congenital esophageal atresia and/or tracheoesophageal fistula. Chest. 2004;126:915-25.
50. Al-Qahtani AR, Almaramhi H. Minimal access surgery in neonates and infants. J Pediatr Surg. 2006;41:910-3.
51. Wu Y, Yan Z, Hong L, Hu M, Chen S. Thoracoscopic repair of congenital esophageal atresia in infants. J Laparoendosc Adv Surg Tech A. 2009;19(3):461-3.
52. Mariano ER, Chu LF, Albanese CT, Ramamoorthy C. Successful thoracoscopic repair of esophageal atresia with tracheoesophageal fistula in a newborn with single ventricle physiology. Anesth Analges. 2005;101:1000-2.
53. Saade E, Setzer N. Anesthetic management of tracheoesophageal fistula repair in a newborn with hypoplastic left heart syndrome. Pediatr Anesth 2006;16:588-90.
54. Dalens B, Labbe A, Haberer JP. Selective endobronchial blocking versus selective intubation. Anesthesiology. 1982;55:555-6.
55. Tobias JD. Anaesthesia for neonatal thoracic surgery. Best Pract Res Clin Anaesth. 2004;18:303-20.
56. Tobias JD. Anaesthetic implications of thoracoscopic surgery in children. Paediatr Anaesth 1999;9:102-10.
57. Ho AM, Wong JCP, Chui PT, Karmakar MK. Case report: use of two balloon-tipped catheters during thoracoscopic repair of a type C tracheoesophageal fistula in a neonate. Can J Anesth. 2007;54:223-6.

# CHAPTER 7

# Nonoperating Room Anesthesia in Pediatrics

*Ranju Singh, Pooja Singh*

## ABSTRACT

Nonoperating room anesthesia (NORA) in pediatrics is a specialized field that is growing rapidly. The administration of NORA should ideally be performed by qualified anesthesiologists and nonanesthesiologists delivering NORA must be adequately trained and have a thorough understanding of the pharmacology of the agents used, as well as the ability to use antagonists for opioids and benzodiazepines. Patient selection for NORA is critical, considering the medical complexity of these patients. Monitoring during NORA is essential and should include pulse oximetry, capnography, noninvasive blood pressure, temperature, and electrocardiograph. Airway assessment for NORA patients is as thorough as general anesthesia, with a focused history, physical examination, and airway examination to identify potential complications and formulate an airway management plan.

Nonoperating room anesthesia in pediatrics demands a high level of skill, adaptability, and resource optimization to navigate the unique challenges of each procedure and ensure the best possible outcomes for pediatric patients.

**Keywords:** Sedation; Pediatric; Monitoring; Airway

## KEY POINTS

- Nonoperating room anesthesia (NORA) can be challenging because it involves managing unpredictable environments, unfamiliar equipment, pediatric patients with complex medical needs, and variable communication.
- Careful patient selection and airway assessment similar to that done before general anesthesia are critical in NORA.
- Prolonged fasting is unnecessary and may be detrimental.
- Resources and equipment needed for NORA include environmental (wall gases, oxygen supply, and safe electricals), anesthetic equipment, monitoring devices, and transport equipment.
- Sedation and regional anesthesia are commonly used in NORA.
- The monitoring standards and quality in NORA should be similar to those in the operating room.
- Special considerations are needed for specific settings such as magnetic resonance imaging (MRI) or endoscopy suites.
- Vigilance for complications, especially airway and respiratory complications, is essential in NORA.
- The pediatric adaptation of the postanesthetic discharge scoring system (PADSS) should be employed, and appropriate discharge instructions must be given to the caregiver.

## ■ INTRODUCTION

Nonoperating room anesthesia (NORA) refers to administering anesthesia or sedation to patients undergoing uncomfortable or painful procedures outside the operating room (OR).[1] NORA in pediatric patients presents a unique set of challenges compared to traditional OR settings. Unlike the controlled environment of the OR, NORA encompasses a wide range of procedural areas, such as radiology and cardiac catheterization suites, dental and fracture clinics, endoscopy rooms, radiation oncology, and emergency departments. Studies have shown an increased risk of airway-related adverse events, complications, and even death outside the OR locations.[2-4] Understanding the distinctive features of NORA is essential for pediatric anesthesiologists to provide safe and effective care.[5]

The landscape of anesthesia administration has been undergoing a significant transformation, with a notable increase in cases occurring outside the traditional OR. Data from the National Anesthesia Clinical Outcomes Registry (NACOR) from 2010 to 2014 revealed a steady rise in NORA cases, from 28 to 36% of all anesthesia encounters. If current trends persist, it is projected that NORA procedures will constitute as much as 50% of all anesthesia encounters within the next decade.[6]

This shift is particularly pronounced in pediatric anesthesia, where diagnostic radiologic imaging has emerged as the leading NORA category requiring anesthesia. Unlike adults, anesthesia is often warranted in children for imaging procedures due to their inability to cooperate with awake protocols. Thus, the anesthesiologist plays a critical role in facilitating necessary medical interventions while ensuring patient comfort and safety. Increase in interventional procedures in sick children with multiple comorbidities is responsible for the exponential increase in NORA cases. Moreover, there has been a notable shift in parental expectations, with an increasing demand for anesthesia or sedation care for pediatric procedures that were historically performed on unsedated children. This growing expectation reflects a broader societal trend toward prioritizing patient comfort and minimizing procedural stress, particularly in vulnerable populations like children.

Many factors make NORA in children a challenge, even for pediatric anesthesiologists. The knowledge and tailored anesthetic management strategies required for the diversity of procedures performed outside the familiar OR environment can be daunting. For instance, sedation for magnetic resonance imaging (MRI) demands meticulous attention to maintaining airway patency and avoiding respiratory depression. At the same time, anesthesia for cardiac catheterization procedures necessitates hemodynamic stability and precise titration of anesthetic agents. The unfamiliarity with advanced technological equipment used by proceduralists can be unnerving. The absence of dedicated anesthesia space and infrastructure, age-appropriate equipment, nonavailability of resuscitative equipment and choice of drugs, and lack of adequately trained support staff in non-OR settings underscore the importance of resource optimization and adaptability. Anesthesiologists must navigate the challenges of limited space, restricted patient access, high ambient noise levels, variable lighting conditions, unsafe electrical connections, and suboptimal ventilation systems while ensuring patient safety and comfort. Most catheterization and radiology suites are commonly situated in the basement of hospitals and are not easily accessible. Communication through mobile phones is also impossible due to the thick walls built for radiation protection, severely limiting the ability to call for help.

## Who Can Give NORA?

In pediatric patients, NORA should preferably be administered by an anesthesiologist with advanced airway management skills and pediatric resuscitation capabilities who can decide when to intervene.[7] Nonanesthesiologists, when delivering NORA, are at a greater risk of making inadvertent errors, inability to identify impending crises, and inability to adequately manage an emergency. The individual administering sedation or analgesia must have a thorough understanding of the pharmacology of the agents used and be well-versed in the use of antagonists for opioids and benzodiazepines. A dedicated individual must be present to monitor the patient throughout the procedure, with the ability to recognize complications early. During deep sedation, this monitor should have no other responsibilities beyond patient observation, while during moderate sedation, they may assist with minor tasks once analgesia and vital signs are stable. At least one person in the procedure room must be capable of establishing an airway and administering positive pressure ventilation. For moderate sedation, an individual with pediatric advanced life support skills should be immediately available within five minutes, and for deep sedation, this individual should be present in the room. Additional assistance should be readily accessible to ensure optimal patient care and safety. Proper training of nonanesthesiologists delivering NORA is needed. Guidelines for administering sedation and analgesia for nonanesthesiologists have been published.[8]

## PATIENT SELECTION AND PREOPERATIVE ASSESSMENT FOR NONOPERATING ROOM ANESTHESIA PROCEDURES

### Preoperative Assessment

Before administering anesthesia for NORA procedures in pediatric patients, thorough patient selection and preoperative assessment are paramount. Unlike scheduled surgeries in the OR, NORA procedures often vary in urgency and complexity, requiring meticulous evaluation to ensure safety and optimal outcomes. Regardless of the anesthesia location or the length of the procedure, all patients scheduled for anesthesia should undergo a thorough preoperative assessment (as for any surgery in the OR), ideally conducted by trained personnel following standardized protocols.[9] It may also be appropriate to optimize the patients, if clinically indicated, before accepting them for operative procedures outside the OR.

Emergency procedures or add-on cases outside regular working hours, more common in NORA, pose particular challenges for preanesthesia assessment due to time constraints, limited availability of laboratory services, and potential limitations in accessing patient records.[9] The centralization of preanesthesia evaluation and scheduling processes can help reduce limitations regarding accessing patient records.[10]

### Patient Selection

Considering the challenges in administering NORA, attention to detail in patient selection is paramount. Also, NORA patients are more medically complex than those in the traditional OR. A comprehensive medical history is essential, including developmental milestones, current illness symptoms, and any respiratory or cardiovascular issues. Previous anesthesia experiences, airway interventions, surgical history, known allergies, medications, and hospital admissions must be thoroughly reviewed to assess potential risks and tailor anesthesia plans accordingly. A comprehensive preoperative assessment must encompass the child's physiological status, developmental stage, cognitive function, and emotional well-being.[11] An integrated approach for risk stratification, risk reduction, and care optimization before the day of the procedure can easily be applied to the NORA patient population.

## Communication

It is important to discuss the plan of anesthesia/sedation, the need for intravenous catheters, and the use of medications to facilitate cooperation, maintain calmness, and prevent pain and discomfort during the procedure. This information helps alleviate anxiety and allows patients and their caregivers to better prepare for the upcoming experience. Information leaflets or videos during preoperative assessments and onsite can be valuable for educating patients and their families about the procedure and anesthesia process. Basic details about the procedure, including its purpose and potential benefits, should be communicated clearly to the patient, considering their age and understanding.

## Consent

Obtaining informed consent from the patient or their legal guardian is fundamental to anesthesia. Documentation of this consent ensures legal and ethical compliance and records the patient's agreement to undergo the proposed procedure and anesthesia plan.

## Fasting

Documenting the time since the patient's last meal is crucial, especially since many patients arrive for procedures in the morning from home. For elective procedures, the standard fasting guidelines typically recommend solids to be avoided for at least 6 hours before the procedure, breast milk for 4 hours (or one missed feed for infants feeding more frequently), and clear fluids for 2 hours before anesthesia administration. The duration of fasting before procedures requiring anesthesia has been a topic of ongoing debate in recent years. There is evidence that, as per current practice, children often fast for durations that are far beyond the recommended time thresholds, with adverse consequences such as irritability, dehydration, and hypoglycemia.[12] In addition, fasting does not guarantee an empty stomach, and there is no observed association between aspiration and compliance with standard fasting guidelines. Current concerns about aspiration are thus out of proportion to the actual risk. Given the lower observed frequency of aspiration and mortality than during general anesthesia, fasting strategies in procedural sedation can reasonably be less restrictive. Green et al. have put forward a consensus-derived algorithm in which each patient is first risk-stratified during their presedation assessment, using evidence-based factors relating to patient characteristics, comorbidities, the procedure, and the anticipated sedation technique.[12] Based upon the categorization of aspiration risk (negligible, mild, or moderate), graded fasting cut-offs for liquids and solids are recommended.

## Airway Assessment

The airway assessment of a patient undergoing NORA should be the same as would have been done if the patient was undergoing general anesthesia. The depth of sedation may increase unexpectedly for various reasons; hence, the team must be prepared to secure the airway if any complications appear. Even if endotracheal intubation or supraglottic device use is not anticipated, a detailed airway assessment remains mandatory to identify any potential complications preemptively. A focused history, a focused general physical examination followed by a focused airway examination is essential to locate any anticipated difficult airway and to quantify the problem areas of airway management precisely. This helps to formulate an airway management plan based on the practitioner's clinical skills and the available equipment and support resources.

## EQUIPMENT AND RESOURCE CONSIDERATIONS FOR NONOPERATING ROOM ANESTHESIA

Nonoperating room anesthesia in pediatric patients requires carefully considering equipment and resources to ensure safe and effective care delivery. Many remote NORA settings may need more infrastructure to support anesthesia requirements than purpose-built ORs.[1] The anesthesia equipment may need to be updated, retrofitted, or transported from other suites, potentially lacking features tailored to pediatric patients.[13] When providing NORA, anesthesia professionals should demand appropriate time to set up and familiarize themselves with the location, equipment, and available staff. Improperly functioning equipment, suboptimal workspace, and inadequate support in the NORA suite are a recipe for disaster.

Furthermore, appropriate sizing of devices and adjuncts for pediatric patients must be prioritized to meet the unique needs of this patient population. Blood pressure, heart rate, and electrocardiography (ECG) monitors are critical for monitoring. Further, the equipment should include those needed for front-of-the-neck airway (FONA) access. This is essential because, in case of any complications and difficulty in securing the airway, FONA can be critical. Hence, the required equipment should be available, such as an ultrasound machine, tracheostomy set, and tracheostomy tube.

Routine maintenance and equipment servicing are essential to ensure optimal functionality and prevent malfunctions during procedures. Portable anesthesia machines, monitors, airway management devices, anesthesia and emergency drugs, and resuscitation equipment tailored to pediatric patients must be readily available. Pediatric-specific dosing guidelines and drug formulations should also be readily available for accurate medication administration.[14]

### Environment
- Adequate lighting
- Oxygen and backup cylinders
- Wall gases (nitrous oxide and medical air)
- Central suction and catheters
- Thermostat control
- Safe electrical outlets

### Equipment
- Anesthesia machine
- Oxygen delivery equipment

- Pediatric airway equipment—appropriately sized
- Difficult airway cart
- Crash cart
- Venous access supplies
- Infusion pumps
- Essential anesthesia drugs and drugs for resuscitation
- Defibrillator with pediatric paddles

## Monitors
- Pulse oximetry with audible pulse tone and low threshold alarm
- Capnograph
- Noninvasive blood pressure
- Temperature probe
- Electrocardiograph with heart rate

## Transport-related Equipment
- Oxygen delivery devices
- Transport trolleys
- Portable monitors

## ANESTHESIA TECHNIQUES AND PHARMACOLOGICAL CONSIDERATIONS FOR PEDIATRIC PROCEDURES

In NORA for pediatric patients, selecting appropriate anesthesia techniques and pharmacological agents is crucial for ensuring safe and effective care. Unlike procedures in the OR, NORA encompasses a diverse range of settings and patient populations, each with unique anesthesia requirements. Pediatric patients undergoing NORA procedures may vary widely in age, developmental stage, and medical comorbidities, necessitating a tailored approach to anesthesia management. Anesthesiologists must consider factors, such as the child's airway anatomy, cardiovascular stability, and neurodevelopmental status when selecting anesthesia techniques.[15]

The goals of sedation or anesthesia for pediatric NORA are as follows:
- To guard the patient's safety and welfare.
- To minimize physical discomfort and pain.
- To control anxiety, minimize psychological trauma, and maximize the potential for amnesia.
- To control movement to allow the successful conduct of the procedure.
- To provide timely discharge from the hospital.

Sedation, regional anesthesia (RA), and general anesthesia are commonly employed in NORA, with the choice depending on patient characteristics, procedural requirements, the anticipated duration of the procedure, and the level of pain involved. Sedation may be appropriate for minimally invasive procedures, providing anxiolysis and analgesia while maintaining spontaneous ventilation. RA techniques, such as nerve blocks or epidurals, offer targeted pain relief and minimize systemic effects, making them suitable for specific surgical and diagnostic procedures.[11]

When general anesthesia is indicated, careful attention must be paid to pharmacological considerations, including drug selection, dosing, titration, patient's overall health status, potential side effects of the chosen agent, and the desired level of sedation or calmness required for the procedure. Pediatric patients exhibit age-dependent pharmacokinetics and pharmacodynamics, requiring meticulous dosing adjustments to achieve the desired anesthetic depth while minimizing side effects and complications.[16]

The ideal drug regimen should have the following desirable characteristics:
- Rapid onset and offset of action
- Predictable duration
- Easy titratability
- Multiple delivery options
- Safe with a wide therapeutic window
- Minimal cardiorespiratory depression and minimally affected by renal or hepatic disease
- Minimal drug interactions

Induction and maintenance of anesthesia can be achieved using intravenous or inhalational agents or a combination. By individualizing the choice of induction agents and routes of administration, anesthesia providers can optimize patient comfort, procedural success, and safety in various clinical scenarios.

Managing children with special needs, especially those with neurologic deficits or significant anomalies, presents unique challenges in anesthesia administration. These patients may require repeat anesthesia and often exhibit increasing anxiety, refusal of drugs, or even combative behavior. Principles of care in such cases involve early recognition of behavioral cues, encouraging parental support, and establishing clear guidelines for perioperative management of uncooperative children. Ethical use of restraint techniques may also be necessary to ensure patient safety and procedural success. Some commonly used drugs are shown in **Table 1**.

## Sedation

The goal of sedation in NORA settings is to achieve a level of sedation that allows the procedure to be performed safely and comfortably while minimizing the risk of adverse events.[17] Patient selection criteria for sedation in NORA settings typically include factors, such as the patient's age, medical history, American Society of Anesthesiologists (ASA) physical status classification, and the complexity and duration of the procedure. Patients with significant comorbidities or airway concerns may not be suitable candidates for sedation outside the OR and may require anesthesia in a controlled environment with advanced airway management capabilities. The anesthesia provider is responsible for assessing the patient, selecting appropriate sedation medications and doses, monitoring the patient throughout the procedure, and managing any sedation-related complications that may arise.[18]

The risk of complications increases with increasing levels of sedation. Further, the child may progress to deeper sedation levels without clinically recognizable signs. Although there are several scales to evaluate the quality and safety of sedation practices in children, clinicians most frequently follow the ASA classification of sedation, which assesses patient responsiveness, airway patency, adequacy of spontaneous ventilation, and cardiovascular function.[19] Cravero et al. have developed and validated a six-point scale called the Pediatric Sedation State Scale (PSSS), which measures the quality and effectiveness of procedural sedation in children.[3] The level of

**TABLE 1:** Commonly used anesthetic agents in nonoperating room anesthesia (NORA).

| Induction agent | Purpose | Dosages | Administration |
|---|---|---|---|
| Midazolam | Provides anxiolysis, sedation, and amnesia. Mostly used for premedication | *Oral:* 0.3–1.0 mg/kg *Intranasal:* 0.2 mg/kg *Intravenous:* 0.05–0.1 mg/kg | Oral, intranasal, and intravenous |
| Propofol | Widely used for intravenous induction. Fast onset and short duration of action. Also has antiemetic effect | 2–4 mg/kg | Intravenous |
| Ketamine | Induction agent with analgesic effect. Useful in asthmatics. Causes tachycardia, hypertension, and excessive secretions | *Intravenous:* 1–2 mg/kg *Intramuscular:* 2–5 mg/kg *Oral:* 5–10 mg/kg (mixed with sweet beverage, administered about 30 minutes before procedure) | Intravenous, intramuscular, and oral |
| Ketofol | Combination of ketamine and propofol. Used for short procedural sedation and analgesia. Provides hemodynamic stability and less respiratory depression | Not specified | Intravenous |
| Fentanyl | Potent analgesic. Can cause hypotension, respiratory depression, muscle rigidity, postanesthetic nausea, and vomiting | 0.5–2 µg/kg | Intravenous |
| Dexmedetomidine | Becoming popular for sedation. Does not cause respiratory depression. Offers hemodynamic stability | 0.1–1 µg/kg (slow infusion or bolus) | Intravenous |

sedation can also be assessed in older children by scores such as the Ramsay sedation scale **(Table 2)**. A Ramsay sedation score of 4 or more may indicate oversedation and require intervention.

The anesthesia provider must be prepared to manage common sedation-related complications in children, such as respiratory depression, airway obstruction, and hemodynamic instability.[20] Regarding the use of oxygen, there is no conclusive evidence either supporting or opposing the use of prophylactic oxygen during procedural sedation and analgesia. Supplemental oxygen might mask signs of

| **TABLE 2:** Ramsay sedation scale. | |
|---|---|
| Score | Description |
| 1 | Patient is anxious and agitated or restless, or both |
| 2 | Patient is cooperative, oriented, and tranquil |
| 3 | Patient responds to commands only |
| 4 | Patient exhibits a brisk response to a light glabellar tap or loud auditory stimulus |
| 5 | Patient exhibits a sluggish response to a light glabellar tap or loud auditory stimulus |
| 6 | Patient exhibits no response to a light glabellar tap or loud auditory stimulus |

respiratory depression by delaying the onset of oxygen desaturation. The rates of hypoxia and respiratory depression appear to be comparable whether supplemental oxygen is used or not. The available data does not demonstrate any clear benefit or a tendency toward a benefit from using supplemental oxygen during moderate sedation.[21] However, withholding oxygen to detect hypoventilation is ill-advised, and anesthesiologists must not disregard using supplemental oxygen if clinically indicated.[22]

## Regional Anesthesia

Regional anesthesia is a valuable complement to general anesthesia in the OR and provides safe and efficient perioperative pain management. With the expertise of experienced anesthesiologists, the availability of ultrasound-guided block equipment, pediatric patient-appropriate equipment, and a well-structured monitoring protocol, more pediatric patients can benefit from RA techniques outside the traditional OR environment. This approach not only offers effective pain relief but also reduces reliance on systemic opioids, thereby minimizing associated side effects,[11] enhancing patient satisfaction, and improving perioperative outcomes. However, careful patient selection and appropriate technique application are crucial considerations in ensuring the safety and efficacy of RA. Providers must remain vigilant for potential complications, such as local anesthetic systemic toxicity (LAST), nerve injury, and block failure.[23]

## ■ MONITORING

Unlike the controlled environment of the OR, NORA settings may lack dedicated anesthesia monitoring equipment and specialized support staff, requiring adaptation to ensure patient safety.[24] Despite the development of monitoring guidelines, nonanesthesiologists have not yet implemented uniform monitoring standards in NORA settings, and basic monitoring principles are inconsistent.[25] The monitoring standards and quality in NORA should be similar to those in the OR. Effective monitoring of pediatric patients undergoing NORA procedures involves continuous vital signs, including pulse oximetry and ECG with heart rate, intermittent blood pressure measurement, and intermittent respiratory rate and depth assessment. Capnography is another handy monitor, particularly in procedures with a risk of hypoventilation or airway obstruction. The sampling of exhaled carbon dioxide is possible in nonintubated patients by using nasal prongs, which simultaneously allow the administration of supplementary oxygen. By delivering oxygen through one

**BOX 1:** Monitoring in nonoperating room anesthesia (NORA).

- Pulse oximetry equipped with an audible pulse tone and a low threshold alarm
- Adequate illumination and exposure of the patient to enable assessment of color
- Anesthesia machine equipped with an oxygen analyzer
- Continuous end-tidal carbon dioxide analysis with an audible alarm
- Continuous electrocardiogram (ECG) and heart rate monitoring
- Temperature monitoring
- Bispectral index (BIS) monitoring (where available)

prong and sampling exhaled gas from the other, the nasal cannula provides end-tidal values comparable to those achieved with intubated patients. Face masks with built-in capnography systems are also available for pediatric use.[26] The patient's temperature should be monitored in locations like the MRI suite, where hypothermia is a known complication. Continuous monitoring of the degree of sedation is also essential. It is usually based on clinical criteria such as consciousness and response to commands. The bispectral index (BIS) is a specialized monitor that provides reliable, objective, and consistent guidance for the sedation depth and helps in the timely identification of oversedation. Although it cannot replace the clinical patient assessment, in well-equipped and specialized centers, BIS monitors can be added to the monitors for NORA. In addition to standard monitoring, anesthesia providers must remain vigilant for signs of respiratory depression, airway obstruction, and hemodynamic instability, which may arise due to factors, such as sedation, anesthesia, or procedural stimuli. Prompt recognition and intervention are critical for preventing adverse events and ensuring patient well-being. A summary of the monitoring requirements is shown in **Box 1**.

# CONSIDERATIONS FOR SPECIFIC PEDIATRIC NONOPERATING ROOM ANESTHESIA PROCEDURES

Understanding the specific requirements and nuances of different NORA procedures is essential for ensuring safe and effective anesthesia delivery.[11] **Table 3** shows the various settings for NORA delivery.

## Nonoperating Room Anesthesia in Gastrointestinal Interventions

Diagnostic endoscopy can often be performed under moderate sedation. However, endoscopic retrograde cholangiopancreatography (ERCP) and therapeutic procedures such as dilatation and stenting of esophageal strictures, treatment of esophageal varices, and peroral endoscopic myotomy typically require deep sedation or general anesthesia. The risk for aspiration in patients with achalasia cardia and gastroesophageal reflux is high, and these patients' trachea should preferably be intubated to protect the airway. ERCP is particularly challenging; deep sedation is needed as a noncooperative patient is at risk of duodenal perforation; and deep sedation may lead to airway compromise and desaturation. Further, as the patient is prone, access to airway procedures is limited. Contrast-related complications such as anaphylactic reactions and nephrotoxicity can also occur.

## Nonoperating Room Anesthesia in Cardiological Interventions

Preanesthetic assessment should gather a history of cyanosis, shortness of breath, signs and symptoms of congestive heart failure, previous surgical or cardiological

**TABLE 3:** Fields and procedures where nonoperating room anesthesia (NORA) is administered.

| Field | Procedures/techniques |
|---|---|
| Endoscopy | Esophagogastroduodenoscopy (EGD), endoscopic retrograde cholangiopancreatography (ERCP), dilatation and stenting of esophageal strictures, treatment of esophageal varices, and peroral endoscopic myotomy |
| Interventional pulmonology | Endobronchial ultrasound, transbronchial needle aspiration, balloon bronchoplasty, airway stents, and bronchoalveolar lavages |
| Interventional cardiology | Defect closure (ASD, VSD, and PDA), valve dilatation, valve implantation, electrophysiological studies, embolization of collaterals, and permanent pacemaker insertion |
| Interventional radiology | Computed tomography (CT) scans, magnetic resonance imaging (MRI), lumbar puncture, bone marrow aspiration (BMA) |
| Dental | Filling, root canal treatment, orthodontic procedures, and dentigerous cyst excision |
| Neurological | Embolization of cerebral and dural arteriovenous malformations, coiling of cerebral aneurysms, thrombolysis, and balloon dilatation of vessels. |

(ASD: atrial septal defect; PDA: patent ductus arteriosus; VSD: ventricular septal defect)

interventions, use of anticoagulant therapy, and other cardiac medications. General anesthesia or sedation should be adjusted according to the level of cardiac dysfunction and the specific cardiac defect. Maintaining adequate perfusion of both systemic and pulmonary circulation and appropriate filling pressures, heart rate, and coronary perfusion pressures is essential. Invasive monitoring and blood gas analysis might be necessary. General anesthesia with endotracheal may be required if transesophageal echocardiography (TEE) is planned, as most children cannot tolerate the TEE probe under sedation.

## Nonoperating Room Anesthesia for Neurological Interventions

Nonoperating room anesthesia in patients undergoing neurological interventions is equally challenging. Maintenance of cerebral perfusion pressure and management of intracranial pressure is essential. Generally, controlled ventilation under general anesthesia is preferred. Preparedness to address hemodynamic instability and immediate access to assistance should be ensured. Measures to maintain normothermia are essential. Major complications encountered include hemorrhage, thromboembolic events, coil occlusion, and cerebral vasospasm, which can exacerbate hypotension and adversely affect hemodynamics.

## Nonoperating Room Anesthesia for Magnetic Resonance Imaging

Monitoring in MRI suites poses significant challenges, primarily due to the need to eliminate ferromagnetic objects. The presence of such objects can lead to interference or malfunction of equipment due to the fluctuating magnetic fields inherent in MRI technology. Various monitoring and medical devices must adhere to specific requirements of the MRI suite to mitigate risks and maintain accuracy during procedures. For instance, ECG monitors with high-impedance graphite electrodes and leads to prevent thermal injury are required. At the same time, blood pressure measurements with oscillometers with nonferrous gauges are needed for accurate readings. Copper stylets are preferred, and endotracheal tubes and laryngeal mask airways are chosen based on nonmagnetic designs to prevent image distortion and ensure patient safety.

The MRI is a noisy and claustrophobic environment with restricted access to the patient. As movement artifacts in MRI can significantly impair the quality of images, immobility is an essential aim of NORA. This has to be achieved while ensuring the safety and comfort of the patient. Anesthesia is induced in a dedicated anesthetic room adjacent to the MRI scanner. This room should permit rapid transfer of the patients to the MRI scanner and quick retrieval in case of any complication. Patients should be transferred into the scanning room on an MRI-safe in a nonferrous trolley. The airway of the patient who goes head first into the magnet is completely inaccessible and should be well secured. During scanning, maintenance of anesthesia can be achieved by intravenous or inhalation techniques using MR-compatible anesthetic machines and ventilators, which can be sited adjacent to the magnet bore, minimizing the length of the breathing system. Now, MRI-safe infusion pumps are also available. In case of hypoventilation or other complications, the scan has to be stopped, the scanning table has to be pulled outside the magnet bore, and the patient needs to be attended to in the same setting. This rescue is time-consuming and requires regular practice to be effective. Defibrillators are not permitted inside the MRI suite; therefore, resuscitation procedures must be conducted outside the magnetic field to avoid interference. Hypothermia is also a significant concern in pediatric patients undergoing MRI.

## COLLABORATION AND COMMUNICATION: MULTIDISCIPLINARY APPROACH IN NONOPERATING ROOM ANESTHESIA

Successful outcomes hinge on effective collaboration and communication among multidisciplinary teams in NORA for pediatric patients. Unlike procedures conducted in the OR, NORA settings often involve diverse healthcare professionals, and anesthesia providers must collaborate closely with proceduralists, including radiologists, cardiologists, and interventional specialists, to coordinate perioperative care and facilitate seamless procedural workflow. Closed-loop communication and clear messages are essential for promoting efficiency and minimizing risks.[10] Clear allocation of roles and responsibilities and effective teamwork between anesthesia providers and other personnel (including technicians and nursing officers) is vital for ensuring patient safety and comfort throughout the perioperative period.[20] Furthermore, a good rapport between the anesthesiologists and the ancillary support personnel, such as respiratory therapists, pharmacists, and child life specialists, enhances the patient's safety and overall procedural experience.

## MANAGING EMERGENCIES AND COMPLICATIONS IN NONOPERATING ROOM ANESTHESIA

Nonoperating room anesthesia for pediatric patients entails potential emergent situations and complications, necessitating vigilant preparedness and prompt intervention from anesthesia providers.[3] Most commonly, near misses or critical

> **BOX 2:** Complications of nonoperating room anesthesia.
>
> *Category:*
> - Airway complications—obstruction and stridor
> - Respiratory complications—laryngospasm, bronchospasm, desaturation, and apnea
> - Hypothermia
> - Agitation and delirium
> - Inadequate or deeper level of sedation
> - Postprocedural nausea and vomiting
> - Blood pressure/heart rate variation
> - Inadequate postoperative analgesia
> - Hypoglycemia
> - Aspiration

events occur due to operator error or lack of rescue systems.[27] The widely seen complications are listed in **Box 2**.[28]

The mortality in NORA is reported to be around 0.02%. The primary complications are hemodynamic instability and a need to upgrade care to either a high-dependency unit (HDU) or an intensive care unit (ICU); these occur in about 0.10% of cases each. The minor complications are postoperative nausea and vomiting, inadequate pain control, and blood pressure and heart rate fluctuations.[29] Respiratory complications, including respiratory depression, are more frequent during NORA, often due to nonvigilance, inappropriate anesthetic techniques, and nonanesthesiologist staff handling complex cases, esophageal intubation during resuscitation, and unexplained bradycardia. About 10% of anesthesiologists lack a backup plan for unanticipated difficult intubation. Thus, familiarity with the difficult airway algorithm and early call for help are crucial. Inadequate oxygenation/ventilation is a common preventable event in NORA, avoidable with vigilant monitoring using pulse oximetry and capnography. Diagnostic suites maintain lower temperatures to prevent equipment overheating, making children particularly vulnerable to hypothermia, which can increase surgical blood loss, delay recovery, and raise oxygen consumption; thus, active warming measures should be used. Patients should fast according to standard guidelines, as sedatives and anesthetic agents can blunt airway reflexes, increasing aspiration risk.

On the other hand, prolonged fasting can cause dehydration, hypovolemia, and hypoglycemia, so maintaining sufficient volume status through prehydration and slow intravenous drug administration is a wise precaution. Nausea and vomiting are also, common but treatable and preventable causes of unplanned hospitalization; at-risk patients should be identified and should receive prophylactic medication. By implementing robust protocols and remaining vigilant, anesthesia providers can mitigate potential complications and enhance patient outcomes in diverse clinical environments.[30]

## POSTANESTHESIA CARE AND DISCHARGE PLANNING FOR NONOPERATING ROOM PEDIATRIC PATIENTS

Unlike the controlled environment of the OR, NORA settings may lack dedicated postanesthesia recovery areas, necessitating adaptation to optimize patient recovery and discharge readiness. Patients must be observed and monitored until they have

**TABLE 4:** Pediatric postanesthetic discharge scoring system.

| Parameter | Score |
|---|---|
| *Vital signs:* Heart rate and blood pressure according to age | |
| • Variation <20% from preoperative level | 2 |
| • Variation between 20 and 40% | 1 |
| • Variation >40% | 0 |
| *Level of activity:* Walking or activity | |
| • Stable gait, no dizziness (normal activity) | 2 |
| • Walking with assistance (or reduced activity) | 1 |
| • Unable to walk (hypotonia) | 0 |
| *Nausea and/or vomiting* | |
| • Minimal | 2 |
| • Moderate | 1 |
| • Severe (despite treatment) | 0 |
| *Pain:* Acceptable and/or controllable with oral analgesics | |
| • Yes | 2 |
| • No | 1 |
| *Surgical bleeding* | |
| • Minimal (no dressing change needed) | 2 |
| • Moderate (one to two dressing changes needed) | 1 |
| • Severe | 0 |

satisfactorily recovered, closely watching for signs of airway obstruction, respiratory depression, or hemodynamic disturbances.[11,31] An anesthesiologist or adequately trained nonanesthesiologist who administered NORA must make the discharge decision.

Postanesthesia care typically focuses on physiologic criteria that must be met for a safe discharge. Initially, the patient is shifted from the OR to the postanesthesia care unit (PACU) when there is complete recovery from anesthesia and the return of vital signs to near baseline using scores such as the modified Aldrete scoring system to assess a patient's readiness. Subsequently, discharge to home is evaluated. Pediatric adaptation of the postanesthetic discharge scoring system (PADSS) can be used to decide on the suitability of discharge. The Ped-PADSS is built on five items, each quoted 0, 1, or 2, as shown in **Table 4**. A score of 9/10 is required for discharge.[32]

When discharged, the patient must be accompanied by a responsible adult. The concerned adult must carefully explain the warning signs, and written instructions must be provided. An emergency contact number must also be provided to the caregiver so they can call and seek advice in case of any complication.

## ■ CONCLUSION

The growing demand for pediatric anesthesia in nonoperating room settings highlights the need for comprehensive systems and protocols to ensure safety and quality care. Establishing clear guidelines for patient selection, enhanced monitoring, and standardized management of complications is essential. Institutional commitment is crucial for providing necessary resources, fostering a safety culture, and ensuring adherence to best practices. Anesthesiologists must take a lead role in the design of NORA services and prioritize patient safety to ensure effective anesthesia delivery. Also, collaborative efforts between anesthesia providers, proceduralists, and healthcare administrators must drive innovation and quality improvement. By embracing advancements in anesthesia technology and care strategies, providers can enhance patient outcomes and advance pediatric anesthesia.[30]

## REFERENCES

1. Landrigan-Ossar M, Setiawan CT. Pediatric Anesthesia Outside the Operating Room: Safety and Systems. Anesthesiol Clin. 2020;38:577-86.
2. Metzner J, Domino KB. Risks of anesthesia or sedation outside the operating room: the role of the anesthesia care provider. Curr Opin Anaesthesiol. 2010;23:523-31.
3. Cravero JP, Blike GT, Beach M, Gallagher SM, Hertzog JH, Havidich JE et al. Incidence and Nature of Adverse Events During Pediatric Sedation/Anesthesia for Procedures Outside the Operating Room: Report From the Pediatric Sedation Research Consortium. Pediatrics. 2006;118:1087-96.
4. Cravero JP. Risk and safety of pediatric sedation/anesthesia for procedures outside the operating room. Curr Opin Anaesthesiol. 2009;22:509-13.
5. Dutton RP. Rapid Growth in NORA Will Continue: Science Must Follow! ASA Monitor. 2022;86:43.
6. Chang B, Kaye AD, Diaz JH, Westlake B, Dutton RP, Urman RD. Interventional Procedures Outside of the Operating Room: Results From the National Anesthesia Clinical Outcomes Registry. J Patient Saf. 2018;14:9-16.
7. Setiawan CT, Landrigan-Ossar M. Pediatric Anesthesia Outside the Operating Room: Case Management. Anesthesiol Clin. 2020;38:587-604.
8. Epstein BS. The American Society of Anesthesiologist's efforts in developing guidelines for sedation and analgesia for nonanesthesiologists: the 40th Rovenstine Lecture. Anesthesiology. 2003;98(5):1261-8.
9. Chang B, Urman RD. Non-operating Room Anesthesia: The Principles of Patient Assessment and Preparation. Anesthesiol Clin. 2016;34:223-40.
10. Chow VW, Hepner DL, Bader AM. Electronic Care Coordination From the Preoperative Clinic. Anesth Analg. 2016;123:1458-62.
11. Wong T, Georgiadis PL, Urman RD, Tsai MH. Non-Operating Room Anesthesia: Patient Selection and Special Considerations. Local Reg Anesth. 2020;13:1-9.
12. Green SM, Leroy PL, Roback MG, Irwin MG, Andolfatto G, Babl FE, et al. An international multidisciplinary consensus statement on fasting before procedural sedation in adults and children. Anaesthesia. 2020;75:374-85.
13. Roberts RJ, Banta L, Verghese ST. Non-Operating Room Anesthesia for Pediatric Surgical Procedures. In: Verghese ST, Kane TD (Eds). Anesthetic Management in Pediatric General Surgery: Evolving and Current Concepts. Cham: Springer International Publishing; 2021. pp. 101-17.
14. Nelson O, Bailey PD. Pediatric Anesthesia Considerations for Interventional Radiology. Anesthesiol Clin. 2017;35:701-14.
15. Shih G, Bailey PD Jr. Nonoperating room anesthesia for children. Curr Opin Anaesthesiol. 2020;33(4):584-8.
16. Maddirala S, Theagrajan A. Non-operating room anaesthesia in children. Indian J Anaesth. 2019;63(9):754-62.

17. Min JY, Lee JR, Kang YS, Ho JH, Byon HJ. Pediatric characteristics and the dose of propofol for sedation during radiological examinations: a retrospective analysis. J Int Med Res. 2021;49:300060521990992.
18. Sirimontakan T, Artprom N, Anantasit N. Efficacy and Safety of Pediatric Procedural Sedation Outside the Operating Room. Anesth Pain Med. 2020;10(4):e106493.
19. American Society of Anesthesiologists Task Force on Sedation and Analgesia by Non-Anesthesiologists. Practice guidelines for sedation and analgesia by non-anesthesiologists. Anesthesiology. 2002;96(4):1004-17.
20. Bellolio MF, Puls HA, Anderson JL, Gilani WI, Murad MH, Barrionuevo P, et al. Incidence of adverse events in paediatric procedural sedation in the emergency department: a systematic review and meta-analysis. BMJ Open. 2016;6:e011384.
21. Deitch K, Chudnofsky CR, Dominici P. The utility of supplemental oxygen during emergency department procedural sedation and analgesia with midazolam and fentanyl: a randomized, controlled trial. Ann Emerg Med. 2007;49(1):1-8.
22. Sheahan CG, Mathews DM. Monitoring and delivery of sedation. Br J Anaesth. 2014;113 (Suppl 2):ii37-47.
23. De Buck F, Devroe S, Missant C, Van de Velde M. Regional anesthesia outside the operating room: indications and techniques. Curr Opin Anaesthesiol. 2012;25:501-7.
24. Routman J, Boggs SD. Patient monitoring in the nonoperating room anesthesia (NORA) setting: current advances in technology. Curr Opin Anaesthesiol. 2021;34:430-6.
25. Fanning RM. Monitoring during sedation given by non-anaesthetic doctors. Anaesthesia. 2008;63:370-4.
26. Nagoshi M, Morzov R, Hotz J, Belson P, Matar M, Ross P, et al. Mainstream capnography system for nonintubated children in the postanesthesia care unit: Performance with changing flow rates, and a comparison to side stream capnography. Paediatr Anaesth. 2016;26:1179-87.
27. Bell C, Sequeira PM. Nonoperating room anesthesia for children. Curr Opin Anaesthesiol. 2005;18:271-6.
28. Hardman B, Karamchandani K. Management of anesthetic complications outside the operating room. Curr Opin Anaesthesiol. 2023;36:435-40.
29. Chang B, Kaye A, Diaz J, Westlake B, Dutton R, Urman R. Complications of Non-Operating Room Procedures: Outcomes From the National Anesthesia Clinical Outcomes Registry. J Patient Saf. 2015; Published Ahead of Print.
30. Herman AD, Jaruzel CB, Lawton S, Tobin CD, Reves JG, Catchpole KR, et al. Morbidity, mortality, and systems safety in non-operating room anesthesia: a narrative review. Br J Anesth. 2021;127:729-44.
31. Youn AM, Ko YK, Kim YH. Anesthesia and sedation outside of the operating room. Korean J Anesthesiol. 2015;68:323-31.
32. Moncel JB, Nardi N, Wodey E, Pouvreau A, Ecoffey C. Evaluation of the pediatric post anesthesia discharge scoring system in an ambulatory surgery unit. Paediatr Anaesth. 2015;25:636-41.

# CHAPTER 8

# Pediatric Thoracic Anesthesia

*Monica Hervias Sanz, Francisco Javier Escriba Alapont*

## ABSTRACT

Pediatric thoracic surgery encompasses many procedures throughout childhood, including open, thoracoscopic, or video-assisted approaches. Anesthesia in pediatric thoracic cases presents unique challenges due to anatomical and physiological differences and potential comorbidities. It requires specialized pediatric anesthesiologists. Understanding pediatric anatomical, physiological, and ventilatory specifics is paramount. One-lung ventilation (OLV) in pediatric patients demands meticulous planning and device selection due to pediatric airway constraints. Radiological imaging aids in device sizing, ensuring optimal fit. This chapter outlines various techniques and considerations focusing on lung isolation. It discusses the importance of selecting appropriate bronchial blockers (BB) based on patient age and size: techniques for both intraluminal and extraluminal approaches are described; additionally, it explores selective bronchial intubation and double-lumen tubes (DLT). The physiology of OLV in pediatric patients needs to be understood in order to manage hypoxemia effectively. This chapter provides a diagnostic and treatment sequence for managing hypoxemia. Furthermore, it covers regional analgesic techniques for pediatric thoracic surgery.

**Keywords:** Pediatric thoracic anesthesia; Video-assisted surgery; One lung ventilation in children

## KEY POINTS

- Pediatric thoracic surgery involves various procedures throughout the pediatric age range and benefits from one-lung ventilation (OLV).
- Performing OLV in younger children presents challenges related to the smaller airway size, the scarcity of age-appropriate devices, and the increased predisposition to hypoxemia.
- The anesthetic plan should include evaluating the tracheobronchial tree and selecting the appropriate endotracheal tube, lung isolation device, and bronchoscope based on the patient's age and size.
- In the event of hypoxemia during OLV, a diagnostic and treatment protocol should be followed, including checking the isolation device, making ventilatory adjustments, and increasing the inspiratory fraction of oxygen ($FiO_2$).
- Regional blocks reduce anesthetic toxicity and ensure effective perioperative pain control.

# INTRODUCTION

Pediatric thoracic surgery includes various surgeries throughout the pediatric age, including open, thoracoscopic, and video-assisted approaches. More minor patients pose an anesthetic challenge due to their anatomo-physiological peculiarities, to which the possible associated comorbidities, which are common in some cases, must be added.

Pediatric anesthesiologists should perform pediatric thoracic anesthesia in centers with specialized pediatric units and professionals accustomed to working in pediatric settings.

The differences between pediatric patients and adults include anatomical differences in the size of the tracheobronchial tree, which determines the need for specific devices, and at a physiological level, which requires knowing the ventilatory needs and pediatric heart-lung interaction.

Finally, each stage of pediatric age is associated with a different type of surgical pathology that must be understood. Pediatric thoracic anesthesia is challenging, even for most pediatric anesthesiologists.

# PEDIATRIC AIRWAY, RESPIRATORY PHYSIOLOGY, AND VENTILATION

Thanks to the possibility of conducting more comprehensive chest studies through computed tomography (CT), the anatomy of the tracheobronchial tree in children is better understood. The most notable anatomical features are as follows:

- The left main bronchus is smaller in diameter than the right one, which requires an endotracheal tube (ETT) size 0.5 smaller if a mainstem left bronchus selective intubation is to be performed.[1]

    The distance from the carina to the origin of the left upper bronchus is three times greater than the distance between the carina and the origin of the right upper lobe bronchus. This means that the left lung offers greater security to maintain isolation in case of changes in the patient's position or surgical manipulations.

- Up to the age of 8 years, the distance of the right upper bronchus origin is ≤1 cm from the carina, which should be considered when performing selective intubation or right lung isolation.

    Physiologically, the pediatric patient has poorer redistribution of West zones, greater diaphragmatic pressure on a mostly cartilaginous rib cage, and lower lung compliance.[2] Neonates, infants, and young children have a higher predisposition to hypoxemia due to their increased oxygen consumption.

## Ventilation in the Pediatric Patient

The anesthetic circuits used during one-lung ventilation (OLV) are particularly relevant due to the compressibility of the system and compliance, which could accumulate a compressed gas volume between 50 and 125 mL depending on the material for a positive pressure of 25 $cmH_2O$. This volume is especially significant in pediatrics, where tidal volumes are small, but circuit pressures are high, given the small diameter of tracheal tubes. According to Boyle's law, this would create an instrumental dead space with a loss of tidal volume, which, if pediatric-compatible anesthesia machines are not used, can generate significant hypoventilation states in the patient by not compensating for the volume compressed by the ventilator circuit. Due to the effects of anesthetic circuit compliance, the higher the pressure generated at the end of inspiration (peak pressure), the greater the volume of gas that will be compressed and retained within the anesthesia machine circuit and not reach the patient.[3] Today, turbine circular systems with precise compensation systems allow us to work well in these complex scenarios. Hence, the auto-check is essential, as the best anesthesia machines for these complex cases are essential.

### Recruitment Maneuvers in Pediatrics

In 2003, Tusman considered recruitment maneuvers through manual ventilation with high peak pressures in pediatric patients to prevent atelectasis[4] and in 2010 described a noninvasive method to monitor optimal lung positive end-expiratory pressure (PEEP) that can be easily applied at the patient's bedside. The process consists of analyzing the behavior of dynamic compliance ($C_{dyn}$), airway resistance (Raw), and $CO_2$ elimination by breathing ($VTCO_2$, br) during the PEEP titration phase. The optimal PEEP coincides with the highest $C_{dyn}$ value and the lowest Raw value during the PEEP titration test.[5]

A more recent update by García—Fernández concludes that to date, the only recruitment maneuver that has proven to be the safest and most effective, even in the neonatal population, are the stepped pressure control maneuvers with a fixed cycling pressure of 15 $cmH_2O$ and progressive PEEP steps of 5 $cmH_2O$. During the opening phase, pediatric patients' maximum inspiratory pressure of 30 $cmH_2O$ and a PEEP of 15 $cmH_2O$ should be reached.[3,6]

## ■ ONE-LUNG VENTILATION

The practice of OLV involves ventilating only one lung, mechanically separating both lungs, and allowing lung isolation to facilitate surgical exposure and minimize lung injury from retractors or surgical tools in pulmonary, mediastinal, esophageal, and aortic surgery, as well as surgery of the chest wall and spine, and some cardiac surgery approaches to close intracardiac defects.[2,7] Additionally, lung isolation is helpful in nonsurgical processes such as empyema and pulmonary hemorrhage or in achieving differential ventilation **(Box 1)**.

The pathologies differ according to the pediatric age group, such that in the neonatal period, the most frequent include tracheal stenosis, pulmonary sequestration, congenital diaphragmatic hernia, tracheoesophageal fistula, congenital lobar emphysema, and vascular ring. Older children usually present with infections,

**BOX 1:** Indications for one-lung ventilation in children.

*Surgical:*
- Pulmonary resection
- Video-assisted thoracoscopic surgery (VATS)
- Mediastinal surgery
- Esophageal surgery
- Thoracic vascular surgery
- Minimally invasive cardiac surgery

*Intensive care unit:*
- Pulmonary hemorrhage
- Purulent pulmonary secretions in unilateral lung infection
- Pulmonary alveolar proteinosis during lung lavage

malignancy, and musculoskeletal deformities. One of the most feared presentations in this latter age group is the anterior mediastinal mass due to possible complications such as total airway compression and cardiovascular collapse under general anesthesia.

## Lung Isolation Techniques in the Pediatric Patient

The general principles of OLV apply to adults and children, but lung isolation is challenging in pediatric patients mainly due to the small airway size. OLV poses a challenge for the anesthesiologist for three reasons that differentiate it from lung isolation in adults: the technical difficulties associated with the small size of the entire tracheobronchial tree, the limited availability of devices adapted to different ages and bronchial sizes, and the greater predisposition to hypoxemia due to anatomical and physiological differences, with patients under 2 years of age presenting the most significant difficulty.

Some open-approach thoracic surgeries and other minimally invasive surgeries can be successfully performed without lung isolation through retraction of structures or $CO_2$ insufflation via thoracoscopic techniques.[8,9] Still, the ability to deflate the ipsilateral lung provides better conditions, and it is desirable to achieve lung isolation for the best surgical exposure.

### Preoperative Evaluation

When considering lung isolation in a pediatric patient, planning is crucial. Several points should be considered, referred to as the ABCD of pediatric lung isolation,[8,10] which, as in adults, includes the evaluation of anatomy (A), the selection of the appropriate bronchoscope size (B), chest imaging evaluation (C), and what differentiates it from adults, the selection of the device relative to the variable diameter of the pediatric airway according to age (D). Patients usually have at least a chest X-ray. However, it is preferable to have a CT scan of the airway in the tiniest patients, which will help determine the size of the device (tube and/or BB) as well as the flexible fiberoptic bronchoscope (FOB) needed for insertion and verification of lung isolation (see the following text).

The trachea has an elliptical shape, with a smaller sagittal diameter than the frontal one, which is the limiting factor when selecting the diameter and length of the ETT.[11] The ratio between the right and left bronchus to the trachea is 0.86 and 0.66, respectively.[11] It should be noted that the right bronchus origin is <1 cm from the carina, which can greatly complicate lung blockade on some occasions. The left mainstem bronchus is significantly smaller than the right one.[9]

Published tables with tracheal and main bronchial diameters relative to age can help select the appropriate ETT and FOB **(Fig. 1)**[9,11] and the lung isolation device depending on their external diameter. However, if available, referring to the patient's radiological images is always recommended to ensure material selection according to the patient's dimensions.

In addition to the study of the patient's airway, a preoperative echocardiogram should be performed due to the high association of congenital heart diseases, such as tracheoesophageal fistula and some congenital thoracic malformations, or due to cardiac dysfunction that other pathologies, like mediastinal masses, may cause.[7] The coexistence of cardiac involvement should be anticipated to tailor the anesthetic plan as it increases the risk of complications.

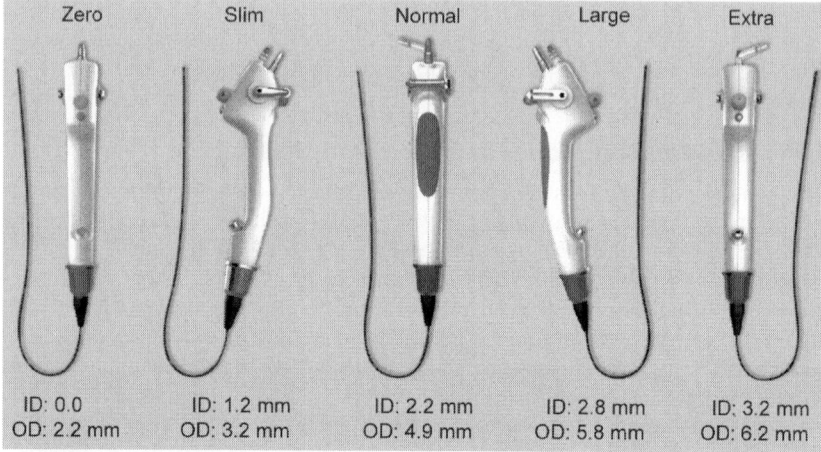

| Model | Zero | SLIM | IP | Normal | Large | Extra |
|---|---|---|---|---|---|---|
| Outside diameter mm | 2.2 | 3.2 | 4.0 | 4.9 | 5.8 | 6.2 |
| Working channel mm | 0.0 | 1.2 | 2.0 | 2.2 | 2.8 | 3.2 |

**Fig. 1:** Pediatric flexible fiberoptic bronchoscopes sizes.
*Courtesy:* Vathin (Hunan Vathin Medical Instrument Co).

Unlike adult patients, where preoperative pulmonary function assessment is essential, these tests have yet to show utility in pediatric patients due to the difficulties in performing them in younger children. They can help predict outcomes in patients with muscular dystrophy or undergoing spinal surgery. Still, in most pediatric populations, pulmonary function will be standard in the medium and long term.[7]

### Selection of the Lung Isolation Technique and Device

To select the lung isolation technique, it is necessary to have a good understanding of the internal diameters (ID) of the ETTs, the outer diameter (OD) of the selected airway devices, and the OD of the FOB required for the technique.[7,8] This is because it is essential not only to ensure smooth passage of the FOB inside the ETT but also to maintain adequate patient ventilation. Refer to **Box 2** for further details.

Fortunately, pediatric FOBs with a diameter of 2 mm are available, although these do not have an internal suction channel or oxygen delivery capability **(Fig. 1)**.

As previously mentioned, it is advisable to review the measurements of the tracheobronchial tree[11] and the patient's CT scan to select the appropriate FBC, ETT, and bronchial blocker (BB). Additionally, it is essential to review the ID of the ET tubes, as slight variations may exist among different manufacturers. It should be noted that cuffed tubes have approximately an additional 0.5 mm OD.[11]

**BOX 2:** Endotracheal tube and bronchoscope diameter relation.

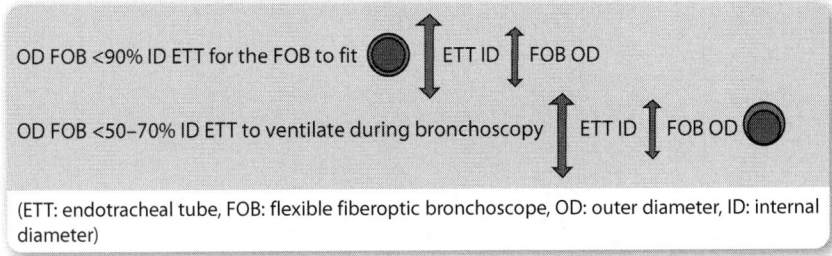

(ETT: endotracheal tube, FOB: flexible fiberoptic bronchoscope, OD: outer diameter, ID: internal diameter)

Considering anatomical limitations and available devices, there are three different techniques for pulmonary blockade depending on the device used: Single lumen ETT, BB, and double lumen tube (DLT).

1. *Single lumen endotracheal tube intubation*

    This is the simplest method to intubate a mainstem bronchus using a conventional single-lumen ETT. This technique is often employed in more minor patients, such as neonates and infants, due to the lack of appropriately sized BBs or DLTs for their small tracheobronchial tree, although in some centers, it is performed up to the age of 5 years.[9] The technique involves advancing the ETT unquestioningly to selectively intubate one of the bronchi, confirming its position with the FOB, and by the absence of breath sounds in the contralateral operative lung.[7]

    This approach has risks and challenges. If a cuffed ETT is used, it must be ensured that the cuff is entirely within the bronchus, so the length from the tip of the tube to the end of the cuff should be shorter than the length of the bronchus.[11] The diameter of the left mainstem bronchus is smaller than that of the right. The median diameter of the left mainstem bronchus in infants under 3 months is 3.9 mm [interquartile range (IQR) 3.7–4.1], which is relevant when choosing the ETT for selective intubation, as the OD of an uncuffed 3.0 ETT can be >4 mm, which may cause bronchial injury or may not be advanced to achieve lung isolation.[9] When intubating the short right mainstem bronchus, whose takeoff is often <1 cm from the carina, it is possible to block the upper lobe bronchus, excluding it from ventilation. This can also occur with the left upper lobe if the tube is advanced too deeply or if the ETT is rotated such that Murphy's eye is opposite to the takeoff of the left upper lobe bronchus, so in both cases, proper placement should be verified with FOB and auscultation, or point-of-care ultrasonography or fluoroscopy if the others are not available or conclusive. Regardless of whether intubation of the right or left mainstem bronchus is planned, the authors recommend using an ETT one size smaller than what would be chosen based on the patient's age and the use of cuffed ETTs whenever possible to allow for a good seal without needing to advance the ETT excessively into the bronchus.[7]

    Other disadvantages of this technique often include incomplete sealing of the bronchus when uncuffed tubes are used and the inability to aspirate or apply $O_2$ to the isolated lung.[7,11]

2. *Bronchial blocker*

    The BB is an airway device consisting of a balloon-tipped catheter whose positioning is facilitated using a FOB or guidance under fluoroscopy and rigid

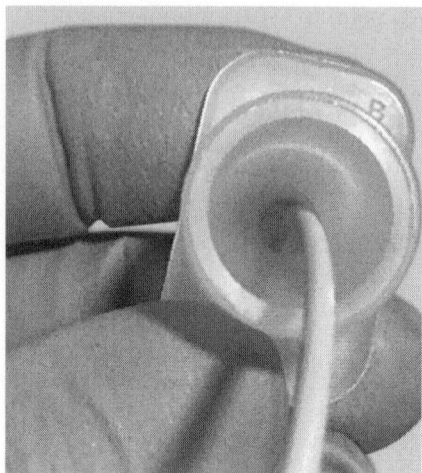

**Fig. 2:** In an intraluminal approach, bronchial blocker (BB) outer diameter and endotracheal tube (ETT) internal diameter relation is <50%.

bronchoscopy.[7] From the age of 6 months, when this technique is more feasible, the use of BB is preferred.[7] The use of BB achieves better sealing and operating conditions than bronchial intubation, as the lung isolation is more predictable.

The technique of placing the tipped balloon catheter will depend on the relationship between the diameters of the ETT and the BB, depending on whether the BB OD is 50% of the ETT ID or not, to allow for proper patient ventilation with the BB. This relationship will determine the position of the BB relative to the ETT, such that if the diameter ratio is <50%, an intraluminal or coaxial approach will be used. If not, an extraluminal approach with the BB parallel to the ETT will be required **(Fig. 2)**.[7]

In addition to the diameter of the BB, the FOB OD must be considered, which will guide the BB position. So, if an intraluminal approach is decided, the sum of the OD of the FOB and BB should be <50% of the ETT ID for correct patient ventilation during BB placement **(Fig. 3)**. If the ETT ID is too small, an extraluminal approach should be chosen **(Fig. 4)**.

Generally, an extraluminal approach with a 4 or 5 Fr BB should be used in children under 2 years of age. Between 3 and 4 years of age, an intraluminal approach with a 5 Fr BB or extraluminal 7 Fr BB may be utilized, although the former often requires overinflation of the balloon, which is not without risks such as mucosal injury or positional instability.[9] For children ≥8 years old, 7-9 Fr BBs can be used intra or extraluminal.

- Extraluminal approach technique

  This can be performed in two different ways:
  1. Some groups temporarily intubate the desired mainstem bronchus with an uncuffed ETT to guide the blocker placement. Afterward, the ETT is withdrawn, and a second ETT (preferably cuffed) is inserted parallel to the blocker. FOB confirms the optimal position of the blocker.[9,12]
  2. The authors perform the insertion of the BB at the time of the patient's permanent intubation. The BB is positioned posterior to the glottis to

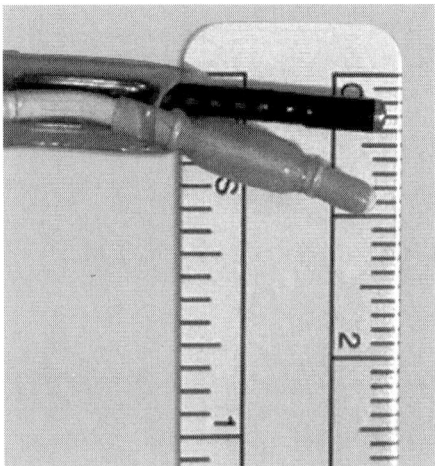

**Fig. 3:** Bronchial blocker (BB) and fiberoptic bronchoscope (FOB) inside the endotracheal tube (ETT).

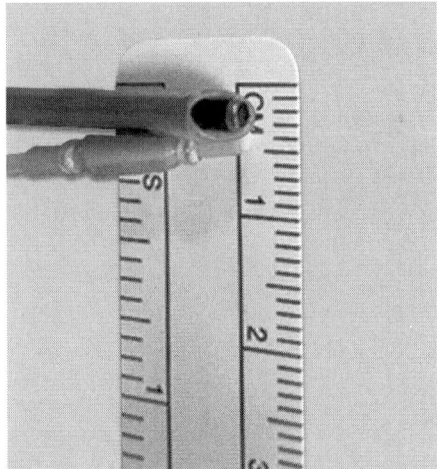

**Fig. 4:** Fiberoptic bronchoscope (FOB) inside endotracheal tube (ETT) and extraluminal bronchial blocker (BB).

minimize glottic and vocal cord injury, and the patient is intubated by placing the ETT in the anterior glottic area. Once intubated and the ETT secured, the FOB is inserted through the ETT, and without fully inflating the ETT cuff to allow for BB mobilization, the BB is advanced guided by FOB visualization until positioned in the selected bronchus. This technique may be challenging to block the left mainstem bronchus due to its natural tendency to pass toward the right mainstem bronchus. The balloon is inflated while maintaining visualization to ensure it does not herniate outward (which promotes mispositioning) and does not block

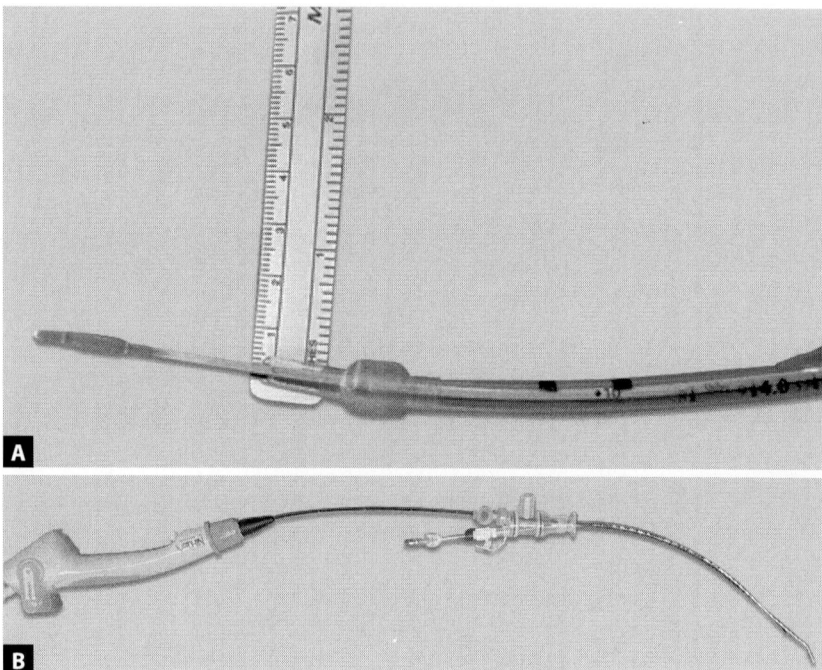

**Figs. 5A and B:** (A) Intraluminal bronchial blocker (BB) insertion before fiberoptic bronchoscope (FOB) insertion. (B) Intraluminal insertion. Note the length of the multiport adaptor that extends the blocker intraluminal path.

the upper lobe. Sometimes, the balloon is not adequate to fully seal, necessitating overinflation, although this increases the risk of blocker displacement.[9]

- Intraluminal approach technique

The BB insertion is directly through the ETT, allowing better tracheal sealing. To select this technique, it must be ensured that the sum of the BB OD and FOB OD is <50–70% of the ETT ID, to allow for adequate ventilation and avoid hypoxemia. Sometimes, it is necessary to introduce the BB first through the supplied multiport adaptor, which has a smaller distal diameter, leaving the balloon in the distal position and subsequently sliding the FOB because the balloon and the FOB cannot fit simultaneously **(Figs. 5A and B)**. If this is not known beforehand, it can pose a problem and delay the execution of the technique and ventilation since sometimes it is necessary to use another larger-sized ETT adaptor. This must be planned before the patient arrives in the operating room. On the other hand, the length of the multiport adaptor must be considered because it can excessively extend the intraluminal route, causing the BB to be short and requiring trimming of the ETT to reduce its path **(Fig. 6)** or switching to the extraluminal approach.

In any chosen approach, all components, including the interior of the ETT, FOB, and BB, should be lubricated to facilitate smooth insertion and movements. All technique steps should be verified in both approaches, and

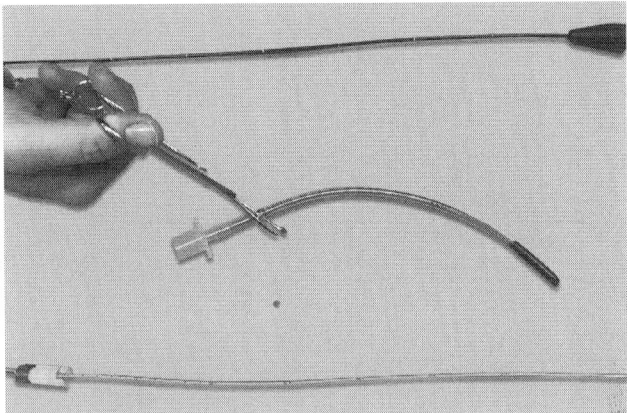

**Fig. 6:** Shortening of the endotracheal tube (ETT). The adaptor is reconnected to the shorter ETT.

necessary connections should be checked before the patient arrives in the operating room. Additionally, prebriefing with assisting staff is advisable to avoid unnecessary delays in unforeseen circumstances that may lead to hypoxemia. It should be ensured that both the FOB and BB slide smoothly in the ETT and that all the accessories needed to facilitate ventilation during the procedure are available.

One of the most common reasons for improper BB placement is poor bronchoscopic visualization due to bronchial secretions or serosanguinous debris in the airway. In these cases, fluoroscopy can help guide BB placement, and there are emerging reports on point-of-care ultrasound imaging to confirm lung isolation.[7]

Regardless of the chosen technique for OLV, it is essential to confirm lung isolation at different steps, before and after placing the patient in the lateral decubitus position or any movement that may suggest loss of lung isolation or malposition of the airway device. Balloon migration during the surgical procedure is common in small patients, either due to surgical manipulations or changes in patient position. If this occurs, it must be confirmed and repositioned under FOB or fluoroscopy guidance. Sometimes, repositioning the balloon is difficult due to the small size of the airway, poor visualization caused by blood or secretions in the airway, or patient positioning. The balloon may migrate proximally into the distal trachea, completely occluding the airway and causing sudden hypoxemia and reduced end-tidal $CO_2$. In this case, the surgeon must be immediately notified to deflate the balloon and reposition it under FOB guidance, resulting in loss of isolation and may briefly pause the surgery. In other cases, the BB may migrate distally, causing loss of isolation in the upper lobe, which is more common in young children on the right side due to the bronchus's close takeoff from the carina **(Fig. 7)**, where minimal movements can result in loss of isolation. Sometimes, overinflating the balloon is necessary, and in all cases, BB movements should be guided by FOB. During repositioning, there may not be sufficient visualization with

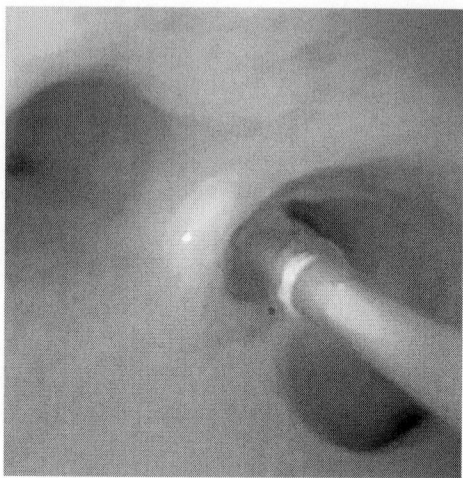

**Fig. 7:** Fiberoptic bronchoscope (FOB) view of the right upper lobe takeoff, very close to the carina, to place the bronchial blocker (BB) balloon correctly before inflating it.

the FOB (due to secretions and blood), or the patient may have less reserve and desaturate during bronchoscopy, requiring blind advancement of the BB with a low success rate, leading again to fluoroscopy for successful BB repositioning.[9]

The initial pulmonary blockades were performed with Fogarty® embolectomy catheters, and other off-label devices are used for lung isolation, such as the Miller® atrioseptostomy catheter (Edward Lifesciences) and pulmonary artery catheters.[7] These devices have low-volume, high-pressure balloons that can injure or even rupture the tracheal mucosa. Additionally, they have the disadvantage of not having an internal channel to permit applying continuous positive airway pressure (CPAP) or aspiration of the isolated lung if necessary. These catheters can be placed with or without bronchoscopic guidance, but the position needs to be confirmed with FOB[11], and their placement can also be extraluminal, as with the Fogarty® sizes 3 or 4F.[12]

Different endobronchial blockers are equipped with low-volume (maximum 3 mL) and low-pressure balloons, with sizes that can be used in pediatric patients. The Arndt Endobronchial Blocker® (Cook Medical, Bloomington) and the Uniblocker™ (Fuji Systems Corporation), which can be used in younger children, and the Univent™ Tube (Fuji Systems Corporation) for older children. The sizes of the Arndt® and Uniblocker™ blockers are 4, 5, 7, and 9 F, allowing for lung isolation in almost all pediatric age groups with different approaches. These blockers are preferable to embolectomy catheters because they have an integrated channel for applying CPAP. Still, the channel dimensions are not sufficient to suck secretions, as can be done when using DLT.[2]

- The Arndt Endobronchial Blocker® is a balloon-tipped blocker with a wire inside an inner lumen and a looped end to insert the FOB to guide its position

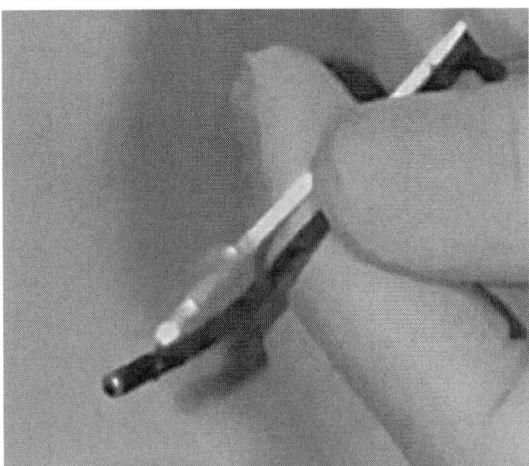

**Fig. 8:** The Ardnt® blocker has a loop attached to the fiberoptic bronchoscope (FOB) for guidance.

into the desired mainstem bronchus **(Fig. 8)**. When the balloon is placed, the wire can be removed to allow suctioning and CPAP application. Balloon dislodgement is a problem due to the difficulty of replacing the wire, which makes its repositioning almost impossible.[13]

- The Uniblocker™ or French Fuji has a rigid axis and an angled tip, facilitating manipulation. If the balloon migrates, it is easy to reposition **(Figs. 9A and B)**.[14] Both the Arndt Endobronchial Blocker® and the Uniblocker™ have a multiport adaptor that allows the introduction of an FOB through one port, the BB through a second port, and the attachment of the ETT to the ventilator through a third port, enabling ventilation during the blocker's placement **(Fig. 10)**.

- The Univent Tube™ is an ETT with a second lumen containing a BB. This BB is a small tube with a low-pressure balloon, and its displacement is less frequent than other BBs. However, the smallest available size has an ID of 3.5, corresponding to an OD of 7.5–8.0 mm.[11]

- The EZ-Blocker™ is a BB with a 7 Fr shaft. Two separate occlusive balloons come off this shaft in a "Y" configuration designed to rest on the carina. There are no EZ-Blockers for smaller patients, and little information is available about its use in children.[15]

The balloons have low pressure and volume, but bronchial mucosal injury can occur due to overdistension or airway rupture. Therefore, bronchoscopic visualization should always be maintained during positioning and manipulation.[12]

3. *Double lumen tube*

    No DLTs smaller than 26F are available, so these tubes are usually used from 8 to 10 years old, with an OD of 9.1 mm, corresponding to a 6.5 cuffed ETT. This diameter is adequate for children ≥8 years old, but it may be too long for some 8–10-year-olds. Radiological images should be reviewed to avoid potential bronchial injuries or faulty isolation.[9] The recommended sizes in children are

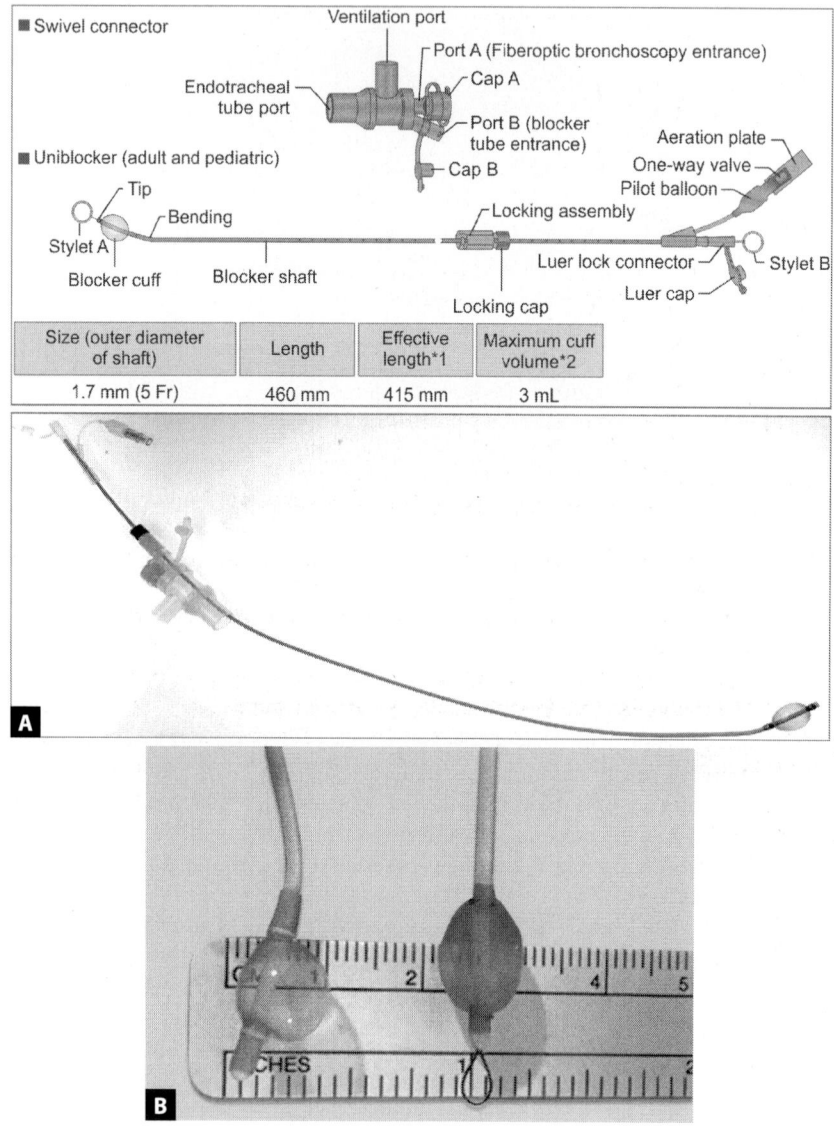

**Figs. 9A and B:** Scheme of Uniblocker™ with specifications (above) and a photo of Uniblocker™ with multiport adaptor (below). With permission of authors.[14] (B) Arndt® and Uniblocker™ 5 Fr balloons. The Uniblocker™ has an angled tip.

based on average values for airway dimensions,[11] and generally, 26–28 Fr DLTs can be used for children aged 10–12 years and 32 Fr DLTs for those aged 12–14 years. Suppose a smaller size than appropriate is chosen. In that case, the DLT tends to migrate distally into the main stem bronchus and will require overinflating the bronchial cuff, which can injure the bronchial mucosa. Differences between boys and girls after puberty should also be considered. Currently, it is recommended

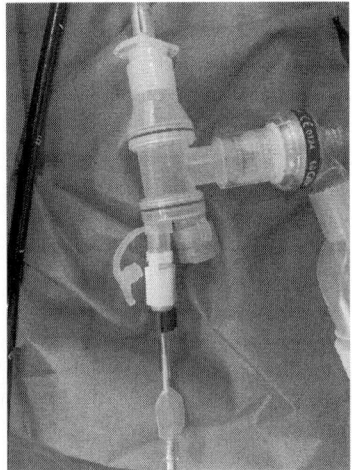

**Fig. 10:** Uniblocker™ multiport adaptor.

for girls with a height <160 cm to use a 35 Fr DLT and 37 Fr for girls >160 cm, 39 Fr for boys <170 cm, and 41 Fr if they are >170 cm tall.[9]

A specially designed DLT, Mararo®, is available for neonates and infants but is not widely available.[12]

The insertion technique is the same as in adults, although the equivalence between the depth of insertion of the DLT and the patient's size is not proportional to the patient's size as in adults. Right DLTs are more challenging to position accurately and have a higher risk of right upper lobe obstruction. Proper DLT placement must be confirmed with FOB visualization. Like other lung isolation techniques, checking the material and compatibility with the FOB and the patient's tracheobronchial tree measurements is advisable before anesthetic induction.

The DLTs provide some advantages over BBs, such as rapid switching between one and two-lung ventilation, allowing positive pressure ventilation to either or both lungs, the possibility of applying CPAP to the blocked lung, the ability to suction both lungs, and protection against contamination of the contralateral lung.[7,11]

The decision tree on the device to be used for lung ventilation in children is shown in **Figure 11**.

## Physiology of One-lung Ventilation

One-lung ventilation involves changes in ventilation and perfusion generated by increased ventilation in the dependent lung and the absence of ventilation in the nondependent lung, leading to atelectasis. Initially, perfusion is maintained in both lungs, resulting in an arteriovenous shunt in the nondependent lung, which, combined with ventilation–perfusion (V/Q) mismatch, causes alveolar hypoxia, reducing the partial pressure of $O_2$ by half within 20–30 minutes.[8] This situation induces vasoconstriction in the nonventilated lung, redirecting blood flow to the ventilated lung (the dependent lung) and improving V/Q matching, a phenomenon known as hypoxic pulmonary vasoconstriction (HPV). Vasoconstriction of hypoxic

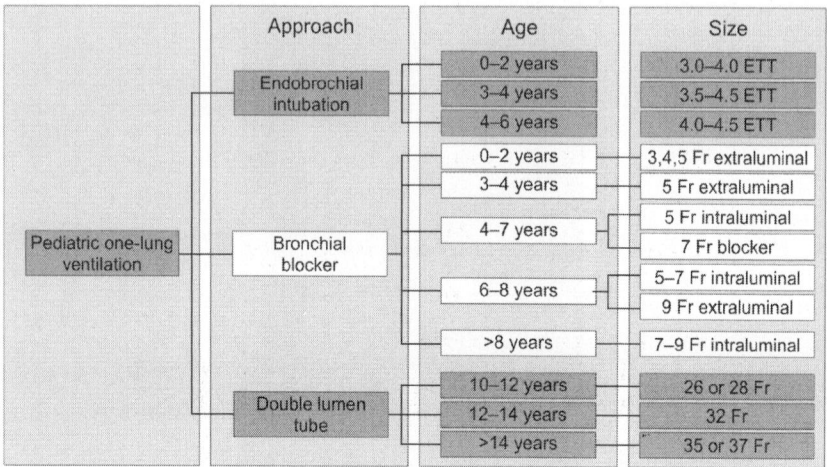

**Fig. 11:** One-lung ventilation decision tree[2,9] (ETT: endotracheal tube, cuffed or uncuffed)

regions occurs due to alveolar hypoxia when $PaO_2$ is <100 mm Hg and is proportional to the level of hypoxemia. The onset of HPV occurs when the alveolar oxygen pressure ($PAO_2$) is 20-40 mm Hg. HPV onset is biphasic. HPV occurs within minutes of initiating OLV, followed by a late phase (which can last hours). The reverse process of restoring perfusion returns to normal when hypoxemia resolves, also following a biphasic pattern, which may take several hours to reestablish normal perfusion.

Despite HPV, there are multiple factors in neonates and infants (<12 months old) that predispose them to hypoxemia:[2,7,9]

- The mostly cartilaginous rib cage is unable to prevent compression of the dependent lung from positioning, in addition to compression of the abdominal contents. This results in a lower functional residual capacity (FRC) close to or below residual volume, predisposing to airway closure in the dependent lung.
- The smaller hydrostatic pressure gradient in proportion to body size in more minor patients does not improve V/Q mismatch as it does in older patients.
- Neonates, infants, and young children have increased oxygen consumption.

Patients with chronic lung disease of the lung to be operated on typically tolerate single-lung ventilation is better than patients with healthy lungs. This is because perfusion in the chronically diseased lung is decreased in these patients, preferentially perfusing the healthy lung. When OLV begins, the intrapulmonary shunt fraction is lower; hence, the initial hypoxemic response is diminished.

The HPV decreases shunt, improving arterial oxygenation, although other factors such as blood pH and alveolar $CO_2$ pressure can reduce or increase the vasoconstrictor response. Situations of acidosis and/or hypercapnia enhance pulmonary vasoconstriction, while alkalosis and/or hypocapnia produce the opposite effect **(Box 3)**. Other factors such as hypothermia also decrease HPV, and inhalational anesthetics at concentrations greater than 1 MAC inhibit HPV, unlike intravenous agents such as Propofol, which do not have such inhibitory effects.[8]

Proper lung ventilation technique prevents volutrauma, barotrauma, or atelectrauma, so it is essential to manage different ventilatory modes and tailor them

> **BOX 3:** Anesthetic factors modifying or influencing hypoxic pulmonary vasoconstriction (HPV).
>
> *Promote HPV:*
> - Metabolic/respiratory acidosis
> - Hypercapnia
> - Hyperthermia
> - Moderate decrease in mixed venous oxygenation
>
> *Decrease HPV:*
> - Metabolic or respiratory alkalosis
> - Hypocapnia
> - Hypothermia
> - Hemodilution
> - Elevated left atrial pressure
> - Administration of volatile inhalational agents at doses >1 minimum alveolar concentration (MAC)

to the patient undergoing OLV. There is a high risk of atelectasis in smaller patients. Time constants differ substantially from those in adults: children under 3 years of age generally have small volumes and maintain their minute volume through high respiratory frequencies, so lung filling and emptying times are faster and shorter, approaching 1:1.2 inspiratory-expiratory time (I:E) ratios compared to the 1:2 ratios in adults. Not modifying the I:E ratio in a neonate could favor the tendency to collapse, as it is during expiration that the newborn has the risk window for collapse and atelectasis to occur.

During OLV in smaller patients, one must be prepared for a high risk of hypercapnia. However, it appears to be well tolerated in most children and returns to baseline levels quickly upon returning to two-lung ventilation.[16,17]

During OLV, there is a decrease in compliance, particularly in older pediatric patients.[17]

In some cases, especially in smaller patients, achieving a tidal volume over 4–5 mL/kg may not be possible, even at high inspiratory peak pressures. Generally, it is preferable to maintain tidal volumes between 4 and 7 mL/kg in smaller patients, with at least 4 cmH$_2$O of PEEP and inspiratory pressures between 21 and 24 cmH$_2$O.[9] Lee et al. found that using 4 mL/kg tidal volumes with 6 cmH$_2$O of PEEP reduced the risk of postoperative complications compared to ventilation with 8 mL/kg.[18] Infants, especially neonates, are always managed with auto-PEEP of 2–3 cmH$_2$O to compensate intrinsically for their tendency to collapse (usually caused by glottic closure before exhalation is complete), and the optimal PEEP for each patient should be calculated and individualized.

Hypoxemia, even with patients ventilated with a fraction of inspired oxygen (FiO$_2$) = 1, is expected during OLV.[9,18] Templeton et al., in a multicenter study in children under OLV, reported that 26% of patients had hypoxemia [Peripheral oxygen saturation (SpO$_2$) <90%], and it persisted for >5 minutes in 18%. The association of using high FiO$_2$ levels with tissue oxidative damage and pulmonary complications is well known. Still, it must be balanced with the risk of hypoxemia when deciding what FiO$_2$ to reach. In a retrospective study in young children undergoing OLV with different lung isolation techniques, tidal volumes <6 mL/kg were not associated with a higher rate of hypoxemia, and the FiO$_2$ needed ranged from 0.72 to 0.8 in patients with left lung isolation and from 0.8 to 0.96 in those with right lung isolation.[19] In procedures where there is a need for sequential bilateral isolation, patients experience more hypoxemia during the isolation of the second lung. If adequate oxygenation cannot be maintained during OLV, there are several diagnostic and interventional steps recommended.[7]

## Sequence of Diagnosis and Treatment of Hypoxemia During One-lung Ventilation

- Verify proper lung isolation. Lung ventilation strategies. Avoid factors that decrease HPV.
- If hypoxemia during OLV ($SpO_2$ <90% or $PaO_2$ <60 mm Hg)

Immediate interventions
- Administer 100% $O_2$. Increase $FiO_2$ as necessary to maintain $SpO_2$ ≥92%.
- Assess ETT or BB position by auscultating respiratory sounds or through FOB, which should be available throughout the procedure. If device migration has occurred, it should be repositioned and verified after each change in patient positioning.
- Perform lung recruitment maneuvers to the dependent lung and search for optimal PEEP in the lung. Remember that excessively generous PEEP could redistribute flow to the nonventilated lung, generating more shunt.
- If using a double-lumen tube or BB with a working channel, suction the tube softly to ensure no secretions obstruct.

If there is improvement but not enough
- Apply CPAP to the nondependent lung. A CPAP level between 5 and 10 mm Hg generally, does not interfere with surgical conditions and will help reduce the shunt fraction. If a BB with a working channel is available, transient jet ventilation techniques can also be implemented.
- Consider passive oxygen insufflation in the nondependent lung.
- Consider high-frequency ventilation.

No improvement, evidence of end-organ ischemia.
- In cases of pneumonectomy, clamp the pulmonary artery as soon as possible to reduce the shunt effect.
- Return to two-lung ventilation and inform the surgeon.
- Consider extracorporeal membrane oxygenation (ECMO) if all mentioned alternatives fail and surgery needs to continue.

## ■ ANALGESIC TECHNIQUES FOR THORACIC SURGERY

Like in adults, regional techniques reduce intraoperative opioid consumption and lower the incidence of pulmonary complications and the endocrine stress response, allowing for reasonable postoperative pain control.[2] In younger ages, regional anesthesia helps decrease the neurotoxic risk of general anesthetics.

Common regional blocks in the pediatric population include intercostal, paravertebral, erector spinae plane block (ESPB), and epidural blocks. The technique selection usually depends on the anesthesiologist's experience, patient factors, and the type of surgery. An essential difference from the adult population is that these blocks are typically performed with the patient under general anesthesia, requiring significant expertise to avoid severe complications in pediatric patients. Ultrasound has shown increased efficacy in block placement, as there is more incredible technical difficulty in children due to the short skin-epidural distance, very narrow space, and softer ligamentum flavum.[2] Thoracic epidural analgesia is adequate for treating postoperative pain in thoracic surgery, preventing atelectasis, and improving pulmonary function. It is considered the gold standard for post-thoracotomy pain relief, although it is not without risks.[20] The widespread use of ultrasound for regional anesthesia has increased the preference for a paravertebral block for intra- and postoperative analgesia, presenting the advantage over an epidural block of lower risk, as the puncture site is farther from the neuroaxis. The thoracic ESPB has gained popularity in recent years due to the simplicity of the technique and the possibility of introducing a catheter for postoperative pain control. However, controversy exists regarding its utility for postoperative pain.[20,21]

Preferred local anesthetics are those with lower toxicity, such as ropivacaine and levobupivacaine. Infants under 3 months have a higher risk of toxicity due to the greater volume of distribution and risk of accumulation in infusions, in addition to the immaturity of organ function and metabolism. Ropivacaine is considered safe in infants under 3 months, with a maximum dose of 0.2 mg/kg/h (between 0.1 and 0.2) in continuous epidural infusion. Paravertebral analgesia requires higher doses compared to epidural analgesia, with a recommended dose of 0.2 mg/kg/h.[2]

For patients with chest deformities undergoing surgery, epidural, and paravertebral analgesia reduces postoperative pain, although cryotherapy has gained prominence in recent years.[8]

## ■ CONCLUSION

Pediatric thoracic anesthesia necessitates meticulous preoperative planning and specialized equipment selection to ensure optimal patient outcomes.

Managing OLV in pediatric thoracic surgery demands careful consideration of multiple factors, including patient age, size, airway anatomy, and surgical requirements. The different techniques for lung isolation have their merits and limitations, with the choice often dependent on individual patient characteristics (age and airway dimensions), the devices available, and procedural considerations.

Performing OLV in pediatric patients is challenging due to the risk of hypoxemia and hypercapnia, which must be carefully managed to minimize adverse outcomes. Strategies such as lung recruitment maneuvers, optimal PEEP settings, and judicious use of oxygen supplementation play crucial roles in maintaining adequate oxygenation and ventilation during OLV.

Regional anesthesia offers advantages by reducing the risk of toxicity and allowing effective pain control in the perioperative period, but mastering the techniques in pediatric patients is essential.

## ■ REFERENCES

1. Hammer GB. Pediatric thoracic anesthesia. Anesthesiol Clin North Am. 2002;20(1):153-80.
2. Semmelmann A, Kaltofen H, Loop T. Anesthesia of thoracic surgery in children. Paediatr Anaesth. 2018;28(4):326-31.
3. Garcia-Fernandez J, Castro L, Belda FJ. Ventilating the newborn and child. Curr Anaesth Crit Care. 2010;21(5-6):262-8.
4. Tusman G, Böhm SH, Tempra A, Melkun F, García E, Turchetto E, et al. Effects of recruitment maneuver on atelectasis in anesthetized children. Anesthesiology. 2003;98(1):14-22.

5. Tusman G, Belda JF. Treatment of anesthesia-induced lung collapse with lung recruitment maneuvers. Curr Anaesth Crit Care. 2010;21(5-6):244-9.
6. García-Fernández J, Romero A, Blanco A, Gonzalez P, Abad-Gurumeta A, Bergese SD. Recruitment manoeuvres in anaesthesia: How many more excuses are there not to use them? Rev Esp Anestesiol Reanim. 2018;65(4):209-17.
7. Murray-Torres T, Winch P, Naguib A, Tobias J. Anesthesia for thoracic surgery in infants and children. Saudi J Anaesth. 2021;15(3):283.
8. Coutinho I, Cristiani F. Anestesia para cirugía torácica en pediatría. In: Cristiani Federico, Motta Pablo, (Eds). Anestesia Pediátrica, primera edicion. Montevideo, Uruguay: Bibliomedica ediciones; 2022. pp. 272-93.
9. Lazar A, Chatterjee D, Templeton TW. Error traps in pediatric one-lung ventilation. Paediatr Anaesth. 2022;32(2):346-53.
10. Letal M, Theam M. Paediatric lung isolation. BJA Educ. 2017;17(2):57-62.
11. Hammer GB, Fitzmaurice BG, Brodsky JB. Methods for single-lung ventilation in pediatric patients. Anesth Analg. 1999;89(6):1426-9.
12. Mohtar S, Hui TWC, Irwin MG. Anesthetic management of thoracoscopic resection of lung lesions in small children. Paediatr Anaesth. 2018;28(11):1035-42.
13. Mohammad S, Cameron S, Jain R, Griffin E, Matuszczak M. Modified technique for endobronchial blocker placement in pediatric patients undergoing thoracic surgery. Pediatric Anesthesia. 2023;33(9):768-70.
14. Fuertes Saez N, Escriba Alepuz F, Argente Navarro P. Selective bronchial block with Uniblocker™ in paediatric pulmonary sequestration. Trends in Anaesthesia and Critical Care. 2019;28:39-42.
15. Templeton TW, Templeton LB, Lawrence AE, Sieren LM, Downard MG, Ririe DG. An initial experience with an Extraluminal <scp>EZ</scp> -Blocker®: A new alternative for 1-lung ventilation in pediatric patients. Pediatric Anesthesia. 2018;28(4):347-51.
16. Templeton TW, Piccioni F, Chatterjee D. An Update on One-Lung Ventilation in Children. Anesth Analg. 2021;132(5):1389-99.
17. Hale JE, Meador MR, Mossad EB. Lung separation in children: Options and impact on gas exchange and lung compliance. Pediatric Anesthesia. 2019;29(9):915-9.
18. Lee JH, Bae JI, Jang YE, Kim EH, Kim HS, Kim JT. Lung protective ventilation during pulmonary resection in children: a prospective, single-centre, randomised controlled trial. Br J Anaesth. 2019;122(5):692-701.
19. Templeton TW, Miller SA, Lee LK, Kheterpal S, Mathis MR, Goenaga-Díaz EJ, et al. Hypoxemia in Young Children Undergoing One-lung Ventilation: A Retrospective Cohort Study. Anesthesiology. 2021;135(5):842-53.
20. Singh S, Andaleeb R, Lalin D. Can ultrasound-guided erector spinae plane block replace thoracic epidural analgesia for postoperative analgesia in pediatric patients undergoing thoracotomy? A prospective randomized controlled trial. Ann Card Anaesth. 2022;25(4):429-34.
21. Luo R, Tong X, Yan W, Liu H, Yang L, Zuo Y. Effects of erector spinae plane block on postoperative pain in children undergoing surgery: a systematic review and meta-analysis of randomized controlled trials. Paediatr Anaesth. 2021;31(10):1046-55.

## ■ RECOMMENDED READING

1. Templeton TW, Piccioni F, Chatterjee D. An Update on One-Lung Ventilation in Children. Anesth Analg. 2021;132(5):1389-99.
2. Ma M, Slinger PD. UpToDate. (2022). One lung ventilation: general principles. Available from: https://pro.uptodatefree.ir/Show/14945. [Last accessed July, 2024].
3. Ma M, Slinger PD. UpToDate. (2022). Lung isolation techniques. Available from: https://pro.uptodatefree.ir/Show/14944. [Last accessed July, 2024].

CHAPTER 9

# Analgesia in Thoracic Surgery

*Himani V Bhatt, John Choi, Ali N Shariat*

## ABSTRACT

Postoperative pain following cardiac and thoracic procedures is a significant concern due to its potential to cause prolonged intubation, increased myocardial oxygen consumption, hemodynamic instability, and long-term disability. Traditional pain management with opioids and neuraxial analgesia has limitations due to risks in anticoagulated patients and inadequate sensory coverage. Regional anesthesia, specifically fascial plane blocks such as the pectoralis (Pecs) I and II, serratus anterior plane (SAP), and erector spinae plane (ESP) blocks, has emerged as a promising alternative. These techniques offer effective pain relief while minimizing the risks of spinal hematoma and hemodynamic compromise. Incorporating these blocks into Enhanced Recovery After Surgery (ERAS) protocols can lead to improved patient outcomes, including reduced opioid consumption, earlier extubation, and shorter intensive care unit (ICU) stays. The ESP block has shown promise as a safe and effective option for pain management in cardiac and thoracic surgeries, especially in patients with anticoagulation requirements.

**Keywords:** Analgesia; Sternotomy; Regional

## KEY POINTS

- Pain from cardiothoracic surgeries and procedures is multifactorial and underappreciated.
- Traditional regional anesthesia techniques, such as neuraxial and paravertebral blocks, are effective but carry risks of spinal hematoma and hemodynamic compromise.
- Novel fascial plane blocks are relatively simple techniques with an excellent safety profile.
- Increasing evidence suggests that fascial plane blocks may provide a safe and reliable method to address pain following cardiothoracic surgery and procedures as part of a multimodal analgesic regimen.

## ■ INTRODUCTION

Multiple factors contribute to pain following cardiac and thoracic procedures, including the incision, chest tube drains, sternal/rib retraction, internal mammary artery harvesting, fascial plane dissection, and vascular catheters. In addition to acute incisional pain, pain related to nerve compression and sustained pressure can lead to a neuropathic pain component. Furthermore, the parietal and visceral pleura are particularly sensitive to this pressure and stretch-related stimuli.[1,2] When postoperative pain is poorly controlled, the resulting splinting can restrict breathing and the ability to cough,[3] leading to prolonged intubation and intensive care unit (ICU) length of stay.[4] Uncontrolled postoperative pain can also cause an increase in myocardial oxygen consumption and hemodynamic instability. Acute pain can also lead to long-term disability due to chronic pain and depression.[5] More importantly, these factors can lead to chronic pain syndromes for which continued opioid use is often required. The incidence of chronic pain after surgery can vary between 21 and 55%.[6] Chronic pain and prolonged hospital length of stay substantially increase healthcare expenditure.[2] Therefore, anesthesiologists have sought effective techniques such as regional anesthesia to mitigate acute postoperative pain after cardiothoracic procedures.

## NEURAXIAL TECHNIQUES IN CARDIAC AND THORACIC SURGERY

Neuraxial techniques have been used in thoracic surgery for many decades. In 1980, Matthews et al.[7] reported the use of intrathecal morphine (L3-4 or L4-5) in patients going for open heart surgery. 36 of 40 patients were extubated in the operating room, and all patients were pain-free through the first 27.5 hours postoperatively. No adverse events were reported, and the minimum interval between injection and heparinization for cardiopulmonary bypass was 50 minutes. In a further study, Chaney and colleagues randomized patients going for coronary artery bypass grafting (CABG) to receive either intrathecal morphine or placebo. Patients receiving intrathecal morphine had a significant decrease in postoperative opioid usage, but the stress response, measured by postoperative epinephrine levels, was unaffected.[8]

Thoracic epidural analgesia (TEA) for pain control can be an option for both cardiac and thoracic surgical patients. Liem and colleagues randomized patients going for CABG to receive either a TEA or no epidural. They found that those receiving an epidural were awake sooner, resumed spontaneous respirations earlier, and were extubated earlier than those who did not. Cardiac output was also significantly higher in the epidural group, and the incidence of tachycardia and MI was higher in the GA group.[9] In a large prospective study, over 1,000 patients going for cardiothoracic surgery were randomized to TEA placed at T1-4 or standard therapy with opioids. TEA was associated with lower 6-month mortality, lower frequency of postoperative dialysis, and lower frequency of myocardial infarction.[10]

Despite studies demonstrating benefits, TEA is not widely accepted in cardiac surgery. On the other hand, TEA is still considered the gold standard for pain management in thoracic surgeries. There are many well-known advantages to use an epidural for thoracic surgery, such as effective and reliable pain control, sympathetic blockage with an increase in myocardial oxygen supply and increased coronary blood flow, and early awakening, immobilization, and extubation secondary to superior pain control.

Despite these advantages, both cardiac and thoracic patients will always be at a higher risk for infection, nerve injury, and, more importantly, bleeding and hematoma. There are no case reports linking spinal hematoma to intraoperative heparinization with epidurals in the context of cardiothoracic surgery. Furthermore, the risk of spinal hematoma in these cases remains speculative. It has been estimated by Ho et al. that between 1:150,000 and 1:1,500 for epidural blockades and 1:220,000 to 1,600 for spinal blockades.[11] However, it can have devastating consequences, especially when other less risky options become available.

Ultrasound-guided regional anesthesia techniques have been critical to the successful management of postoperative pain in various settings.[12-14] Recently described fascial plane blocks, including Pecs I and II, serratus anterior plane block (SAPB), and erector spinae plane block (ESPB), may successfully treat postoperative cardiac pain while eliminating the risks of spinal hematoma and hemodynamic compromise due to sympathectomy.[15] The fascial plane blocks target nerves by depositing local anesthesia into intermuscular planes where the target nerves are located.[16]

These blocks can be incorporated into the Enhanced Recovery after Surgery (ERAS) protocol, designed to facilitate early recovery, reduce hospital length of stay, and improve patient outcomes and satisfaction after cardiothoracic surgery.[17,18]

## ■ CHEST WALL ANATOMY

Innervation of the chest wall consists of T1-T11 spinal nerves and T12 subcostal nerves. The anterior chest wall and sternum are supplied by the anterior divisions of the second to the sixth thoracic intercostal nerves (T2-6). The abdominal and thoracic walls are supplied by intercostal nerves 7-11. Initially, the intercostal nerves lie between the pleura and endothoracic fascia and then pierce the fascia to lie between the internal and innermost intercostal muscles. At the angle of the rib, they give rise to the terminal nerves—lateral anterior and collateral cutaneous branches. The lateral cutaneous branches pierce the intercostal and serratus anterior muscle complex to supply the skin and subcutaneous tissues over the anterolateral and posterolateral thorax. The anterior cutaneous branches continue in the intercostal groove and remain between the internal and innermost intercostal muscles. At the lateral border of the sternum, they pass through the internal intercostal membrane, external intercostal membrane, and pectoralis major to supply the anterior chest wall. The anterior cutaneous branches then divide into medial and lateral branches at the lateral border of the sternum, where they innervate the parasternal area and midline with significant crossover innervation from the contralateral side. Intercostal nerves also supply the parietal pleura, mammary gland, and periosteum of the ribs. Other nerves that supply the chest wall include supraclavicular nerves (C3-4) which are branches of the cervical plexus and provide sensation to the anterior-superior aspect of the thorax and the "cape" of the shoulder, the medial (C8-T1) and lateral (C5-7) pectoral nerves, the thoracodorsal nerve (C6-8) supplying the latissimus dorsi, and the long thoracic nerve (C5-7) which supplies the serratus anterior muscle.[19]

## ■ TECHNIQUES

Regional anesthesia techniques such as paravertebral block (PVB), deep and superficial parasternal intercostal fascial plane blocks, SAPB, and ESPB, have been used for postoperative analgesia in sternotomy and thoracotomy. Notably, these fascial plane blocks can easily cover the dermatomal distribution of the incision and port placement in thoracic procedures, such as video-assisted thoracoscopy (VATS), robotic VATS, and thoracotomy **(Fig. 1)**. The fascial plane blocks target nerves that are too small to visualize directly with ultrasound. These blocks require bulk volume

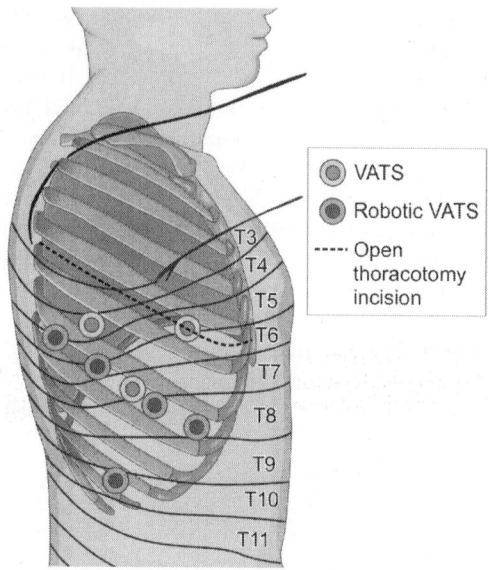

**Fig. 1:** Site of thoracotomy incision and port sites for video-assisted thoracic surgery (VATS) and robotic video-assisted thoracic surgery.
*Source:* Gregory J, @2024 Mount Sinai, Health System.

spread of local anesthesia within the targeted fascial plane. The extent of local anesthetic spread through these planes may vary considerably due to anatomical differences between patients, resulting in unpredictable sensory coverage.[20] Profound sensory blockade is also rare with fascial plane blocks instead of neuraxial and PVBs. Therefore, fascial plane blocks are utilized primarily as part of a multimodal analgesic regimen rather than as the primary anesthetic. Inadvertent intramuscular injection is also possible and may be avoided by observing "hydrolocation" or the sonographic appearance of the anechoic injectate, peeling the muscle from the adjacent bony structure or muscle **(Figs. 2A to C)**.[21]

## Paravertebral Block

The paravertebral blockade has a significantly lower risk of spinal hematoma than neuraxial anesthesia; however, American Society of Regional Anesthesia and Pain Medicine (ASRA) guidelines recommend that the same standards for neuraxial anesthesia be applied to deep plexus blocks.[22] Moreover, the unilateral nature of sensory coverage by a PVB is most useful for cardiac surgery utilizing a unilateral approach by anterior thoracotomy. The use of a unilateral paravertebral catheter is as effective as TEA at the T4–5 level for postoperative analgesia in patients undergoing minimally invasive direct coronary artery bypass surgery.[23] Procedures utilizing a midline sternotomy incision would require bilateral PVBs, which can result in local anesthetic systemic toxicity even when utilizing dosages under those commonly recommended.[24]

Gulbahar et al. randomized patients undergoing thoracotomy to receive either thoracic epidural block or PVB and found no difference in postoperative VAS pain

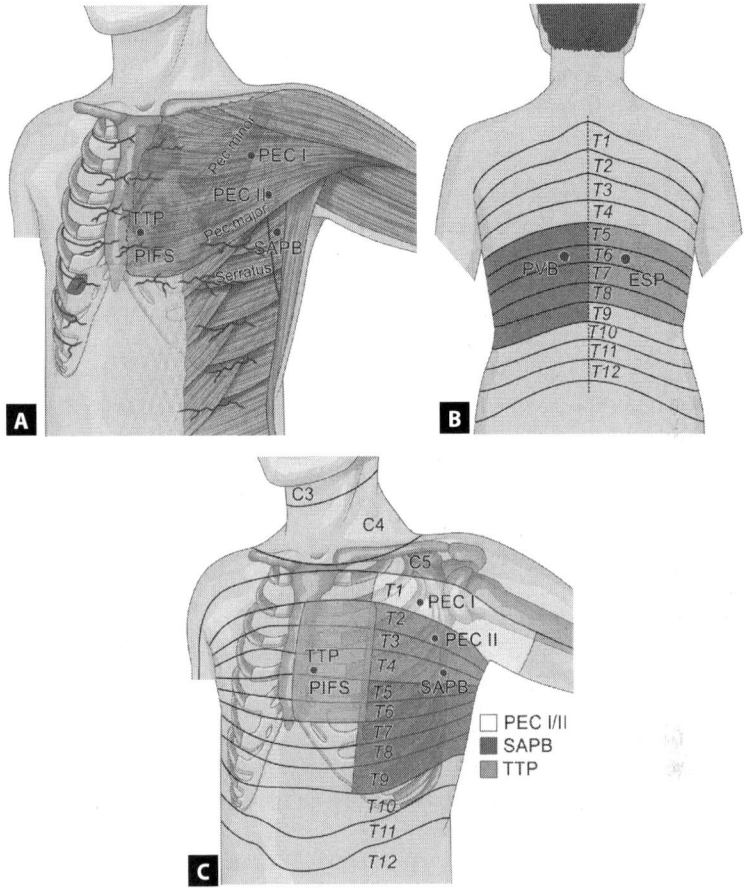

**Figs. 2A to C:** Dermatomal distribution of thoracic fascial plane blocks. (ESP: erector spinae plane; PEC: pectoral nerve block; PIFS: pectoral interfascial superficial block; PVB; paravertebral block; SAPB: serratus anterior plane block; TTP: transversus thoracic plane)

scores and morphine consumption on postoperative days 1-3.[25] In a significant meta-analysis, Yeung et al. found that PVB was comparable to thoracic epidural for analgesic efficacy in thoracic procedures and had a lower incidence of hypotension, nausea, vomiting, pruritus, and urinary retention.[26]

## Interpectoral (Pecs I) and Pectoserratus Nerve Blocks (Pecs II)

Pecs blocks provide analgesia to the pectoral, mammary, inframammary, and axillary regions and are commonly performed for procedures involving the anterior chest wall. In the Pecs I block, local anesthetic is injected between the pectoralis major and minor muscles to anesthetize the lateral (C5-7) and medial (C8-T1) pectoral nerves. These nerves provide innervation to the lateral and medial pectoral nerves. Some applications of the Pecs I block include the insertion of implantable defibrillators/pacemakers, anterior thoracotomies, and breast surgeries such as the insertion of breast expanders and submuscular prostheses.[27-29]

In Pecs II blocks, in addition to performing a Pecs I block, local anesthetic is injected between the pectoralis minor and serratus anterior muscles. It is utilized in procedures involving the anterior and lateral chest walls. This block is designed to open the "axillary corridor" to reach the lateral branches of the intercostal nerves from T2–T6, the intercostobrachial nerve (lateral cutaneous branch of T2), the long thoracic nerve, and the thoracodorsal nerve. Pecs II blocks are equivalent to PVBs for postoperative pain control and opioid consumption in patients undergoing VATS.[30]

Pecs blocks have successfully provided anesthesia for inserting a cardiac resynchronization therapy device (CRTD). Mavarez et al. reported the use of Pecs II block as the sole anesthetic for pacemaker insertion for a patient with severe aortic stenosis and sick sinus syndrome. The patient required no additional intraoperative and postoperative opioids for 24 hours or more.[31] Fujiwara et al. reported the use of Pecs I block supplemented with intercostal nerve block and dexmedetomidine for the implantation of a CRTD in an anticoagulated patient with New York Heart Association (NYHA) 4 congestive heart failure and <20% ejection fraction.[32] The same Pecs and intercostal nerve block combination has been utilized for automatic implantable cardioverter-defibrillator (AICD) insertion in children with Duchenne muscular dystrophy (DMD).[33] Children with DMD often have compromised cardiac and respiratory function with a potential risk of significant morbidity and mortality during the induction and maintenance of general anesthesia. Pecs blocks have been successfully used in supermorbidly obese patients with limited cardiac and respiratory reserve.[34] Pecs blocks helped maintain hemodynamic stability, limit opioid use, and avoid airway manipulation. Yalamuri et al. successfully utilized Pecs I and II blocks to provide analgesia in a chronic pain patient who underwent right anterior thoracotomy for minimally invasive mitral valve repair. To extend the benefits, the authors repeated the block with liposomal bupivacaine, which provided another 48 hours of pain relief and significantly improved pulmonary mechanics to facilitate weaning from oxygen.[4] Pecs blocks have the potential to be included as nonopioid analgesia to promote faster recovery from minimally invasive surgeries associated with significant post-thoracotomy pain. Kumar et al. performed a randomized controlled study comparing Pecs blocks versus control on patients undergoing CABG through midline sternotomy. Bilateral single injection Pecs I and II blocks were provided to one group of patients in the immediate postoperative period. Pecs blocks significantly improved pain scores for up to 24 hours and enhanced peak inspiratory flow in spirometry. Improved spirometry facilitates fast tracking and extubation; thus, patients with Pecs blocks require a significantly lesser duration of ventilator support (108.5 ± 24.34 minutes) in comparison to the control group (206.3 ± 47.05) with a $p$ <0.0001.[35]

In summary, Pecs blocks are safe and effective techniques used as part of a multimodal analgesic regimen in minimally invasive cardiac and thoracic procedures and, in exceptional cases, as a primary anesthetic for device implantation.

## Serratus Anterior Plane Block

The SAPB is a valuable technique for analgesia in patients undergoing thoracic surgery, particularly VATS. It involves the injection of local anesthetic, either superficial or deep, into the serratus anterior muscle to block the lateral cutaneous branches of the intercostal nerves from T2 to T9. This block offers technical simplicity and a minimal risk of complications.[36,37] Several studies have demonstrated its efficacy, where one study found that patients receiving SAPB had significantly lower postoperative pain scores and reduced opioid consumption compared to standard intravenous opioid therapy, with fewer incidences of postoperative nausea and vomiting (PONV).[38,39] When SAPB was compared to local anesthetic infiltration in patients going for thoracoscopic surgery, the use of SAPB resulted in lower opioid use and postoperative pain scores.[40,41] SAPB, when compared to TEA and other fascial plane blocks such as PVB,[42-46] is noninferior in treating postoperative pain following VATS and has fewer complications and higher patient satisfaction.[47] The advantages of SAPB include technical simplicity, minimal risk of complications such as pneumothorax or nerve injury, and adequate analgesia, reducing the need for opioids. However, the extent of local anesthetic spread can be unpredictable, and the duration of analgesia may be limited, necessitating additional doses or continuous infusion techniques. SAPB is an effective and safe regional anesthesia technique for managing postoperative pain following thoracic surgery, particularly VATS, enhancing patient outcomes and satisfaction.

## SUPERFICIAL AND DEEP PARASTERNAL INTERCOSTAL PLANE BLOCKS

The superficial and deep parasternal intercostal plane (SPIP and DPIP) blocks both target the anterior cutaneous branches of T2-6, which innervates the sternum and a small skin area over the sternum. This block is done with a single or multiple injection(s) performed at the parasternal border, and local anesthetic is injected between the pectoralis major and external intercostal muscle for SPIP block and the internal intercostal muscle and transversus thoracis muscle for the DPIP block. The SPIP block has gained more popularity due to its superficial approach and, therefore, less risk of injury to the internal mammary artery and lung pleura. Case reports are documented demonstrating the use of parasternal intercostal plane (PIP) blocks for rib pain and chest wall trauma as a pain management technique.[48] However, due to its coverage of the anterior cutaneous distribution, most of the literature on PIP blocks is for sternotomy-related pain versus thoracotomy-related pain.[5,49-54]

### Erector Spinae Plane Block

The erector spinae muscle spans the entire spine from the skull's base to the sacrum's medial crest. It comprises three muscles: (1) the spinalis, (2) longissimus thoracis, and (3) iliocostalis. The erector spinae plane (ESP) is a myofascial plane located deep and ventral to the ESM and posterior to the transverse processes.[55] Advantages include technical simplicity and a favorable safety profile.

The ESPB is most commonly performed in the thoracic region with the intent to block ventral and dorsal rami of spinal nerves T2-T9 with a sensory distribution from the posterior thoracic wall posteriorly to the midclavicular line anteriorly. ESPB may also block the rami communicantes that supply the sympathetic chain.[56] The local anesthetic may also variably diffuse anteriorly to the paravertebral spaces through the costotransverse foramina, the intertransverse complex, and laterally along the intercostal spaces, possibly providing visceral and somatic analgesia. For this reason, some researchers argue that the analgesic effects of ESPB are essentially due to the spread of local anesthetic into the paravertebral space and hence call the block "paravertebral by proxy".[57] This theory has been controversial, with further cadaveric studies challenging the notion that local anesthetic reliably enters the paravertebral space following the performance of ESPB.[58] Furthermore, a study involving healthy volunteers has shown a sensory distribution for the ESPB limited to the posterior thorax.[46] Nevertheless, evidence has accumulated on the ESPB's efficacy in various settings, including cardiac and thoracic procedures.

When patients going for thoracotomy were randomized to receive either single-shot ESPB or TPVB, both methods had similar postoperative opioid usage. However, patients who received ESPB had less hypotension and bradycardia.[59] In patients undergoing VATS, when ESPB was compared to SAPB, patients in the ESPB had a significantly longer time to request analgesic and lower dynamic pain scores than patients who received SAPB.[60] When patients going for minimally invasive thoracic surgery were randomized to receive either ESPB or SAPB, ESP provided superior quality of recovery at 24 hours, lower morbidity, and better analgesia.[61] ESPB was noninferior in the analgesic effect on the PVB for VATS regarding pain score, analgesic rescue consumption, and quality of recovery.[62] In a case series, ESPB was used to treat post-thoracotomy pain syndrome, resulting in excellent short-term and, in some cases, long-term improvement of symptoms.[55] ESPB was shown to be inferior to TEA for analgesia in patients following VATS. However, ESP had a better side-effect profile.[63]

The ESPB can be provided either as a single-shot block or a continuous infusion. Kelava et al. presented a successful case of continuous ESP catheters without the risk of sympathectomy-related hypotension and the risk of hematoma postanticoagulation for lung transplant patients.[64] Krishna et al. found that patients going for cardiac surgery via a midline sternotomy who received a single-shot ESPB had significantly lower pain scores and opioid consumption in the first 12 hours postextubation, were extubated earlier, and were discharged earlier from the ICU than those who did not receive a block.[65] Nagaraja et al. compared bilateral continuous ESPB with traditional TEA in patients undergoing cardiac surgery through sternotomy. Patients in the ESPB group had significantly less pain at 24, 36, and 48 hours. They were equivalent to the epidural group in terms of intraoperative fentanyl consumption, ventilator duration, and length of ICU stay. This study implies that the continuous ESPB technique is superior to the thoracic epidural technique due to its better safety profile in anticoagulated patients.[66] Macaire et al. compared the bilateral continuous ESPB technique at the T5 level in patients undergoing cardiac surgery through sternotomy to retrospective controls who did not receive a block and found that the ESPB required significantly fewer opioids, had a shortened time to extubation, earlier mobilization, and a decreased ICU length of stay.[67] Adhikary et al. reported an excellent safety margin when a unilateral continuous ESPB catheter was performed as rescue analgesia in a series of anticoagulated patients undergoing left ventricular assist device (LVAD) implantation through a thoracotomy incision.[68] Therefore, ESPB shows promise as a safe alternative to epidural and paravertebral analgesia in cardiac surgeries involving thoracotomy and midline sternotomy.

## ■ CLINICAL IMPLICATIONS

The utility of regional techniques and their incorporation into a multimodal analgesia regimen for thoracic procedures has become an essential facet of pain management. Also, the continued interest in the development and systemic implementation of evidence-based perioperative care protocols or ERAS models makes incorporating these techniques more useful. Multiple recent guidelines recommend incorporating fascial plane blocks within enhanced recovery care models. The 2019 ERAS guidelines for enhanced recovery after lung surgery recommend the use of regional anesthesia for opioid reduction with equivalent efficacy when compared to TEA with a high level of evidence.[69] In addition, the Society of Cardiovascular Anesthesiologists (SCA) 2023 practice advisory recommends using PVBs and fascial plane blocks alone or in combination as part of a multimodal pain regimen for acute pain management in patients undergoing thoracic surgery.[70]

The PROSPECT recommendations for post-thoracotomy analgesia recommend paravertebral and ESPB blocks as first-line analgesic methods and SAPB as second-line therapy. TEA, however, is not recommended despite its proven record of providing reliable analgesia due to its higher potential for severe complications during needle and catheter insertion, as well as the possibility of hypotension, urinary retention, and/or lower extremity weakness.[71]

## CONCLUSION

The management of postoperative pain following cardiac and thoracic surgery is critical for patient recovery, and regional anesthesia offers a promising alternative to traditional opioid-based pain management when added to a multimodal regimen. Regional anesthesia techniques, such as fascial plane blocks, are effective in reducing postoperative pain, opioid consumption, and ICU stay duration. When integrated into ERAS protocols, these techniques can lead to better patient outcomes, faster recovery, and higher satisfaction rates.

Incorporating these regional anesthesia techniques into multimodal analgesic regimens can significantly enhance pain management strategies in thoracic and cardiac surgery, offering patients a safer, more effective, and opioid-sparing approach to postoperative care. As the field of anesthesiology continues to evolve, adopting and refining these techniques will be crucial in improving the quality of care and patient outcomes in cardiothoracic surgery.

## REFERENCES

1. Mueller XM, Tinguely F, Tevaearai HT, Revelly JP, Chioléro R, Von Segesser LK. Pain location, distribution, and intensity after cardiac surgery. Chest. 2000;118(2):391-6.
2. Choinière M, Watt-Watson J, Victor JC, Baskett RJ, Bussières JS, Carrier M, et al. Prevalence of and risk factors for persistent postoperative nonanginal pain after cardiac surgery: A 2-year prospective multicentre study. Can Med Assoc J. 2014;186(7):E213-23.
3. Sasseron AB, Figueiredo LCD, Trova K, et al. A dor interfere na função respiratória após cirurgias cardíacas? Revista Brasileira de Cirurgia Cardiovascular. 2009;24(4):490-496.
4. Yalamuri S, Klinger RY, Bullock WM, Glower DD, Bottiger BA, Gadsden JC. Pectoral Fascial (PECS) I and II Blocks as Rescue Analgesia in a Patient Undergoing Minimally Invasive Cardiac Surgery. Reg Anesth Pain Med. 2017;42(6):764-6.
5. Liu SS, Wu CL. Effect of postoperative analgesia on major postoperative complications: a systematic update of the evidence. Anesth Analg. 2007;104(3):689-702.
6. Lahtinen P, Kokki H, Hynynen M. Pain after cardiac surgery: a prospective cohort study of 1-year incidence and intensity. Anesthesiology. 2006;105(4):794-800.
7. Mathews ET, Abrams LD. Intrathecal morphine in open heart surgery. Lancet. 1980;2(8193):543.

8. Chaney MA, Smith KR, Barclay JC, Slogoff S. Large-dose intrathecal morphine for coronary artery bypass grafting. Anesth Analg 1996;83(2):215-22.
9. Liem TH, Booij LH, Gielen MJ, Hasenbos MA, van Egmond J. Coronary artery bypass grafting using two different anesthetic techniques: Part 3: Adrenergic responses. J Cardiothorac Vasc Anesth. 1992;6(2):162-7.
10. Stenger M, Fabrin A, Schmidt H, Greisen J, Erik Mortensen P, Jakobsen CJ. High thoracic epidural analgesia as an adjunct to general anesthesia is associated with better outcome in low-to-moderate risk cardiac surgery patients. J Cardiothorac Vasc Anesth. 2013;27(6):1301-9.
11. Ho AM, Chung DC, Joynt GM. Neuraxial blockade and hematoma in cardiac surgery: Estimating the risk of a rare adverse event that has not (yet) occurred. Chest. 2000;117(2):551-5.
12. Smith LM, Barrington MJ. Ultrasound-guided blocks for cardiovascular surgery: Which block for which patient? Curr Opin Anaesthesiol. 2020;33(1):64-70.
13. Bignami E, Castella A, Pota V, Saglietti F, Scognamiglio A, Trumello C, et al. Perioperative pain management in cardiac surgery: a systematic review. Minerva Anestesiologica. 2018;84(4):488-503.
14. Bigeleisen PE, Goehner N. Novel approaches in pain management in cardiac surgery. Curr Opin Anaesthesiol. 2015;28(1):89-94.
15. Abu Elyazed MM, Mostafa SF, Abdelghany MS, Eid GM. Ultrasound-guided erector spinae plane block in patients undergoing open epigastric hernia repair: a prospective randomized controlled study. Anesth Analg. 2019;129(1):235-40.
16. Helander EM, Webb MP, Kendrick J, Montet T, Kaye AJ, Cornett EM, et al. PECS, serratus plane, erector spinae, and paravertebral blocks: a comprehensive review. Best Prac Res Clin Anaesthesiol. 2019;33(4):573-81.
17. Salenger R, Morton-Bailey V, Grant M, Gregory A, Williams JB, Engelman DT. Cardiac enhanced recovery after surgery: a guide to team building and successful implementation. Semin Thorac Cardiovasc Surg. 2020;32(2):187-96.
18. Noss C, Prusinkiewicz C, Nelson G, Patel PA, Augoustides JG, Gregory AJ. Enhanced recovery for cardiac surgery. J Cardiothor Vasc An. 2018;32(6):2760-70.
19. Loukas M, Hullett J, Louis RG, Holdman S, Holdman D. The gross anatomy of the extrathoracic course of the intercostobrachial nerve. Clin Anat. 2006;19(2):106-11.
20. Dautzenberg KHW, Zegers MJ, Bleeker CP, Tan ECTH, Vissers KCP, van Geffen GJ, et al. Unpredictable injectate spread of the erector spinae plane block in human cadavers. Anesth Analg. 2019;129(5):e163-6.
21. Mittnacht AJC. Fascial Plane blocks in cardiac surgery: Same but different. J Cardiothor Vasc An. 2019;33(2):426-7.
22. Horlocker TT, Vandermeuelen E, Kopp SL, Gogarten W, Leffert LR, Benzon HT. Regional anesthesia in the patient receiving antithrombotic or thrombolytic therapy: American Society of Regional Anesthesia and Pain Medicine Evidence-Based Guidelines (Fourth Edition). Reg Anesth Pain Med. 2018;43(3):263-309.
23. Dhole S, Mehta Y, Saxena H, Juneja R, Trehan N. Comparison of continuous thoracic epidural and paravertebral blocks for postoperative analgesia after minimally invasive direct coronary artery bypass surgery. J Cardiothorac Vasc Anesth. 2001;15(3):288-92.
24. Balan C, Bubenek-Turconi SI, Tomescu DR, Valeanu L. Ultrasound-guided regional anesthesia-current strategies for enhanced recovery after cardiac surgery. Medicina (Kaunas). 2021;57(4):312.
25. Gulbahar G, Kocer B, Muratli SN, Yildirim E, Gulbahar O, Dural K, et al. A comparison of epidural and paravertebral catheterisation techniques in post-thoracotomy pain management. Euro J Cardiothorac Surg. 2010;37:467-72.
26. Yeung J, Gates S, Naidu B, Wilson M, Gao Smith F. Paravertebral block versus thoracic epidural for patients undergoing thoracotomy (Review). Cochrane Database Syst Rev. 2016;2(2):CD009121.

27. Bashandy GMN, Abbas DN. Pectoral nerves I and II blocks in multimodal analgesia for breast cancer surgery: a randomized clinical trial. Reg Anesth Pain Med. 2015;40(1):68-74.
28. Kulhari S, Bharti N, Bala I, Arora S, Singh G. Efficacy of pectoral nerve block versus thoracic paravertebral block for postoperative analgesia after radical mastectomy: a randomized controlled trial. Br J Anaesth. 2016;117(3):382-6.
29. Versyck B, Van Geffen GJ, Chin KJ. Analgesic efficacy of the Pecs II block: a systematic review and meta-analysis. Anaesthesia. 2019;74(5):663-73.
30. Yildirim K, Sertcakacilar G, Hergunsel GO. Comparison of the results of ultrasound-guided thoracic paravertebral block and modified pectoral nerve block for postoperative analgesia in video-assisted thoracoscopic surgery: a prospective, randomized controlled study. J Cardiothorac Vasc Anesth. 2022;36(2):489-96.
31. Mavarez AC, Ripat CI, Suarez MR. Pectoralis plane block for pacemaker insertion: a successful primary anesthetic. Front Surg. 2019;6:64.
32. Fujiwara A, Komasawa N, Minami T. Pectoral nerves (PECS) and intercostal nerve block for cardiac resynchronization therapy device implantation. Springerplus. 2014;3(1):409.
33. Froyshteter A, Bhalla T, Tobias J, Cambier G, Mckee C. Pectoralis blocks for insertion of an implantable cardioverter defibrillator in two patients with Duchenne muscular dystrophy. Saudi J Anaesth. 2018;12(2):324.
34. Pai BHP, Shariat AN, Bhatt HV. PECS block for an ICD implantation in the super obese patient. J Clin Anesth. 2019;57:110-1.
35. Kumar K, Kalyane R, Singh N, Nagaraja PS, Krishna M, Babu B, et al. Efficacy of bilateral pectoralis nerve block for ultrafast tracking and postoperative pain management in cardiac surgery. Ann Card Anaesth. 2018;21(3):333-8.
36. Blanco R, Parras T, McDonnell JG, Prats-Galino A. Serratus plane block: a novel ultrasound-guided thoracic wall nerve block. Anaesthesia. 2013;68(11):1107-13.
37. Kunigo T, Murouchi T, Yamamoto S, Yamakage M. Injection volume and anesthetic effect in serratus plane block. Reg Anesth Pain Med. 2017;42(6):737-40.
38. Kunhabdulla NP. Serratus anterior plane block for multiple rib fractures. Pain Physician. 2014;5;17(5;9):E651-62.
39. Ökmen K, Ökmen BM. The efficacy of serratus anterior plane block in analgesia for thoracotomy: a retrospective study. J Anesth. 2017;31(4):579-85.
40. Semyonov M, Fedorina E, Grinshpun J, Dubilet M, Refaely Y, Ruderman L, et al. Ultrasound-guided serratus anterior plane block for analgesia after thoracic surgery. J Pain Res. 2019;12:953-60.
41. Chen G, Li Y, Zhang Y, Fang X. Effects of serratus anterior plane block for postoperative analgesia after thoracoscopic surgery compared with local anesthetic infiltration: a randomized clinical trial. J Pain Res. 2019;12:2411-17.
42. Wang L, Wang Y, Zhang X, Zhu X, Wang G. Serratus anterior plane block or thoracic paravertebral block for postoperative pain treatment after uniportal video-assisted thoracoscopic surgery: a retrospective propensity-matched study. J Pain Res. 2019;12:2231-8.
43. Khalil AE, Abdallah NM, Bashandy GM, Kaddah TAH. Ultrasound-Guided serratus anterior plane block versus thoracic epidural analgesia for thoracotomy pain. J Cardiothor Vasc An. 2017;31(1):152-8.
44. Kim S, Bae CM, Do YW, Moon S, Baek SI, Lee DH. Serratus anterior plane block and intercostal nerve block after thoracoscopic surgery. Thorac Cardiovasc Surg. 2021;69(06):564-9.
45. Saad F, El Baradie S, Abdel Aliem MW, Ali M, Kotb TM. Ultrasound-guided serratus anterior plane block versus thoracic paravertebral block for perioperative analgesia in thoracotomy. Saudi J Anaesth. 2018;12(4):565.

46. Zhang Y, Fu Z, Fang T, Wang K, Liu Z, Li H, et al. A comparison of the analgesic efficacy of serratus anterior plane block vs paravertebral nerve block for video-assisted thoracic surgery: a randomized controlled trial. Wideochir Inne Tech Maloinwazyjne.2022;17(1):134-42.
47. Wang Y, Shi M, Huang S, Fe X, Gu X, Ma Z. Ultrasound-guided serratus anterior plane block versus paravertebral block on postoperation analgesia and safety following the video- assisted thoracic surgery: a prospective, randomized, double-blinded non-inferiority clinical trial. Asian J Surg. 2023;46:4215-21.
48. López-Matamala B, Fajardo M, Estébanez-Montiel B, Blancas R, Alfaro P, Chana M. A new thoracic interfascial plane block as anesthesia for difficult weaning due to ribcage pain in critically ill patients. Med Intensiva. 2014;38(7):463-5.
49. Fujii S, Vissa D, Ganapathy S, Johnson M, Zhou J. Transversus thoracic muscle plane block on a cadaver with history of coronary artery bypass grafting. Reg Anesth Pain Med. 2017;42(4):535-7.
50. Murata H, Hida K, Hara T. Transverse thoracic muscle plane block: tricks and tips to accomplish the block. Reg Anesth Pain Med. 2016;41(3):411-2.
51. Raza I, Narayanan M, Venkataraju A, Ciocarlan A. Bilateral subpectoral interfascial plane catheters for analgesia for sternal fractures: a case report. Reg Anesth Pain Med. 2016;41(5):607-9.
52. Bhatt HV, Hernandez N, Shariat A. Successful use of serratus and transversus thoracic plane blocks for subcutaneous implantable cardioverter-defibrillator placement. J Cardiothor Vasc An. 2018;32(1):e22-3.
53. Barr AM, Tutungi E, Almeida AA. Parasternal intercostal block with ropivacaine for pain management after cardiac surgery: a double-blind, randomized, controlled trial. J Cardiothor Vasc An. 2007;21(4):547-53.
54. Saini K, Chauhan S, Kiran U, Bisoi AK, Choudhury M, Hasija S. Comparison of parasternal intercostal block using ropivacaine or bupivacaine for postoperative analgesia in patients undergoing cardiac surgery. World J Cardiovasc Surg. 2015;05(06):49-57.
55. Forero M, Adhikary SD, Lopez H, Tsui C, Chin KJ. The erector spinae plane block: a novel analgesic technique in thoracic neuropathic pain. Reg Anesth Pain Med. 2016;41(5):621-7.
56. Chin KJ, Malhas L, Perlas A. The erector spinae plane block provides visceral abdominal analgesia in bariatric surgery: a report of 3 cases. Reg Anesth Pain Med. 2017;42(3):372-6.
57. Costache I, Pawa A, Abdallah FW. Paravertebral by proxy-time to redefine the paravertebral block. Anaesthesia. 2018;73(10):1185-8.
58. Ivanusic J, Konishi Y, Barrington MJ. A cadaveric study investigating the mechanism of action of erector spinae blockade. Reg Anesth Pain Med. 2018;43(6):567-71.
59. Fang B, Wang Z, Huang X. Ultrasound-guided preoperative single-dose erector spinae plane block provides comparable analgesia to thoracic paravertebral block following thoracotomy: a single center randomized controlled double-blind study. Ann Transl Med. 2019;7(8):174.
60. Gaballah KM, Soltan WA, Bahgat NM. Ultrasound-guided serratus plane block versus erector spinae block for postoperative analgesia after video-assisted thoracoscopy: a pilot randomized controlled trial. J Cardiothor Vasc An. 2019;33(7):1946-53.
61. Finnerty D, McMahon A, McNamara J, Hartigan S, Griffen M, Buggy D. Comparing erector spinae plane block with serratus anterior plane block for minimally invasive thoracic surgery: a randomised clinical trial. Br J Anaesth. 2020;5(125):802-10.
62. Zhao H, Xin L, Feng Y. The effect of preoperative erector spinae plane vs. paravertebral blocks on patient-controlled oxycodone consumption after video-assisted thoracic surgery: a prospective randomized, blinded, non-inferiority study. J Clin Anesth. 2020;62:109737.

63. Hong JM, Kim E, Jeon S, Lee D, Baik J, Cho AR, et al. A prospective double-blinded randomized control trial comparing erector spinae plane block to thoracic epidural analgesia for postoperative pain in video-assisted thoracic surgery. Saudi Med J. 2023;44(2):155-63.
64. Kelava M, Anthony D, Elsharkawy H. Continuous erector spinae block for postoperative analgesia after thoracotomy in a lung transplant recipient. J Cardiothor Vasc An. 2018;32(5):e9-e11.
65. Krishna SN, Chauhan S, Bhoi D, Kaushal B, Hasija S, Sangdup T, et al. Bilateral erector spinae plane block for acute post-surgical pain in adult cardiac surgical patients: a randomized controlled trial. J Cardiothorac Vasc Anesth. 2019;33(2):368-75.
66. Nagaraja P, Ragavendran S, Singh N, Asai O, Bhavya G, Manjunath N, et al. Comparison of continuous thoracic epidural analgesia with bilateral erector spinae plane block for perioperative pain management in cardiac surgery. Ann Card Anaesth. 2018;21(3):323.
67. Macaire P, Ho N, Nguyen T, Nguyen B, Vu V, Quach C, et al. Ultrasound-guided continuous thoracic erector spinae plane block within an enhanced recovery program is associated with decreased opioid consumption and improved patient postoperative rehabilitation after open cardiac surgery—a patient-matched, controlled before-and-after study. J Cardiothor Vasc An. 2019;33(6):1659-67.
68. Adhikary SD, Prasad A, Soleimani B, Chin KJ. Continuous erector spinae plane block as an effective analgesic option in anticoagulated patients after left ventricular assist device implantation: a case series. J Cardiothor Vasc An. 2019;33(4):1063-7.
69. Batchelor TJP, Rasburn NJ, Abdelnour-Berchtold E, Brunelli A, Cerfolio RJ, Gonzalez M, et al. Guidelines for enhanced recovery after lung surgery: recommendations of the Enhanced Recovery After Surgery (ERAS®) Society and the European Society of Thoracic Surgeons (ESTS). Euro J Cardiothorac Surg. 2019;55(1):91-115.
70. Makkad B, Heinke TL, Sheriffdeen R, Khatib D, Brodt JL, Meng ML, et al. Practice advisory for preoperative and intraoperative pain management of thoracic surgical patients: Part 1. Anesth Analg. 2023;137(1):2-25.
71. Feray S, Lubach J, Joshi GP, Bonnet F, Van de Velde M. PROSPECT guidelines for video-assisted thoracoscopic surgery: a systematic review and procedure-specific postoperative pain management recommendations. Anaesthesia. 2022;77:311-25.

# CHAPTER 10

# Anesthesia for Pulmonary Endarterectomy

*Palesa Motshabi Chakane, Muhammad Farooq, Palesa Mogane*

## ABSTRACT

Chronic thromboembolic pulmonary hypertension (CTEPH) is a rare debilitating disease potentially curable by surgical pulmonary endarterectomy (PEA). The procedure is performed on cardiopulmonary bypass (CPB) and deep hypothermic circulatory arrest (DHCA). Major complications include pulmonary hemorrhage, reperfusion pulmonary edema, and residual pulmonary hypertension with RV failure. Patients with severe pulmonary hypertension may necessitate institution of extracorporeal membrane oxygenation (ECMO)—central venous-arterial in biventricular failure and venous-venous ECMO in right ventricular (RV) failure. Limiting circulatory arrest times may reduce the incidence of cognitive impairment post-PEA. Intractable vasoplegia may in very sick patients after prolonged CPB with DHCA, in the face of RV failure may be managed with addition of noncatecholamine vasopressors that do not exacerbate PH. We aim to give an overview of the perioperative management of PEA for CTEPH.

**Keywords:** Pulmonary endarterectomy; Chronic thromboembolic pulmonary hypertension; Deep hypothermic circulatory arrest; Anesthesia; Complications

## KEY POINTS

- Chronic thromboembolic pulmonary hypertension remains a rare disease with lethal consequences.
- Pulmonary endarterectomy (PEA) for chronic thromboembolic pulmonary hypertension is potentially curative.
- Interdisciplinary expert team decision-making is essential, including pulmonologists, cardiologists, radiologists, anesthesiologists, and surgeons.
- Patients on pulmonary hypertension-specific treatment preoperatively are at risk of worse outcomes due to delay between diagnosis and surgery pretreated patients.
- Anesthesia entails the maintenance of stable hemodynamic and organ protection.
- Postoperative complications include reperfusion pulmonary edema, residual pulmonary hypertension, hypoxic pulmonary vasoconstriction, and cognitive impairment post-PEA.

## ■ INTRODUCTION

### History

Pulmonary endarterectomy (PEA) is a complex procedure indicated for chronic thromboembolic pulmonary hypertension (CTEPH). It is undertaken to clear pulmonary arteries of accumulated clots and fibrotic tissue that has blocked pulmonary blood flow to the lungs to different degrees due to often repeated deposits of thrombi. The procedure has a history that dates back to the 1950s when initial reports of chronic pulmonary thrombosis were reported.[1] In the 1960s, the first reports of pulmonary endarterectomies surfaced.[2] The approach was initially through unilateral thoracotomies with numerous abandoned procedures and a belief that the condition was not operable,[3,4] progressing to transverse "clamshell" incisions.[5]

Early reports of successful PEA with cooling and cardiopulmonary bypass (CPB) on standby were reported from the University of California San Diego (UCSD) in the early 1960s.[6,7]

A report of a PEA using CPB surfaced in the early 1960s from Massachusetts[8] and other reports later from UCSD.[9] By the 1980s, Daily et al.[10] reported the UCSD experience with CPB and deep hypothermic circulatory arrest (DHCA). A review in 1984 found only 85 reported surgical cases worldwide.[11] By 2003, Jameson et al. reported 1,500 cases from UCSD, emphasizing the importance of sternotomy, CPB, and DHCA.[12] This center developed a risk stratification for patients with CTEP presenting for PEA. In the 1990s, more extensive programs were then developed in Europe and elsewhere in the world.

## Epidemiology

The CTEPH is a rare disease reportedly diagnosed in 3–30 per million and is associated with high mortality.[13] It occurs equally in men and women. Approximately, 0.4–4.8% of these patients are a progression from acute pulmonary embolism. Commonly identified risk factors include prior thromboembolic disease, hypercoagulable states, chronic inflammation, splenectomy, a history of malignancy, and contraceptive pills. The hypercoagulable states include elevated factor VIII levels, factor V Leiden mutation, protein C deficiency, and lupus anticoagulant/antiphospholipid antibodies.[13] Early recognition of this disease and appropriate treatment are the key to improving outcomes. Pulmonary artery endarterectomy is the recommended treatment for patients and is considered curative.[13]

## Pathophysiology

The pathology is reflective of nonresolving emboli in the pulmonary vasculature. This is followed by proliferation, inflammation, scarring, and the development of an organized fibrous layer that replaces the normal intima of the arterial wall.[14] The changes are limited to large vessels and extend to smaller vessels. This phenomenon is essential in the perioperative period and informs the management of pulmonary hypertension (PH) before and after surgery.[15] Studies have reported residual episodes of PH post-PEA and postulate it to be due to this phenomenon.[16,17] A category of patients with chronic pulmonary thromboembolic phenomena not meeting the criteria due to lower pulmonary artery pressures (PAP), ≤25 mm Hg at rest, has been described. This group has been termed "chronic thromboembolic (pulmonary vascular) disease" (CTED or CTEPVD) and is managed similarly.[18]

## ■ DIAGNOSIS

Diagnosis of CTEPH is made through a combination of clinical presentation and confirmation through imaging tests. The V/Q scan can be used as an initial investigation to exclude CTEPH. Other imaging modalities employed in the preparatory face for surgery include pulmonary angiography to confirm [digital subtraction angiography (DSA)]. 3D dynamic contrast-enhanced lung perfusion magnetic resonance imaging (MRI) has been used. Single photon emission computed tomography (SPECT) and other advanced CT modes delineate the diseased vessels, such as CT pulmonary angiogram (CTPA). Echocardiography is used to assess the effects of PH on the right heart and assist in diagnosing the severity of right ventricular (RV) failure. There is invariably always a presence of tricuspid regurgitation. Cardiac catheterization confirms pulmonary artery (PA) pressures and pulmonary vascular resistance (PVR).[19]

## ■ RISK PREDICTION

Physiological factors associated with high risk are the presence of PH-specific drug treatment (sildenafil, bosentan, riociguat, macitentan, and anticoagulants) at the time of surgery, poor effort tolerance at the time of surgery, and PVR postoperatively.[20] A surgical risk stratification system developed by UCSD emphasizes the location of disease in the vascular system, graded from level 0 to 4.

- *Level 0:* No evidence of thromboembolic disease in either lung
- *Level 1:* Chronic thromboembolism (CTE) starting in the main pulmonary arteries (level C: complete occlusion of one main pulmonary artery with CTE)
- *Level 2:* CTE beginning at the level of lobar arteries or in the main descending pulmonary arteries
- *Level 3:* CTE beginning at the level of the segmental arteries
- *Level 4:* CTE starting at the level of the subsegmental arteries.

It is based predominantly on the burden of disease and the level of vascular involvement and does not include other factors that were found to affect risk clinically. A multidisciplinary team, including pulmonologists, cardiologists, radiologists, and anesthesiologists, is involved in team decision-making.[21]

## ■ PERIOPERATIVE MANAGEMENT

### Preoperative Management

Patients often present with some dependency on oxygen supplementation and should be maintained on oxygen preoperatively. Continuation of PH-specific medication in the preoperative period is essential. Long-acting anticoagulants such as direct oral anticoagulants (DOACs) and warfarin should be stopped appropriately and bridged with anticoagulants with short half-lives (enoxaparin or unfractionated heparin). Preoperative anxiolytics are best avoided as they may lead to sedation and episodes of hypoxemia and hypercarbia. This would exacerbate PH. Patients with poor cardiac output necessitating inotropic support should be nursed in an intensive care environment preoperatively on infusions of inotropes.

### Intraoperative Management

Life-saving medication and oxygen should be continued into the theatre environment. A large bore intravenous line in a patient that came from the ward environment would be inserted for drug administration. Depending on the patient's condition, inserting awake invasive intravenous lines such as the arterial and central venous catheter may be necessary. Special consideration should be paid to patients with high baseline central venous pressure (CVP) or right atrial pressures. In some centers, a pulmonary artery catheter is part of the routine in these cases.

Standard American Society of Anesthesiologists (ASA) monitoring extended with a 12-lead electrocardiogram (ECG) is applied. A continuous cardiac output monitor such as the Edwards Life Sciences EV1000 may be beneficial for use intraoperatively and as a continuation of care in the ICU. It provides essential hemodynamic values such as CO, CI, mean arterial pressure (MAP), mean PA pressure, CVP, systemic vascular resistance (SVR), SVR index, PVR, and PVR index, stroke volume variation, and pulse pressure variation. Neuromonitoring in the form of bispectral index analysis (BIS) and near-infrared spectrometry (INVOS) provide a trend and is imperative during CPB and DHCA.

The patients should be allowed a comfortable bed position preinduction. A very careful, slow induction with a combination of an opioid (sufentanil or fentanyl) and a small dose of midazolam (1 mg at a time) often presents stable induction conditions. Other induction agents, such as propofol and etomidate, can be used. Given the prolonged procedure, adequate muscle relaxation can be attained with rocuronium. Post induction, a transesophageal echocardiogram probe is inserted. Two temperature probes (esophageal and urinary) are essential, particularly when cooling and rewarming.

In hemodynamic challenges, catecholamine vasoactive agents should be started preinduction (adrenaline, noradrenaline, and dobutamine). Phenylephrine, with vasopressor effects that affect the pulmonary circulation, is best avoided. Inotropic support aims to maintain coronary perfusion to both the left and right ventricles. Combining norepinephrine and an inodilator such as dobutamine or milrinone often achieves the desired hemodynamic stability. In cases of intractable low cardiac output states exacerbating poor coronary perfusion, additional vasopressor agents (noncatecholamine) may be added **(Table 1)**. Lung protective ventilation with tidal volumes of 4–6 mL/kg and peak end-expiratory pressure ~6–8 mm Hg to avoid hypo or hyperventilation. Respiratory alkalosis and a higher $FiO_2$ may assist in reducing RV afterload in the short term.[22]

## Cardiopulmonary Bypass

A routine CPB institution with heparinization to achieve activated coagulation time (ACT) of >400 seconds is instituted. Routine antibiotics and tranexamic acid should be administered. Maintenance of anesthesia during CPB is through infusions

**TABLE 1:** Noncatecholamine vasopressors.

| Noncatecholamine vasopressor | Dose |
|---|---|
| Vasopressin | 1.2–6 U/h |
| Terlipressin | 1.3 µg/kg/h |
| Methylene blue | 1.5–2 mg/kg bolus |
| Hydroxocobalamin | 5 g over 5 minutes |
| Angiotensin II | 20 ng/kg/min |
| Corticosteroids | 50 mg q 6 hourly |
| Vitamin C | 6 g/day |

of propofol, opioids (remifentanil/sufentanil/fentanyl), and/or dexmedetomidine. Attention to neurological protection is essential and is achieved through monitoring using the BIS and INVOS trends and infusions of propofol and dexmedetomidine.[23] Reductions in cerebral oxygenation should be managed appropriately, including vasodilation by permissive hypercarbia on CPB. At the initiation of DHCA, ice packs are wrapped around the patient's head, taking care to avoid frostbite. The patient is cooled to 18°C core temperature. Timed DHCA intervals of 20–25 with resumption of flow are managed in conjunction with cerebral oximetry.[24]

## Surgical Treatment

Surgery is through a median sternotomy. A pulmonary arteriotomy exposes the operation site. Almost always, the disease is bilateral, even if preoperative workup shows unilateral disease. Opening of both pulmonary arteries is mandatory. A circulatory arrest or very low flow on deep hypothermia is essential to PEA. There is a difference between embolectomy for a fresh clot and TEA, which is harder due to fibrotic tissue. Dissecting the occluding tissue to remove it as a whole **(Fig. 1)** is imperative. For surgical success, access to the correct tissue plane is crucial and avoids incomplete removal or vascular injury leading to lethal complications. After the removal of the chronic clot, the pulmonary arteries are closed, rewarming is commenced, and preparation to come off the CPB is started.

## Separation from Cardiopulmonary Bypass

Preparation for separation from CPB includes removal of ice packs from the head and rewarming. Lung protective ventilation is resumed, and the surgeon performs surveillance to see any bubbling that may indicate communication between the lungs and the vascular structures, which may lead to catastrophic intrapulmonary bleeding. Once the airway bleeding is cleared, ventilation with tidal volumes of approximately 4 mL/kg is started with an inhaled pulmonary vasodilator (iloprost), and a steroid is added to the nebulizer chamber. This is continued during rewarming and separation from the bypass—echocardiographic assessment of both ventricles. A systemic steroid is administered (methylprednisolone 1 g). Electrolyte abnormalities are corrected, and once off CPB, heparin is reversed with protamine. Suitable inotropic support

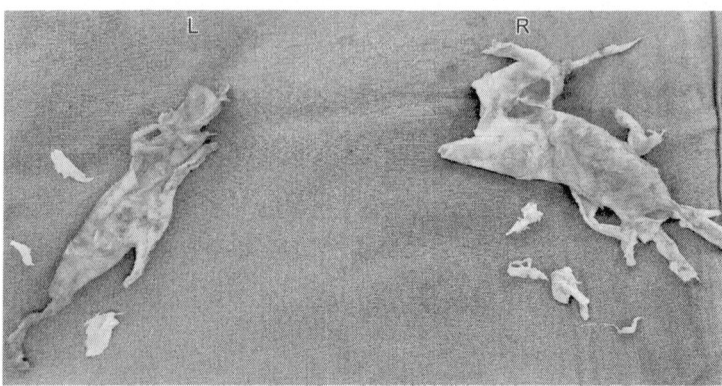

**Fig. 1:** Left (L) and right (R) chronic clot removed whole.

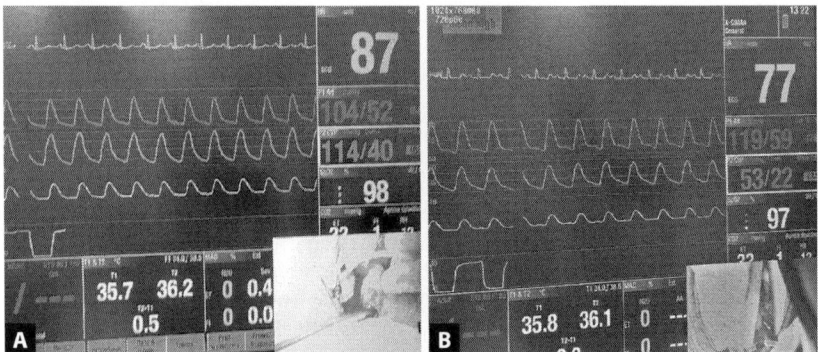

**Figs. 2A and B:** (A) Preoperative: Arterial blood pressure and (B) Postoperative: Pulmonary blood pressure.

such as milrinone/dobutamine and noradrenaline is instituted. Surgery is potentially curative, and pulmonary pressures, which are often suprasystemic, drop to half or lower compared to systemic pressures **(Figs. 2A and B)**.

## Management of Complications

Significant complications include pulmonary hemorrhage, reperfusion pulmonary edema, and residual PH with RV failure. Pulmonary hemorrhage should be excluded early before rewarming. Reperfusion pulmonary edema is managed with restriction of fluids, aggressive use of diuretics, and avoidance of high cardiac output.[25]

Residual PH is a consequence of superimposed small vessel vasculopathy, reversible postoperative pulmonary vasoconstriction because of CPB, mechanical injury, and ischemia-reperfusion injury. At a cellular level, there are reduced levels of nitric oxide and prostacyclin and increased levels of endothelin. Early reinstitution of PH-sensitive medication is therapeutic.[20] Failure to reverse severe PH may lead to cardiac failure necessitating extracorporeal membrane oxygenation (ECMO)—central venous-arterial in biventricular failure and venous-venous ECMO in RV failure.[26] Patients are prone to cognitive impairment post-PEA due to insults from circulatory arrest and hypothermia. Limiting circulatory arrest times may reduce the incidence of this complication.[27] Intractable vasoplegia may occur in very sick patients after prolonged CPB with DHCA in the face of RV failure. It should be managed with vasopressors that do not exacerbate PH. It may be necessary to add noncatecholamine vasopressors to achieve desired hemodynamic goals.

## Postoperative Management

Patients are recovered in the ICU. A common practice is to keep the patients intubated for more than 24 hours to allow for the settlement of residual vascular complications. In patients with persistent PH in inaccessible arteries, balloon pulmonary angioplasty (PBA) may be performed, mainly in established expert centers.

## CONCLUSION

Management of PEA for CTEPH has come a long way since the era of very high mortality rates. Expert centers are reporting <1% mortality. Pharmacological agents and surgical skills have evolved to mitigate risk. Surgery is deemed curative and dependent predominantly on the surgeon's skill. Combination therapy with PBA is feasible in expert centers.

## ■ REFERENCES

1. Hollister LE, Cull VL. The syndrome of chronic thrombosis of the major pulmonary arteries. Am J Med. 1956;21(2):312-20.
2. Houk VN, Hufnagel CA, McClenathan JE, Moser KM. Chronic thrombotic obstruction of major pulmonary arteries. Report of a case successfully treated by thrombendarterectomy, and a review of the literature. Am J Med. 1963;35:269-82.
3. Owen WR, Thomas WA, Castleman B, Bland EF. Unrecognized emboli to the lungs with subsequent cor pulmonale. The New England journal of medicine. 1953;249(23):919-26.
4. Carroll D. Chronic obstruction of major pulmonary arteries. Am J Med. 1950;9(2):175-85.
5. Hurwitt ES, Schein CJ, Rifkin H, Lebendiger A. A surgical approach to the problem of chronic pulmonary artery obstruction due to thrombosis or stenosis. Ann Surg. 1958;147(2):157-65.
6. Snyder WA, Kent DC, Baisch BF. Successful endarterectomy of chronically occluded pulmonary artery. Clinical report and physiologic studies. J Thoracic Cardiovasc Surg. 1963;45:482-9.
7. Moser KM, Rhodes PG, Hufnagel CC. Chronic unilateral pulmonary-artery thrombosis: successful thrombendarectomy with thirty-month follow-up observation. N Engl J Med. 1965;272:1195-9.
8. McBay AJ. Case records of the massachusetts general hospital. CASE 32-1964. N Engl J Med. 1964;271:40-50.
9. Moser KM, Braunwald NS. Successful surgical intervention in severe chronic thromboembolic pulmonary hypertension. Chest. 1973;64(1):29-35.
10. Daily PO, Johnston GG, Simmons CJ, Moser KM. Surgical management of chronic pulmonary embolism: surgical treatment and late results. J Thoracic Cardiovasc Surg. 1980;79(4):523-31.
11. Chitwood WR Jr, Sabiston DC Jr, Wechsler AS. Surgical treatment of chronic unresolved pulmonary embolism. Clin Chest Med. 1984;5(3):507-36.
12. Jamieson SW, Kapelanski DP, Sakakibara N, Manecke GR, Thistlethwaite PA, Kerr KM, et al. Pulmonary endarterectomy: experience and lessons learned in 1,500 cases. The Ann Thoracic Surg. 2003;76(5):1457-62;discussion 62-4.
13. Medrek S, Safdar Z. Epidemiology and pathophysiology of chronic thromboembolic pulmonary hypertension: Risk factors and mechanisms. Methodist Debakey Cardiovasc J. 2016;12(4):195-8.
14. Lang I. Chronic thromboembolic pulmonary hypertension: a distinct disease entity. Eur Respir Rev. 2015;24(136):246-52.
15. Peacock A, Simonneau G, Rubin L. Controversies, uncertainties, and future research on the treatment of chronic thromboembolic pulmonary hypertension. Proc Am Thorac Soc. 2006;3(7):608-14.
16. Sanchez O, Helley D, Couchon S, Roux A, Delaval A, Trinquart L, et al. Perfusion defects after pulmonary embolism: risk factors and clinical significance. J Thromb Haemost. 2010;8(6):1248-55.
17. Meneveau N, Ider O, Seronde MF, Chopard R, Davani S, Bernard Y, et al. Long-term prognostic value of residual pulmonary vascular obstruction at discharge in patients with intermediate- to high-risk pulmonary embolism. Euro Heart J. 2013;34(9):693-701.
18. Delcroix M, Kerr K, Fedullo P. Chronic thromboembolic pulmonary hypertension. epidemiology and risk factors. Ann Am Thoracic Soc. 2016;13(Suppl 3):S201-S6.
19. Pepke-Zaba J, Delcroix M, Lang I, Mayer E, Jansa P, Ambroz D, et al. Chronic thromboembolic pulmonary hypertension (CTEPH): Results from an international prospective registry. Circulation. 2011;124(18):1973-81.

20. Godinas L, Verbelen T, Delcroix M. Residual pulmonary hypertension after pulmonary thromboendarterectomy: Incidence, pathogenesis and therapeutic options. Ann Cardiothorac Surg. 2022;11(2):163-5.
21. Kim NH, Delcroix M, Jais X, Madani MM, Matsubara H, Mayer E, et al. Chronic thromboembolic pulmonary hypertension. Euro Respir J. 2019;53(1): 1801915.
22. Navaratnam M, DiNardo JA. Peri-operative right ventricular dysfunction—the anesthesiologist's view. Cardiovascular Diagnosis and Therapy. 2020;10(5):1725-34.
23. Yuan HX, Zhang LN, Li G, Qiao L. Brain protective effect of dexmedetomidine vs. propofol for sedation during prolonged mechanical ventilation in non-brain injured patients. World J Psychiatry. 2024;14(3):370-9.
24. Conolly S, Arrowsmith JE, Klein AA. Deep hypothermic circulatory arrest. Contin Educ Anaesth Crit Pain. 2010;10(5):138-42.
25. Sanada TJ, Tanabe N, Ishibashi-Ueda H, Ishida K, Naito A, Sakao S, et al. Involvement of pulmonary arteriopathy in the development and severity of reperfusion pulmonary edema after pulmonary endarterectomy. Pulm Circ. 2019;9(2):2045894019846439.
26. Perrot Md, McRae K, Donahoe L, Abdelnour-Berchtold E, Thenganatt J, Granton J. Pulmonary endarterectomy in severe chronic thromboembolic pulmonary hypertension: the Toronto experience. Ann Cardiothorac Surg. 2022;11(2):133-42.
27. Kamenskaya OV, Klinkova AS, Loginova IY, Porotnikova SS, Habarov DV, Lomivorotov VN, et al. Impairment of cognitive functions in patients with chronic thromboembolic pulmonary hypertension before and after surgical treatment. Zh Nevrol Psikhiatr Im S S Korsakova. 2023;123(2):126-31.

# CHAPTER 11

# Anesthetic Considerations and Management of Traumatic Brain Injury

*V Bhadri Narayan*

## ABSTRACT

Traumatic brain injury is a leading cause of death in young people and is a silent epidemic. In India, it is said about 150,000 individuals die, and many more are disabled, leading to a significant social burden on the families. Early diagnosis, rapid transport to hospitals and intervention will play a key role in improving outcomes in TBI. Healthcare facilities should have essential infrastructure to resuscitate and treat these victims so that they have a reasonable chance to reenter society early. Emphasis should be laid on preventing secondary brain injury by identifying both intracranial and systemic causes and implementing the Brain Trauma Foundation guidelines universally. Irrespective of the nature of the injury, whether it is mild, moderate, or severe, they will have some permanent deficit with disturbances in memory, behavior, emotion, balance, and cognition. Treatment in the hospital should be centered around reducing intracranial pressure, maintaining cerebral perfusion, and adopting multi-modal monitoring modalities where available with rapid interventions. Educating the public about the dangers of traumatic brain injury and its consequences, and implementing preventive strategies, including safe driving habits, wearing helmets, avoid risk-taking behavior in young people, will greatly impact the management and outcomes of TBI.

**Keywords:** Anesthesia; Intracranial pressure; Hypotension; Hypoxia; Ischemia; Secondary brain injury; Cerebral perfusion

## KEY POINTS

- Reduce intracranial pressure and maintain cerebral perfusion.
- Rapid resuscitation to prevent secondary brain damage.
- Early implementation of multimodal monitoring will improve outcomes in these patients.
- Avoid hypotension and hypoxia.
- Careful management of the airway plays a crucial role in these patients.
- Rapid transport, early diagnosis of intracranial lesions, and treatment are the key factors.

## ■ INTRODUCTION

Traumatic brain injury (TBI) is one of the leading causes of morbidity and mortality in individuals under 45 years and contributes to a significant socioeconomic burden on society. Though significant advances have been made in the management of TBI, mortality has not changed much over the last decade and remains a cause of great concern. TBI was recently defined by a consensus panel of experts as an alteration in brain function, or other evidence of brain pathology, caused by an external force.[1] TBI may result from blunt or penetrating trauma to the head, indirect acceleration, and the deceleration of troops or blasts. These forces might temporarily or permanently disrupt the functioning of the brain. The consequences of TBI may range from permanent physical disabilities to long-term cognitive, behavioral, psychological, and social defects, which may affect their early re-entry into society. It is said that irrespective of whether TBI is mild, moderate, or severe, all of them will have some degree of permanent disability. An estimated 2.14 million Americans sustain TBI, and approximately 69,000 persons died in the United States in 2021 as a result of their brain injury.[2] An estimated 80,000–90,000 patients will experience long-term disability. TBI contributes to about 30% of all injury-related deaths in the USA.[3] The common causes of TBI are falls, motor vehicle accidents, recreational injuries, assault, and combat injuries. In India, it is said that one person dies every 10 minutes due to TBI, and this will probably triple by 2020, and the mortality from TBI is >150,000 annually.[4] The epidemic must be recognized, and urgent preventive measures must be instituted to decrease the number of persons affected.

## ■ CONSEQUENCES OF TRAUMATIC BRAIN INJURY

Traumatic brain injury can lead to significant and long-term consequences, which can affect the quality of life. The injury affects multiple organ systems, leading to medical complications that will need therapy. The complications that can follow TBI are cognitive impairment, memory, disturbances of emotion and behavior, visual disturbances, coordination, balance, and executive dysfunction. In the gastrointestinal tract (GIT), dysphagia, gastroparesis, and bowel incontinence can affect the nutrition of the individual. About 15% will develop hypertension. Patients are often bedridden for long periods. They are particularly at risk of developing deep vein thrombosis. Neuroendocrine dysfunction is well known after TBI and, if undiagnosed, can affect recovery. In addition, they may have features of dysautonomia and also develop seizure disorders.[5]

## ■ PATHOPHYSIOLOGY

Intracranial pressure (ICP) and cerebral perfusion management are the mainstay for managing TBI patients. It is well documented that increased ICP is associated with increased mortality;[6-8] however, despite controlling the ICP well, there have been no significant changes in the mortality rates. There may be factors outside the cranial cavity that could influence the outcomes. Recently, it has been shown that intra-abdominal pressure (IAP) and intrathoracic pressure (ITP) are associated with ICP elevation, so there may be a relationship between intracranial, intrathoracic, and intra-abdominal compartments.[9] Hence, the concept of a multiple compartment syndrome evolved, and strategies to reduce pressures in other compartments may successfully decrease the elevated ICP. It has been shown now that decompressive laparotomy in patients with concurrent elevations in IAP and measures adopted to reduce ITP do reduce ICP. However, the ideal ventilator management strategy in TBI patients still needs to be determined. It is not routine clinical practice now to measure intra-abdominal and ITPs in managing patients with TBI. Then, have we missed a trick in all these years in management that could strongly influence the outcomes?

If it is true, does it signal that we need a change in strategy? Therefore, comprehensive care of TBI patients involves the management of not only the primary intracranial disorder but also the optimization of the other organ systems in the body, as they could significantly influence the outcome.

## ■ CLASSIFICATION

Traumatic brain injury can be classified into mild [Glasgow Coma Scale (GCS) 13-15], moderate (GCS 9-12), and severe TBI (GCS <8). It can also be classified as penetrating injury versus blunt injury, focal lesions, and diffuse injury. Focal lesions are extradural hematoma, subdural hematoma (SDH), intracranial hematoma, contusions, diffuse axonal injury, and traumatic subarachnoid hemorrhage **(Figs. 1 to 5)**.

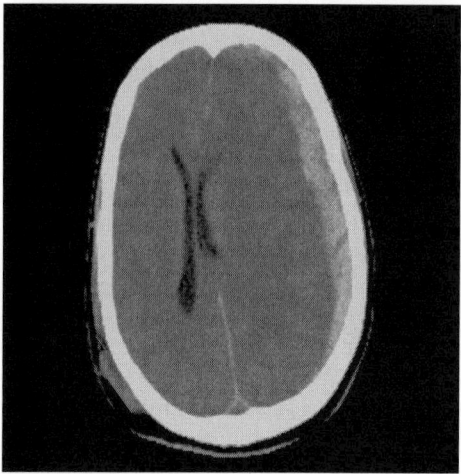

**Fig. 1:** Subdural hematoma.

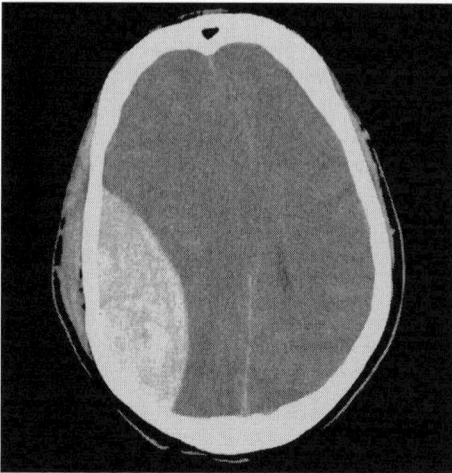

**Fig. 2:** Extradural hematoma.

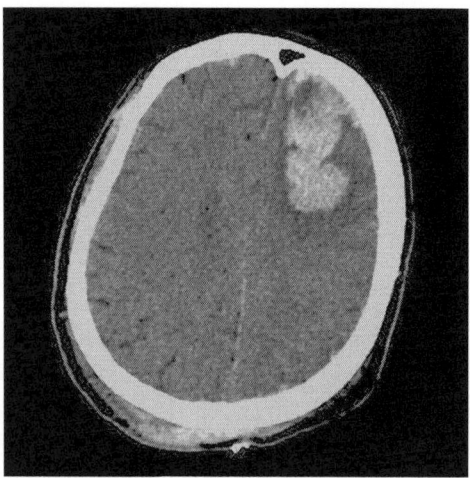

**Fig. 3:** Intracerebral hemorrhage.

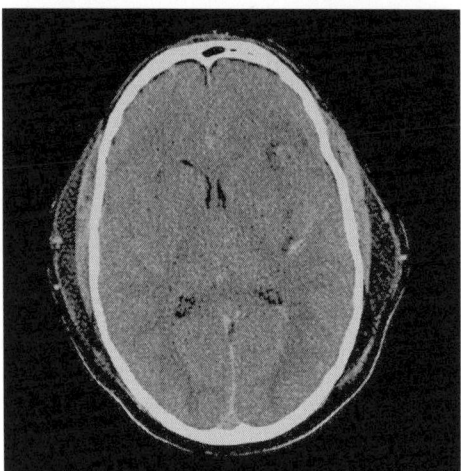

**Fig. 4:** Diffuse axonal injury.

## ■ PATHOPHYSIOLOGY OF TRAUMATIC BRAIN INJURY
### Changes in Cerebral Blood Flow
A triphasic response of changes in blood flow is observed following TBI. An initial phase of decreased blood flow in the first 12 hours is followed by a phase of hyperemia lasting 3–5 days, and then a gradual reflow is seen. Patients whose blood flow returns to near normal levels have better outcomes, whereas those whose flow remains low have a poor prognosis.[10,11]

### Cerebral Autoregulation
Cerebral autoregulation is a pressure-flow relationship and a regulatory process that maintains cerebral blood flow (CBF) constant across a range of blood pressures

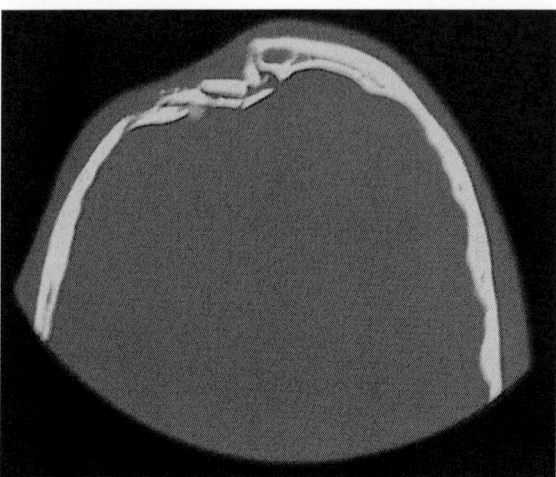

**Fig. 5:** Depressed fracture.

between 50 and 150 mm Hg. This mechanism ensures that as blood flow decreases, there is vasodilation and increased flow to maintain cerebral perfusion pressure (CPP). In contrast, when perfusion pressure increases, there is vasoconstriction and a decrease in blood flow. However, the autoregulation can be impaired, asymmetric, or lost following injury. The mechanisms that control autoregulation are myogenic, neurogenic, metabolic, and endothelial.[12,13]

## Cerebral Metabolism

The metabolic changes following injury can be described in two phases: An initial hyperglycolysis followed by a period of hypometabolism. Multiple pathways are activated, leading to changes in metabolism, inflammation, excitotoxic injury, and axonal injury, leading to secondary brain injury.[14-16] Changes in glucose metabolism play an important role in recovery following injury; there is a metabolic crisis, and if an alternate energy source is not available, the injury is likely to be more serious. Hyperglycemia is seen in moderate to severe injury and is an independent predictor of outcome. The role of lactate is being looked at with interest as it could be an alternate source to ensure normal metabolism in the face of a glycolytic crisis.[9] There is very little glycogen stored in the astrocytes, which gets depleted following TBI; recent studies have shown that there may be a significant role for lactate in the early management of patients.[17]

## Intracranial Hypertension

Traumatic brain injury is associated with increased ICP, resulting in edema, ischemia, hypoxia, and mass lesions. Untreated, this will result in secondary brain injury. In adults, normal ICP is considered 5–15 mm Hg and an ICP >22 mm Hg is considered high and must be treated. Elevations in ICP are detrimental as this can lead to decreased CPP and a decrease in CBF, which may result in cerebral ischemia. Elevated ICP can result in herniation syndromes, leading to neurological deficits and adversely affecting outcomes. When ICP becomes refractory to treatment, the prognosis is very poor. The CPP must be maintained between 60 and 70 mm Hg to avoid further injury.

## Cerebral Edema

Cerebral edema is a clinical state resulting from an excessive accumulation of fluid in the intracellular or extracellular spaces of the brain, causing a volumetric increase in brain tissue. There is the excess accumulation of fluid within the brain resulting from ischemia; hypoxia, which causes increased ICP, accounts for 50% of deaths in severe head injuries.[18] The types described are cytotoxic, interstitial, and vasogenic edema. Cytotoxic edema results in water accumulation in cells and is caused by disruption in the glial cell membrane and $Na^+$ and $K^+$ pump, leading to cellular swelling. The swollen cells alter neuronal and oligodendrocyte function.

Water retention and ions can adversely affect cell function and even lead to apoptosis. The blood–brain barrier (BBB) remains intact in cytotoxic edema.[19] Vasogenic edema results in water accumulation in the extracellular space and is caused by the tight BBB breakdown, which allows proteins and fluid to penetrate the parenchymal extracellular space. The edema spreads and moves extracellularly along fiber tracts and the gray matter. Vasogenic edema is associated with elevated ICP, tissue swelling, changes in blood flow, and compression of brain structures.[20]

## Excitotoxic Injury and Oxidative Stress

In the healthy brain, there is a delicate balance between reactive oxygen species (ROS) and antioxidants. Various ROS have been described; however, following injury, the excessive production of ROS following brain injury overwhelms the antioxidant systems and disrupts this balance, leading to lipid peroxidation, oxidation of proteins, deoxyribonucleic acid (DNA) break, and inhibition of the mitochondrial respiration, which leads to cell death **(Fig. 6)**. The endogenous antioxidant system comprises glutathione (GSH), glutathione reductase (GR), glutathione-S-transferase (GST), glutathione peroxidase (GPx), catalase (CAT), and superoxide dismutase (SOD). The antioxidant systems perform the task of eliminating the ROS from the body.[21-24]

## Intrathoracic Pressure

Patients with TBI often have associated lung injury and thoracic trauma. These injuries will usually require ventilator manipulation with high pressures and positive end-expiratory pressure (PEEP).[25] Concurrent pulmonary issues, such as pulmonary edema from fluid resuscitation, pneumonia, and acute respiratory distress syndrome can increase ventilator pressure requirements. High-pressure ventilation may harm ICP due to the effects of multiple chemical sensitivity (MCS). The impact of ITP on ICP is still unclear in humans, with studies showing increased ICP, whereas other studies have not shown similar effects. Various parameters, such as high-volume ventilation and high PEEP levels may influence the pressure. Inverse ratio ventilation and low tidal volume ventilation benefit the ICP. Still, they may increase the carbon dioxide levels, which can be deleterious in patients with already elevated ICP.[26] Airway pressure release ventilation (APRV), another ventilation mode with a prolonged inspiratory time, similarly did not increase ICP. In patients unable to maintain oxygenation, recruitment maneuvers, when performed with escalating PEEP, increased ICP in 75% of patients with TBI, with a resolution of the ICP elevation at recruitment maneuver completion.[27] However, ICP optimization may be sacrificed for increased ITP in patients with difficulty oxygenating or ventilating, as poor oxygenation is also

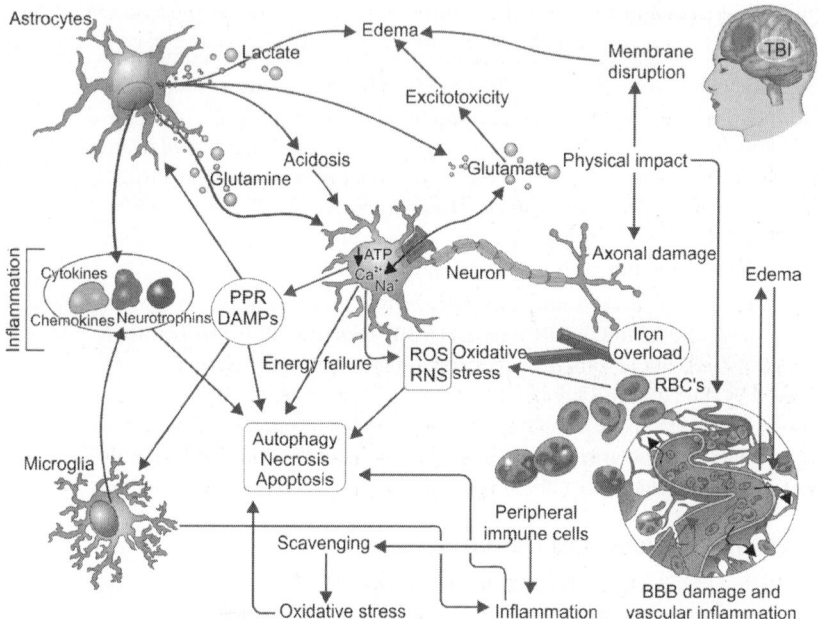

**Fig. 6:** Pathophysiology of traumatic brain injury (TBI). (BBB: blood–brain barrier; DAMPs: damage-associated molecular patterns; RBC: red blood cell; RNS: reactive nitrogen species; ROS: reactive oxygen species)

detrimental to TBI patients.[28] No specific recommendations are made for TBI patients in the intensive care unit (ICU) regarding ventilator strategies or settings.

## MANAGEMENT

### Goals for Anesthetic Management
- Adequate oxygenation
- Control of carbon dioxide
- Maintain or reduce ICP
- Maintain CPP and CBF
- Adopt strategies for neuroprotection

### Preoperative Evaluation and Stabilization
The anesthetic concerns are:
- Raised ICP
- Concurrent medical disease—hypertension, ischemic heart disease (IHD), asthma, and tuberculosis
- Difficult airway
- Effects of concomitant drug therapy
- Pregnancy
- Emergency procedure
- Other injuries—rib fractures, lung contusion, aspiration, and long bone fractures.

There is usually limited time for preanesthetic evaluation, which is often brief and relies on the history given. Information on premorbid medical conditions and previous anesthetic history must also be obtained if available. Rapid assessment of the cardiorespiratory system is done, and all must go through all available investigations such as complete blood count (CBC), glucose, urea, creatinine, sodium, and potassium levels, and liver function tests, if done, are noted. One must carefully examine chest and C-spine imaging studies and X-rays to rule out pulmonary aspiration, contusion, pneumothorax, hemothorax, rib fractures, and effusions **(Figs. 7 and 8)**. About 10% of patients with TBI also have associated spine injuries, and this must be ruled out before induction of anesthesia, either with X-rays of anteroposterior (AP), lateral, and mouth open views of the neck to rule out fractures, subluxation of the spine and odontoid process. Usually, when the CT of the brain is done, the spine is included in patients with TBI to rule out cervical spine injury **(Fig. 8)**.

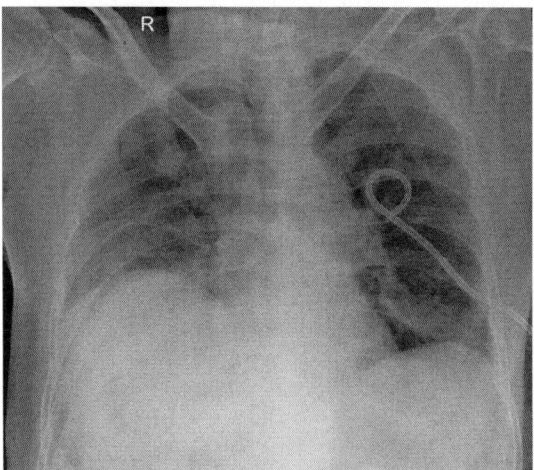

**Fig. 7:** Pneumothorax.

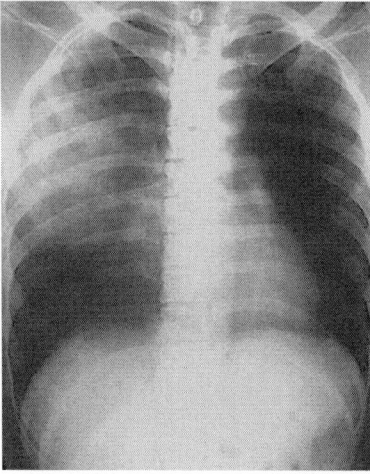

**Fig. 8:** Rib fractures and contusions.

## Induction of Anesthesia

All TBI patients should be considered full stomach, and measures to prevent aspiration must be taken, especially when in altered sensorium. Before induction of anesthesia, patients must be preoxygenated for 3–5 minutes. They are premedicated with fentanyl 2–3 µg/kg or morphine 0.15 mg/kg intravenously (IV). Anesthesia is induced with thiopental in the dose of 3–5 mg/kg or propofol at 2 mg/kg IV. Neuromuscular blockade is achieved with vecuronium 0.08–0.1 mg/kg or rocuronium in a 1 mg/kg IV dose. Succinylcholine can be used if a difficult airway is anticipated, even though there may be a transient increase in the ICP, and should be avoided if contraindicated. Rapid sequence induction (RSI) with manual in-line cervical spine stabilization should be done with cricoid pressure and endotracheal intubation after 3 minutes and achieving a minimum alveolar concentration (MAC) of −1 to 1.2. Lignocaine 1–1.5 mg IV is given 1 minute before intubation to attenuate the pressor response to intubation. Tracheal intubation is confirmed with capnography, and the tube is fixed after bilateral air entry is confirmed. The patient is positioned depending on the procedure, and all precautions must be taken to avoid pressure injuries. Surgery can be performed in the supine, lateral, or prone position.

## Airway Management

- Patients with severe TBI come to the operating room for surgery with their airways secured. The goals of airway management are adequate oxygenation, elimination of $CO_2$, gastric aspiration, increases in ICP, and aggravation of cervical spine injury. Cervical spine injury has to be ruled out before induction of anesthesia. All patients with TBI are assumed to have a C-spine injury, and precautions should be taken to avoid cord injury. The criteria to clear the C-spine when the patient is conscious are:[29]
- Absence of posterior midline cervical tenderness
- The patient is fully conscious and alert
- No evidence of intoxication
- Absence of neurologic deficits
- No painful distracting injuries

Radiological investigations are needed to clear the spine when the patient is unconscious. X-rays of the neck are taken AP, lateral, open mouth, right oblique, and left oblique views. A CT scan of the neck is done to diagnose instability in the form of fractures, dislocations, and the integrity of the three columns **(Fig. 9)**.

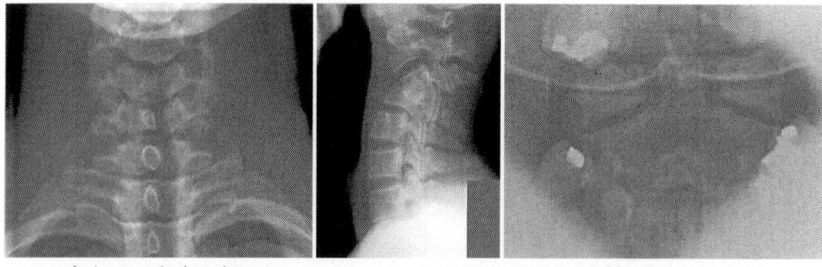

Anteroposterior view     Lateral view     Mouth open view

**Fig. 9:** Cervical spine—anteroposterior, lateral, and mouth open view.

## ■ INTRAOPERATIVE CONSIDERATIONS

- There is no single superior technique. Both inhalation agents and intravenous techniques are used in TBI patients. The methods commonly used are air + oxygen + narcotic + inhalation agent, or a total intravenous technique can be adopted. Intravenous fluids should be chosen to maintain euvolemia and avoid hyperglycemia. Intraoperative blood loss is managed with blood products based on the requirement. If there is brain swelling, hyperosmolar solutions can be used; 20% mannitol or hypertonic saline effectively produces the desired result. Ventilation is adjusted to maintain arterial partial pressure of carbon dioxide ($PaCO_2$) level of 30–35 mm Hg.
- *Hemodynamic management:* The management in TBI patients requires fluids, blood products, vasopressors, and inotropes to maintain CPP and cerebral blood to avoid ischemia. The intracranial causes of secondary brain injury are hematomas such as extradural, subdural, intracerebral, intraventricular and subarachnoid hemorrhage, brain swelling, infection, abscess, and seizures. The extracranial conditions that can lead to secondary brain injury are hypoxia, hypotension, hyponatremia, hypernatremia, hypercarbia, hyperglycemia, and hypoglycemia. Efforts must be made to avoid these conditions and treat them when they occur rapidly.

The major intraoperative complications seen are bleeding and brain swelling. Careful examination of imaging findings will guide the management as edema, midline shift, and mass effect will determine aggressive management to reduce ICP and produce a lax brain to improve operating conditions. The recommended targets for ICP and CPP are <22 mm Hg and a CPP target of 60–70 mm Hg. Intraoperative hypotension is defined as any systolic blood pressure (SBP) <90 mm Hg. Risk factors for intraoperative hypotension are low admission GCS score, preoperative tachycardia, hypertension, delayed surgery,[19] SDH, multiple lesions on CT, and longer duration of anesthesia. Intraoperative hypotension is an independent predictor of poor outcomes, and numerous episodes will only aggravate the situation.[30]

### Tracheal Extubation

The decision to extubate depends on multiple factors: Preoperative GCS, associated injuries, intraoperative complications, and recovery. In patients whose GCS is <8, it is better to leave the tube and ventilate in case the condition of the patients improves postoperatively; the decision to extubate can be taken.

### Monitoring

In addition to routine monitoring such as electrocardiogram (ECG), pulse oximetry, noninvasive blood pressure (NIBP), End-tidal carbon dioxide ($EtCO_2$), and temperature, special monitoring is available in jugular venous oxygen saturation, near-infrared spectroscopy (NIRS), and electroencephalogram (EEG), which can be used when needed. Multimodal monitoring will be more useful in the ICU.

## ■ CONCLUSION

Traumatic brain injury is a significant cause of morbidity and mortality and is of concern as it affects a very young population. The primary injury is not amenable to treatment. The emphasis has to be on preventing secondary brain injury by managing both intracranial and systemic causes. Prevention strategies must be used to educate the public about safe driving and change risk-taking behavior. Early diagnosis and treatment are the keys to making any meaningful difference in the management of TBI.

## ■ REFERENCES

1. Menon DK, Schwab K, Wright DW, Maas AI; Demographics and Clinical Assessment Working Group of the International and Interagency Initiative toward Common Data Elements for Research on Traumatic Brain Injury and Psychological Health. Position statement: Definition of traumatic brain injury. Arch Phys Med Rehabil. 2010;91(11):1637-40.
2. Centers for Disease Control and Prevention. National Center for Health Statistics: Mortality Data on CDC WONDER. Available from: https://wonder.cdc.gov/mcd.html. [Last accessed July, 2024].
3. Faul M, Xu L, Wald MM, Coronado VG. Traumatic brain injury in the United States: Emergency department visits, hospitalizations, and deaths. Atlanta (GA): Centers for Disease Control and Prevention, National Center for Injury Prevention and Control; 2010.
4. Veerappan VR, Nagendra B, Thalluri P, Manda VS, Rao RN, Pattisapu JV. Reducing the Neurotrauma Burden in India—A National Mobilization. World Neurosurg. 2022;165:106-13.
5. Langlois JA, Rutland-Brown W, Wald MM. The Epidemiology and Impact of Traumatic Brain Injury—A Brief Overview. J Head Trauma Rehabil. 2006;21(5):375-8.
6. Juul N, Morris GF, Marshall SB, Marshall LF. Intracranial hypertension and cerebral perfusion pressure: influence on neurological deterioration and outcome in severe head injury. The Executive Committee of the International Selfotel Trial. J Neurosurg. 2000;92:1-6.
7. Miller JD, Butterworth JF, Gudeman SK, Faulkner JE, Choi SC, Selhorst JB, et al. Further experience in the management of severe head injury. J Neurosurg. 1981;54:289-99.
8. Narayan RK, Greenberg RP, Miller JD, Enas GG, Choi SC, Kishore PR, et al. Improved confidence of outcome prediction in severe head injury. A comparative analysis of the clinical examination, multimodality evoked potentials, CT scanning, and intracranial pressure. J Neurosurg. 1981;54:751-62.
9. Scalea TM, Bochicchio GV, Habashi N, McCunn M, Shih D, McQuillan K, et al. Increased intra-abdominal, intrathoracic and intracranial pressure after severe brain injury: multiple compartment syndrome. J Trauma. 2007;62:647-56.
10. Marion DW, Darby J, Yonas H. Acute regional cerebral blood flow changes caused by severe head injuries. J Neurosurg. 1991;74:407-14.
11. Bouma GJ, Muizelaar JP, Stringer WA, Choi SC, Fatouros P, Young HF. Ultra-early evaluation of regional cerebral blood flow in severely head-injured patients using xenon-enhanced computerized tomography. J Neurosurg. 1992;77:360-8.
12. Drummond JC. The lower limit of autoregulation: time to revise our thinking? Anesthesiology. 1997;86:1431-3.
13. Lassen LA. Control of cerebral circulation in health and disease. Circ Res. 1974;34:749-60.
14. Ng SY, Lee AYW. Traumatic Brain Injuries: Pathophysiology and Potential Therapeutic Targets. Front Cell Neurosci. 2019;13:528.
15. Leichtle SW, Sarma AK, Strein M, Yajnik V, Rivet D, Sima A, et al. High-Dose Intravenous Ascorbic Acid: Ready for Prime Time in Traumatic Brain Injury? Neurocrit Care. 2020;32(1):333-9.
16. Demers-Marcil S, Coles JP. Cerebral metabolic derangements following traumatic brain injury. Curr Opin Anaesthesiol. 2022;35(5):562-9.

17. Brooks GA, Martin NA. Cerebral metabolism following traumatic brain injury: new discoveries with implications for treatment. Front Neurosci. 2015;8:408.
18. Marmarou A. Pathophysiology of traumatic brain edema: Current concepts. Acta Neurochir Suppl. 2003;86:7-10.
19. Badaut J, Ashwal S, Obenaus A. Aquaporins in cerebrovascular disease: a target for treatment of brain edema? Cerebrovasc Dis. 2011;31:521-31.
20. Nirula R, Millar D, Greene T, McFadden M, Shah L, Scalea TM, et al. Decompressive craniectomy or medical management for refractory intracranial hypertension: an AAST-MIT propensity score analysis. J Trauma Acute Care Surg. 2014;76:944-52.
21. Ansari MA, Roberts KN, Scheff SW. Oxidative stress and modification of synaptic proteins in hippocampus after traumatic brain injury. Free Radic Biol Med. 2008;45:443-52.
22. Cornelius C, Crupi R, Calabrese V, Graziano A, Milone P, Pennisi G, et al. Traumatic brain injury: Oxidative stress and neuroprotection. Antioxid. Redox Signal. 2013;19:836-53.
23. Readnower RD, Chavko M, Adeeb S, Conroy MD, Pauly JR, McCarron RM, et al. Increase in blood-brain barrier permeability, oxidative stress, and activated microglia in a rat model of blast-induced traumatic brain injury. J Neurosci Res. 2010;88:3530-9.
24. Jarrahi A, Braun M, Ahluwalia M, Gupta RV, Wilson M, Munie S, et al. Revisiting Traumatic Brain Injury: From Molecular Mechanisms to Therapeutic Interventions. Biomedicines. 2020;8:389.
25. Huynh T, Messer M, Sing RF, Miles W, Jacobs DJ, Thomason MH, et al. Positive end-expiratory pressure alters intracranial and cerebral perfusion pressure in severe traumatic brain injury. J Trauma. 2002;53:488-93.
26. Clarke JP. The effects of inverse ratio ventilation on intracranial pressure. Intensive Care Med. 1997;23:106-9.
27. Zhang XY, Yang ZJ, Wang QX, Fan HR. Impact of positive end-expiratory pressure on cerebral injury patients with hypoxemia. Am J Emerg Med. 2011;29:699-703.
28. Chesnut RM, Marshall LF, Klauber MR, Blunt BA, Baldwin N, Eisenberg HM, et al. The role of secondary brain injury in determining outcome from severe head injury. J Trauma. 1993;34:216-22.
29. Hoffman JR, Mower WR, Wolfson AB, Todd KH, Zucker MI. Validity of a set of clinical criteria to rule out injury to the cervical spine in patients with blunt trauma. National Emergency X-Radiography Utilization Study Group. N Engl J Med. 2000;343(2):94-9.
30. Sharma D, Brown MJ, Curry P, Noda S, Chesnut RM, Vavilala MS, et al. Prevalence and risk factors for intraoperative hypotension during craniotomy for traumatic brain injury. J Neurosurg Anesthesiol. 2012;24:178-84.

# CHAPTER 12

# Remifentanil: An Update

*Gaurav Kakkar*

## ABSTRACT

Remifentanil is a potent ultrashort-acting synthetic used in modern anesthetic practice for pain relief and as an adjunct to hypnotic anesthetic drugs. Remifentanil is a specific mu-type-opioid receptor agonist causing profound analgesia and sedation alongside a decrease in sympathetic tone and respiratory depression. It is metabolized rapidly by nonspecific plasma esterases and, therefore, has a rapid clearance and short duration of action. It is a crucial ingredient in practicing total intravenous anesthesia (TIVA). The drug is best used using the target-controlled infusion (TCI) pharmacokinetic model, which uses individual patient variables to calculate and safely deliver the estimated plasma or effect site concentrations. It can cause respiratory depression and bradycardia if given rapidly or in increased doses; hence, manual boluses are strongly discouraged. Appropriate training and robust patient monitoring are critical to its safe use in clinical anesthesia.

**Keywords:** Remifentanil; TCI Minto model; Context-sensitive half-life; Effect site concentration; Ultrashort-acting opioid; Plasma esterases

## KEY POINTS

- Ultrashort-acting opioid metabolized by plasma esterases
- Rapid onset and rapid offset have revolutionized anesthetic practice.
- Fixed context-sensitive half-life is independent of duration.
- No dose modifications for renal or liver impairment
- Best used through TCI pump using pharmacokinetic modeling
- Key synergistic drug for TIVA alongside propofol

## ■ INTRODUCTION

### Overview of Remifentanil

Remifentanil is a potent, ultrashort-acting synthetic opioid analgesic widely used in clinical settings, particularly in anesthesia. It belongs to the anilidopiperidine class of opioid analgesics, which also includes drugs such as fentanyl and alfentanil. Due to its unique pharmacokinetic properties, remifentanil allows for precise control over the duration and depth of analgesia, making it a valuable tool in modern anesthetic practice.[1]

Remifentanil is distinctive because it is metabolized by nonspecific esterases in blood and tissues rather than by the liver. This feature leads to a rapid onset and offset of action, which is particularly advantageous in surgical settings where quick adjustments to the depth of anesthesia are required.

## Historical Background

Remifentanil was first synthesized in the early 1990s and received approval from the US Food and Drug Administration (FDA) in 1996. Its development was driven by the need for an opioid that could be precisely controlled and adjusted in response to rapidly changing clinical conditions, such as those encountered during complex surgical procedures. Since its introduction, remifentanil has become a cornerstone in anesthetic practice due to its efficacy and versatility.

## Importance in Modern Medicine

The unique pharmacokinetic profile of remifentanil has revolutionized anesthetic practice, providing anesthesiologists with an unparalleled degree of control. Its rapid onset and offset make it ideal for use in procedures where quick recovery is essential, such as day surgeries and surgeries where patients need to be assessed promptly postsurgery. Also, its use in intensive care units (ICUs) for sedation and pain management highlights its broad indications in modern clinical practice.

# ■ CHEMICAL AND PHARMACOLOGICAL PROPERTIES

## Chemical Structure

Remifentanil has a chemical structure that distinguishes it from other opioids. It is classified chemically as 1-(2-methoxycarbonylphenyl)-4-(methoxymethyl)-4-piperidinecarboxylic acid methyl ester. *This structure includes an ester linkage, which is crucial for its rapid metabolism by nonspecific esterases and distinguishes it from opioids such as fentanyl, sufentanil, and alfentanil* **(Fig. 1)**.

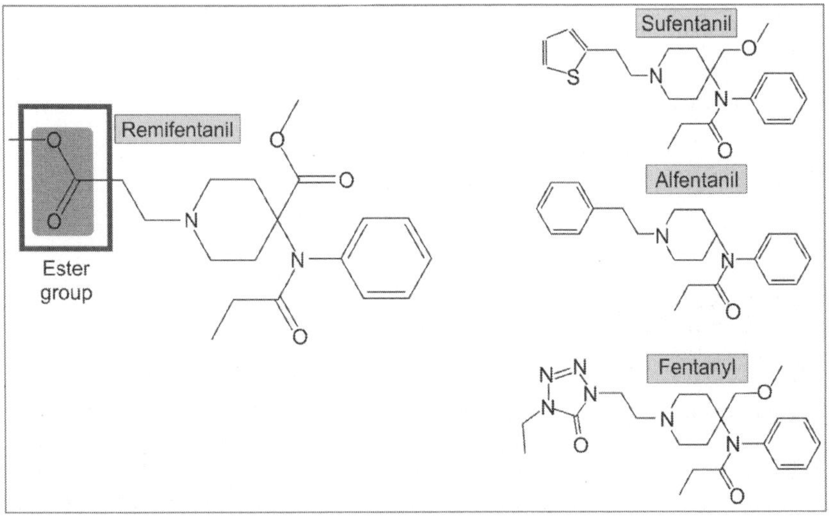

**Fig. 1:** Remifentanil structural comparison with sufentanil, alfentanil, and fentanyl.

## ■ MECHANISM OF ACTION

Like other opioids, remifentanil exerts its effects by binding to the μ-opioid receptors in the central nervous system (CNS). This binding results in the inhibition of ascending pain pathways, alteration of the emotional response to pain, and modulation of descending inhibitory pathways.[2] The high affinity of remifentanil for μ-opioid receptors ensures potent analgesic effects. It has minimal binding at κ, σ, and δ receptors. The kidney removes its active metabolite (minimal amount), remifentanil acid **(Figs. 2 and 3)**. Renal impairment has no consequence on the duration of action or residual drug.

### Pharmacokinetics and Pharmacodynamics

Rapid distribution and elimination phases characterize the pharmacokinetics of remifentanil. Its half-life is approximately 3–10 minutes, significantly shorter than other opioids, due to its rapid metabolism by nonspecific esterases.[3] This rapid clearance leads to a quick offset of action once the infusion is stopped, allowing precise analgesia control. Upon intravenous administration, it distributes quickly to the brain and other tissues, leading to an almost immediate onset of action. Fundamental pharmacokinetic properties include **(Table 1)**:

- *Half-Life:* Remifentanil's half-life is short, approximately 3–10 minutes, due to its rapid metabolism by nonspecific esterases.
- *Clearance:* It is cleared from the plasma rapidly, resulting in a quick offset of action once the infusion is stopped.
- *Volume of distribution:* It has a relatively small volume of distribution, indicating that it remains mainly in the bloodstream and readily accessible tissues.

Remifentanil's pharmacodynamics is consistent with those of other potent opioids. It provides analgesia and sedation **(Table 2)**. Its potency is approximately 100–200 times that of morphine. However, due to its rapid metabolism, the effects are short-lived, necessitating continuous infusion for sustained analgesia.

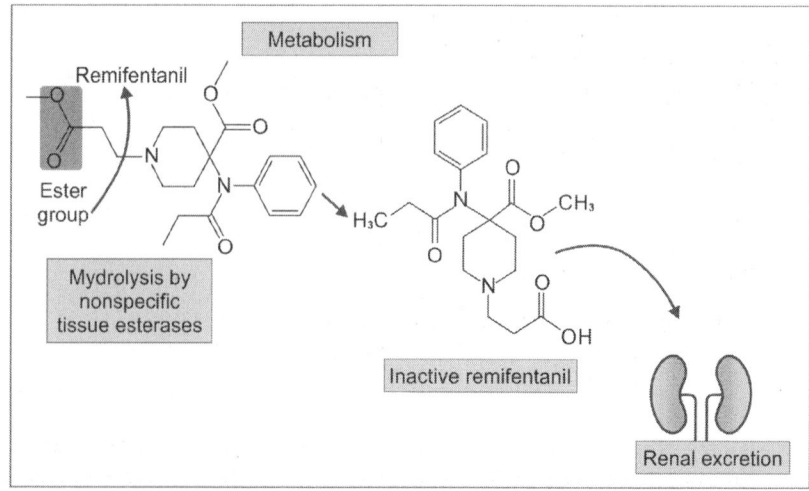

**Fig 2:** Metabolism of remifentanil by nonspecific tissue esters.

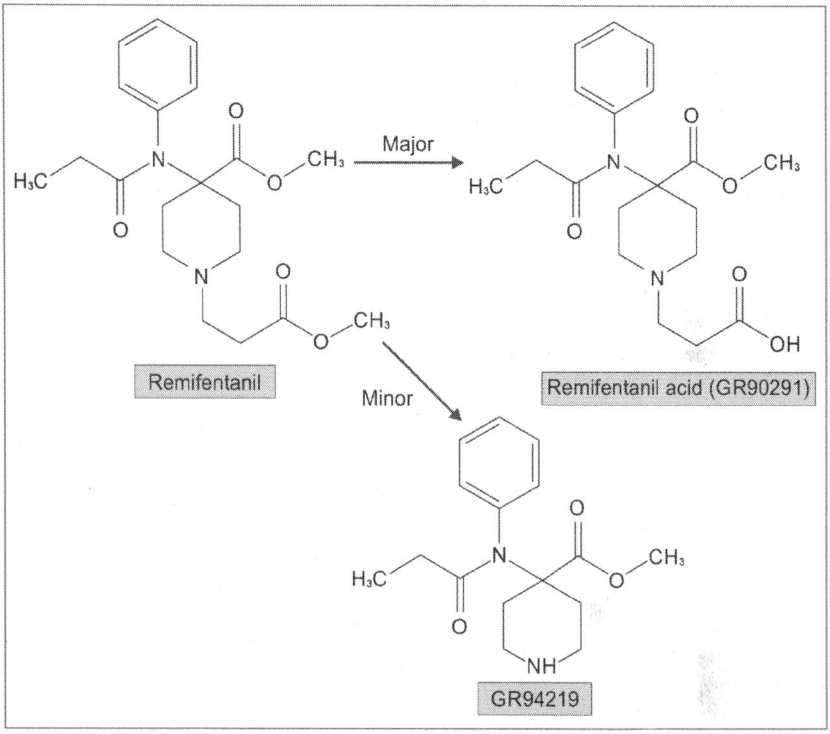

**Fig. 3:** Major and minor metabolites of remifentanil, namely remifentanil acid and GR94219, respectively.

| TABLE 1: Pharmacokinetic comparison of fentanyl and remifentanil. | | | | | | |
|---|---|---|---|---|---|---|
| Agent | Metabolite | Excretion | Protein binding (%) | Distribution (L/kg) | Half Life | Plasma clearance (mL/kg/min) |
| Fentanyl | Liver | Kidney | 84 | 4.1 | 3–4 hours | 13.3 |
| Remifentanil | Plasma | Kidney | 70 | 0.39 | 9.1 minutes | 2,800 |

| TABLE 2: Pharmacodynamic comparison of fentanyl and remifentanil. | | | | |
|---|---|---|---|---|
| Agent | Route of administration | Onset of action | Tmax | Duration of action |
| Fentanyl | IV | 1–2 minutes | 3–4 minutes | 30 minutes |
| Remifentanil | IV | 30 seconds | 1 minute | 5–7 minutes |
| (Tmax: time taken to reach the maximum concentration) | | | | |

- *Rapid onset:* Due to its high lipid solubility, Remifentanil quickly crosses the blood-brain barrier, leading to a rapid onset of analgesia within one minute of administration.[4]

- *Short duration:* The rapid metabolism by esterases leads to a swift decline in drug concentration once the infusion is stopped, making the duration of action very short **(Table 1)**.

These properties make remifentanil an excellent choice for procedures requiring rapid and precise control over analgesia **(Table 3)**.

## Context-sensitive Half-life

Context-sensitive half-life is defined as the time taken for the plasma concentration of a drug to decline by one-half after the infusion that is maintaining its steady state is stopped. The "context" is the duration of infusion **(Figs. 4 and 5)**. The outstanding feature of remifentanil is that there is no accumulation even after prolonged infusion. Its blood concentration decreases to 50% in 3–6 minutes, and recovery from the effects occurs rapidly within 5–7 minutes.[5]

In contrast to other opioids, remifentanil has a short and steady context-sensitive half-life of 3 minutes, which does not change with the increasing duration of infusion. This contrasts with alfentanil, which has a context-sensitive half-life that increases to 1 hour after a 4-hour infusion. Remifentanil is highly lipid soluble with a steady-state volume of distribution of around 30 liters. Unlike other opioids, the termination of action of remifentanil depends on rapid metabolic clearance rather than on redistribution.

**TABLE 3:** Significance of different half-lives of remifentanil.

| Remifentanil half-lives | Value in minutes | Significance |
|---|---|---|
| Rapid distribution half-life | 1 | Immediate onset |
| Slower distribution half-life | 6 | Easier dose titration |
| Terminal elimination half-life | 10–20 | Rapid clearance, Less accumulation |
| Effective biological half-life | 3–10 | Rapid recovery |
| Context-sensitive half-life | 3–6 | Independent duration of infusion |

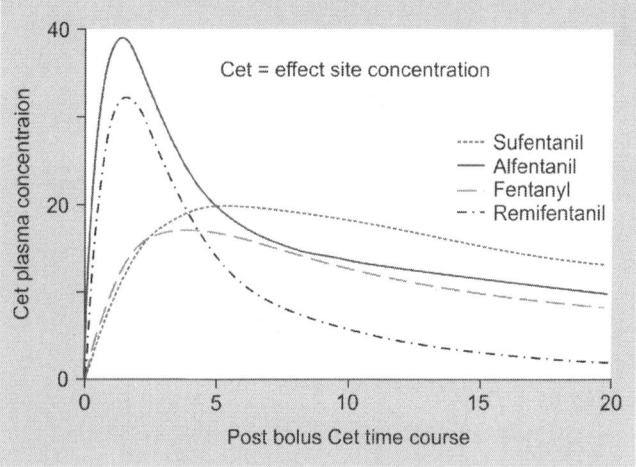

**Fig. 4:** Postbolus effect site plasma concentration-time course after various opioids.

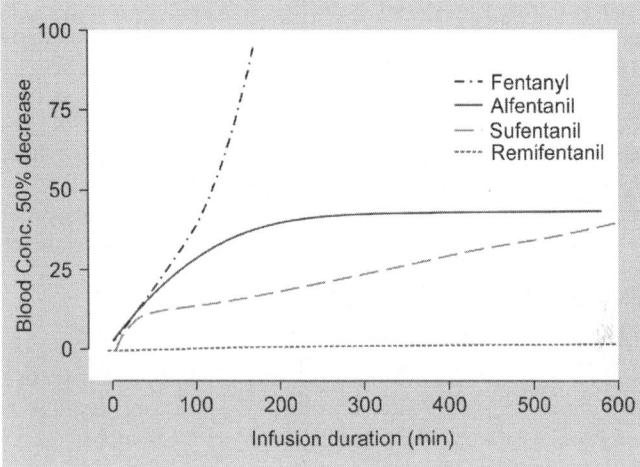

**Fig. 5:** Comparative context-sensitive half-lives of various opioids.

## ■ CLINICAL APPLICATIONS
### Use in Anesthesia
Remifentanil is widely used in balanced anesthesia techniques, providing the analgesic component. Its rapid onset and offset make it ideal for procedures requiring high precision in anesthetic depth. It is often used in combination with other anesthetics such as propofol or sevoflurane.
- *Induction of anesthesia:* Remifentanil induces anesthesia quickly due to its rapid onset.
- *Maintenance of anesthesia:* Continuous infusion during surgery allows for stable and adjustable analgesia.
- *Emergence from anesthesia:* Its rapid offset facilitates quick recovery and assessment postsurgery.

### Pain Management
Remifentanil is used in settings where precise pain control is necessary, such as during labor or in postoperative pain management. Its rapid onset and offset allow for titration to effect and quick cessation when no longer needed.
- *Labor pain:* Continuous infusion provides effective pain relief during childbirth with minimal drug accumulation.
- *Postoperative pain:* Short-term uses postsurgery for immediate pain relief.

## ■ INTENSIVE CARE
In the ICU, remifentanil is used for sedation and analgesia in mechanically ventilated patients. Its rapid clearance is particularly beneficial in this setting, allowing daily "sedation holds" to assess neurological status and readiness for weaning from mechanical ventilation.

### Comparative Effectiveness with Other Opioids
Compared to other opioids, remifentanil offers distinct advantages due to its pharmacokinetic properties, especially context-sensitive half-life **(Fig. 5)**. Unlike

morphine or fentanyl, it does not accumulate in the body, making it ideal for procedures requiring quick recovery. Its predictability and ease of titration provide a significant advantage over other opioids in many clinical scenarios.
- *Fentanyl:* While fentanyl is also potent and used in similar settings, it has a longer half-life and can accumulate, leading to prolonged effects.
- *Morphine:* It has a more prolonged onset and duration of action, making it less suitable for procedures requiring rapid adjustments in analgesia.

The ability to rapidly titrate remifentanil and its quick recovery profile make it superior in scenarios where precise control and quick return to baseline are crucial.

## ADMINISTRATION AND DOSAGE

### Availability and Reconstitution

Remifentanil for injection is available as a lyophilized white powder in glass vials containing 1 mg or 2 mg of remifentanil base. When reconstituted, it becomes a clear and colorless solution containing 1 mg/mL of remifentanil base as remifentanil hydrochloride for intravenous injection.

Remifentanil should be diluted, preferably in 0.9% saline, and given as an intravenous infusion, preferably through dedicated remifentanil target-controlled infusion (TCI) pumps, using three-compartment model such as the Minto model. The delivery through standard syringe drivers/models requires a deep understanding of its pharmacokinetic and pharmacodynamic properties and demands a continuous rate adjustment for the entire duration of its administration. Hence, manual infusion without TCI pumps is not without errors and human factor risks, especially when there is limited or no exposure to remifentanil. Manual boluses of this drug are to be strictly discouraged since profound bradycardia due to advertent fast or dosage errors can be fatal.

The most common dilution is the 50 µg/mL dilution, which requires 1 mg of the drug to be diluted in 19 mL. This can be increased to 2 mg in 40 mL of the diluent or 3 mg in 60 mL **(Table 4)**. Various other concentrations can be used, but it is recommended that a single individual/department have a single concentration policy to reduce potential drug-related errors.

### Guidelines for Different Procedures

The administration of remifentanil requires careful consideration of the clinical context. The dosage and rate of infusion are tailored based on the type and duration of the procedure and patient-specific factors.
- *General surgery:* For major surgeries, an infusion rate of 0.1–0.2 µg/kg/min is standard, with adjustments made based on the depth of anesthesia required.

**TABLE 4:** Remifentanil drug constitution and dilution table.

| Target concentration | Remifentanil vial strengths | Total volume of recommended diluent required | Volume of diluent required for reconstitution | Volume of diluent required for dilution |
|---|---|---|---|---|
| 50 µg/mL | 1 mg | 20 mL | 1 mL | 19 mL |
| 50 µg/mL | 2 mg | 40 mL | 2 mL | 38 mL |
| 20 µg/mL | 1 mg | 50 mL | 1 mL | 49 mL |

- *Short procedures:* For brief procedures, a bolus dose of 1 µg/kg followed by an infusion of 0.05–0.1 µg/kg/min may be used.
- *Labor and delivery:* An infusion rate of 0.025–0.05 µg/kg/min provides effective pain relief during labor.

## Remifentanil in Total Intravenous Anesthesia

Remifentanil is the most suitable opioid for total intravenous anesthesia (TIVA) and is routinely used in the TIVA practice along with propofol due to its synergistic action. A high remifentanil and low dose propofol TCI technique is usually the most popular technique followed by TIVA enthusiasts and results in rapid awakening and intraoperative stability.[6]

The usual effect site dose (Cet) for remifentanil is 6–7ng/mL, and that for propofol is 3–4 µg/mL, respectively. Higher doses may be required for younger or more anxious patients or painful procedures requiring careful titration.

The Minto model is the most commonly used TCI model for TIVA. It incorporates a three-compartment pharmacokinetic model of the drug.

It is named after Dr Charles Minto and is a model for predicting remifentanil concentration in plasma and the effect site (e.g., the brain).

It is advantageous to use TCI models like the Minto model since it has advantages over the "manual" or "µg.kg-1.min-1" practice where only the patient's weight is considered and no other parameters like age, height, and sex. This helps in reliable estimations of the pharmacokinetics of remifentanil in individual patients. It can only be used for patients over 12 years of age with a weight >30 kg. The pharmacokinetics of remifentanil play an essential role in the advancing age. Elderly patients significantly reduce the volume of distribution of remifentanil and the clearance rate compared to young patients. Thus, caution must be exercised during the use of remifentanil for elderly patients to reduce respiratory and cardiovascular side effects. Hence, a TCI model that has in-built safeguards is a preferred technique than to use the same drug via a manual syringe driver using a µg/kg/min regimen.

## ■ REMIFENTANIL IN SPECIAL POPULATIONS

### Use in Pediatric Anesthesia

Remifentanil is increasingly used in pediatric anesthesia due to its rapid onset and offset, allowing precise control over anesthesia depth.
- *Neonates and infants:* Lower infusion rates and careful titration are necessary due to the increased sensitivity of this population.
- *Older children:* Similar dosing strategies to adults, with adjustments based on weight and response.

### Use in Obstetrics

Remifentanil is used for pain relief during labor, offering an alternative to epidural analgesia in specific scenarios where the epidural might be contraindicated.[7] Studies comparing epidural and remifentanil patient-controlled analgesia (PCA) have shown similar patient outcomes and satisfaction scores.

Although remifentanil crosses the placenta, its quick redistribution and rapid metabolism ensure no residual actions in the fetal circulation, even in preterm neonates. To provide a safe PCA remifentanil service, there must be a 1:1 monitoring in the labor ward for continuous monitoring of the mother along with 1–2 L/min of oxygen to ensure no hypoxemia secondary to remifentanil's suppression of the respiratory system. It is always deemed good practice to inform the neonatology team regarding the use of remifentanil PCA by the mother in case the neonate requires any extra resuscitative measures.[8]

Remifentanil is of immense use even in cesarean sections where laryngoscopy response must be blunted, especially in preeclampsia and eclampsia. A TCI infusion with an effect site of 4–6 ng/mL is usually required at induction.[9] It is, however, advised to refrain from giving a manual bolus to achieve the same result as there can be rapid and overdelivery of the drug with severe complications of respiratory depression and rigidity, as compared to TCI infusion.

## Use for Sedation in Critical Care

Remifentanil infusion in the ICU perfectly meets the requirements of analgesia and sedation. Its short context sensitivity, half-life, and minimum or no residual effects are essential for use in the ICU. This further aids in the concept of daily sedation hold and spontaneous breathing trials of ICU patients, now a key performance indicator in critical care practice.[10] Also, no dose adjustment is required in liver or renal failure, which is a significant advantage with conventional opioids that are accumulated to multiple half-lives. A high dose of remifentanil over a prolonged period can cause hyperalgesia, so care should be taken to limit its dose and duration. The other disadvantage is its use in nonintubated patients in critical care, where careful titration and patient selection may be required to minimize respiratory depression and bradycardia/hypotension.

The usual dose in ventilated patients with or without propofol: 0.1–0.15 µg/kg/min or (4–6 ng/mL Cet).

The usual dose in non-ventilated patients: 0.05–0.1 µg/kg/min.

## Use for Conscious Sedation

Remifentanil is a drug of choice for a variety of procedures requiring conscious sedation. However, familiarity with the drug, its delivery matrix, and side effects is essential. Careful selection of patients and availability of complete monitoring and resuscitative equipment are always necessary with this drug. Sedation should always be given using a TCI pump with the Minto model with the usual initial effect side dose (Cet) of 2 ng/mL, which can be titrated carefully to the desired effect. The various procedures that benefit from conscious sedation by remifentanil are bronchoscopy, endoscopy, vertebroplasty, dressing change, biopsy procedures, fracture reductions, etc.

## Use for Awake Fiberoptic Intubation

Awake fiberoptic intubation is a crucial skill required for every anesthetist, and remifentanil provides suitable conditions for skilled hands to achieve this. Drug plasma concentration of 3–4 ng/mL at a dose of approximately 0.15 µg/kg/min is usually enough to facilitate intubation, keeping the patient calm and relaxed. Slow titration in aliquots of 0.1–0.5 ng/mL increases the level in sensitive patients. Concomitant use of oxygen via either nostril, glycopyrrolate to prevent bradycardia, and nasal phenylephrine/lignocaine spray are helpful strategies to supplement the technique. Complete monitoring should be applied as routine. This technique requires careful planning and patience at every step for the drug to have its desired effects on the patient.

## Use in Patients with Chronic Pain

Although less common, remifentanil can be used in specific chronic pain scenarios, particularly where rapid titration and control are required.
- *Acute on chronic pain:* Used in controlled settings to manage severe exacerbations of chronic pain.
- *Procedural pain:* Provides adequate analgesia for procedures in patients with chronic pain conditions.

## Safety and Side Effects

### Common Side Effects

Like all opioids, remifentanil is associated with side effects, most of which are dose-dependent and can be managed with appropriate monitoring and intervention.
- *Nausea and Vomiting:* Common, particularly during the postoperative period.

### Serious Adverse Effects

While serious adverse effects are less common, they can occur, particularly with improper dosing or lack of monitoring.
- *Severe respiratory depression:* This can lead to hypoxia and require immediate intervention.
- *Muscle rigidity:* Particularly at high doses or rapid administration
- *Severe bradycardia or asystole:* With rapid bolus administration. Requires prompt treatment.
- *Hyperalgesia:* Some patients report a hyperalgesia response after prolonged use of high-dose remifentanil, but this is not seen in routine cases.[11]

## Patient-specific Considerations

Several patient-specific factors must be considered when administering remifentanil, including age, weight, and overall health status.
- *Pediatric patients:* Dosage adjustments are necessary based on age and weight, with lower infusion rates typically used.
- *Geriatric patients:* Elderly patients may require lower doses due to increased sensitivity to opioids.
- *Renal or hepatic impairment:* Although the liver or kidneys do not metabolize remifentanil, caution is advised, although dose adjustment is usually unnecessary.
- *Patients with cardiovascular disease:* Careful titration is necessary to avoid hemodynamic instability.
- *Patients with respiratory disease:* Close monitoring is essential due to the risk of respiratory depression.

## ■ CONTRAINDICATIONS

It is not approved for *epidural or intrathecal* use in clinical practice because it contains glycine as an acidic buffer.

## STRATEGIES FOR MITIGATION, MONITORING, AND MANAGEMENT

To minimize the risk of side effects, several strategies can be employed:
- *Titration to effect:* Adjusting the dose based on patient response
- *Continuous monitoring:* Using pulse oximetry, capnography, and electrocardiogram (ECG) to detect early signs of adverse effects
- *Use of TCI pumps:* TCI pumps and plasma and effect site concentrations reduce the chances of the above complications.

Effective management of side effects involves proactive monitoring and prompt intervention. Anesthetists should be prepared to manage respiratory depression, cardiovascular instability, and other potential complications. Continuous monitoring of respiratory rate, oxygen saturation, and end-tidal $CO_2$ should be used to adjust the infusion rate based on respiratory parameters and can help prevent severe respiratory depression. Regular blood pressure and heart rate assessment and use of vasopressors or fluid administration may be required to manage hypotension. Assessing for signs of muscle rigidity and adjusting the infusion rate or administering muscle relaxants may be needed occasionally.

### Remifentanil and Technology

#### Role in Modern Surgical Techniques

Remifentanil plays a crucial role in modern surgical techniques, particularly those requiring rapid changes in anesthetic depth.
- *Minimally invasive surgery:* Allows for precise control over analgesia, facilitating rapid recovery.
- *Robotic surgery:* Used with advanced monitoring techniques to ensure optimal patient outcomes.

#### Integration with Anesthesia Machines and Monitors

Modern anesthesia machines are equipped to deliver remifentanil infusions with high precision, integrating advanced monitoring capabilities.
- *Target-controlled infusion:* Systems allow for precise control over drug delivery, adjusting based on pharmacokinetic models.
- *Automated infusion devices:* Enhance safety and efficacy by providing continuous feedback and adjustment.

## RESEARCH AND FUTURE DIRECTIONS

### Current Research Trends

Ongoing research focuses on optimizing the use of remifentanil in various clinical settings and exploring new applications.
- *Enhanced recovery protocols:* Studies on the role of remifentanil in facilitating rapid recovery postsurgery.
- *Combination therapies:* Research the synergistic effects of remifentanil with other anesthetic agents.

## Potential New Applications

Innovations in drug delivery and new clinical protocols may expand the use of remifentanil.

- *Noninvasive delivery systems:* Development of novel delivery methods, such as transdermal systems.
- *Extended indications:* Exploration of remifentanil's use in new areas, such as chronic pain management and emergency medicine.

## Innovations in Delivery Systems

Technological advancements may lead to more efficient and safer methods of administering Remifentanil.

- *Smart infusion pumps:* Devices that adjust dosing based on real-time patient data.
- *Biodegradable drug carriers:* Development of carriers that provide controlled release of Remifentanil.

## ■ CONCLUSION

Remifentanil has transformed the landscape of anesthetic practice, providing unparalleled control over analgesia with its unique pharmacokinetic properties. Its rapid onset, offset, and potent analgesic effects make it an invaluable tool in modern medicine.

Emphasis should be placed on initiating mandatory training and competencies before novice practitioners use the drug. Although it has been in use for the last 25 years worldwide, its recent entry into India makes it a novel drug for us. This precludes ample training, appropriate infusion, and monitoring equipment for safe patient outcomes.[12]

## ■ REFERENCES

1. Egan TD. Pharmacokinetics and pharmacodynamics of remifentanil: an update in the year 2000. Curr Opin Anaesthesiol. 2000;13:449-55.
2. Breen D, Wilmer A, Bodenham A, Bach V, Bonde J, Kessler P, et al. Offset of pharmacodynamic effects and safety of remifentanil in intensive care unit patients with various degrees of renal impairment. Crit Care. 2004;8:R21-R30.
3. Komatsu R, Turan AM, Orhan-Sungur M, McGuire J, Radke OC, Apfel CC. Remifentanil for general anaesthesia: a systematic review. Anaesthesia. 2007;62:1266-80.
4. Mertens MJ, Engbers FHM, Burm AGL, Vuyk J. Predictive performance of computer-controlled infusion of remifentanil during propofol/remifentanil anaesthesia. Br J Anaesth.2003;90(2):132-41.
5. Minto CF, Schnider TW, Egan TD, Youngs E, Lemmens HJ, Gambus PL, et al. Influence of age and gender on the pharmacokinetics and pharmacodynamics of remifentanil. Model development. Anesthesiology. 1997;86(1):10-23.
6. Mertens MJ, Olofsen E, Engbers FH, Burm AG, Bovill JG, Vuyk J. Propofol reduces perioperative remifentanil requirements in a synergistic manner: response surface modeling of perioperative remifentanil-propofol interactions. Anesthesiology. 2003; 99(2):347-59.
7. Freeman LM, Bloemenkamp KW, Franssen MT, Papatsonis DN, Hajenius PJ, Hollmann MW, et al. Patient controlled analgesia with remifentanil versus epidural analgesia in labour: randomized multicenter equivalence trial. Br Med J. 2015;350:h846.

8. Douma MR, Verwey RA, Kam-Endtz CE, van der Linden PD, Stienstra R. Obstetric analgesia: a comparison of patient-controlled meperidine, remifentanil, and fentanyl in labour. Br J Anaesth. 2010;104(2):209-15.
9. Yoo KY, Kang DH, Jeong H, Jeong CW, Choi YY, Lee J. A dose-response study of remifentanil for attenuation of the hypertensive response to laryngoscopy and tracheal intubation in severely preeclamptic women undergoing caesarean delivery under general anaesthesia. Inter J Obstet Anaesth. 2013;22:10-8.
10. Reade MC, Finfer S. Sedation and delirium in the Intensive Care Unit. N Engl J Med. 2014;370:444-54.
11. Fletcher D, Martinez V. Opioid-induced hyperalgesia in patients after surgery: a systematic review and a meta-analysis. Br J Anaesth. 2014;112(6):991-1004.
12. Checketts MR, Alladi R, Ferguson K, Gemmell L, Handy JM, Klein AA, et al.; Association of Anaesthetists of Great Britain and Ireland. Recommendations for standards of monitoring during anaesthesia and recovery 2015: Association of Anaesthetists of Great Britain and Ireland. Anaesthesia. 2016;71(1):85-93.

# CHAPTER 13

# Anesthesia for Geriatric Cancer Patients

*Uma Hariharan, Rajiv Chawla, Shagun Bhatia Shah*

## ABSTRACT

With the rise in life expectancy and advancements in medical science, there is a more significant senior population that is exposed to cancer risk, warranting that anesthesiologists be prepared for newer challenges. For better perioperative outcomes, a detailed geriatric assessment, risk stratification, nutritional support, and tailored anesthesia for these elderly cancer patients are required. In addition to preexisting comorbid conditions and polypharmacy, the major perioperative concerns include malnutrition, delirium, frailty, postoperative cognitive dysfunction, postoperative pulmonary complications, chronic pain, thromboembolic phenomenon, and chemotherapy-induced toxicity in these older age group patients. Both prehabilitation and rehabilitation play a prime role in positive outcomes and early return to activities of daily living. The senior population's anatomical, physiological, and pharmacological changes must be considered while planning their anesthesia and analgesia.

**Keywords:** Geriatric population; Chronological age; Society of Geriatric Oncology; American Geriatric Society; Polypharmacy; Malnutrition in elderly cancer patients (MECP); Sarcopenia; Comprehensive geriatric assessment; Delirium; Postoperative cognitive dysfunction; WHO analgesic ladder; Charlson comorbidity index; Beers criteria; Immunonutrition; Bispectral index (BIS)

## KEY POINTS

- More and more older age group patients are presenting for onco-surgeries with possible chemoradiotherapy and concurrent problems.
- In addition to anatomical, physiological, and pharmacological changes, geriatric patients have multiple comorbidities, frailty, cognitive decline, malnutrition, elder abuse, and polypharmacy.
- Assessment, prevention, and treatment of malnutrition in elderly cancer patients are essential aspects of perioperative care, along with risk stratification and optimization of comorbid conditions.
- Tailor-made anesthesia regimen with titrated drug doses, bispectral index (BIS) monitoring, and curated analgesia techniques form the cornerstone of perioperative management, in addition to maintenance of hemodynamic profile, normothermia, normoxia, and normocarbia.
- There is an urgent need to revamp the country's senior oncology services and follow the "comprehensive geriatric assessment" model, which includes palliative care.

## INTRODUCTION

The incidence of cancers is rising globally, and the older age group is not immune. As per the International Society of Geriatric Oncology (SIOG),[1] the older age group is >70 years old. The American Society of Clinical Oncology (ASCO) recommendations are for persons aged 65 years and older. Both chronological and physiologic factors are encompassed in the term "elderly". There are two separate groups in chronological component:[2] "young old" (65–80 years of age) and "older old" (>80 years of age). Functional capacity and organ system reserve regarding pathophysiologic parameters define physiologic age. Geriatric cancer rates are increasing, and there is a growing need to optimize the perioperative care of such patients. With advancements in geriatric oncology and cancer surgery, the anesthesiologist must be geared up to circumvent the challenges of geriatric onco-anesthesia. In addition to the possibility of preexisting comorbid conditions, these patients will be on multiple drugs (polypharmacy), which have perioperative implications and interactions. Other pertinent concerns include delirium, postoperative cognitive dysfunction, frailty, nutritional deficiencies, chronic pain, elder abuse, venous thromboembolism, pressure sores, and advance directives. Survival alone is not the prime goal but providing optimal quality of life after the onco-surgery is paramount. Except for testicular cancer, the incidence rate of cancers is significantly higher among the elderly than among any groups of younger and middle-aged persons. Older age-group men have an almost double cancer incidence rate compared with older women. The most commonly diagnosed[3] cancers are of the lung (16%), prostate (13%), and urinary bladder (13%) in men >80 years old, and breast (19%), colorectum (14%), and lung (14%) in women older than 80 years.

## ANATOMICAL AND PHYSIOLOGICAL CHANGES IN THE ELDERLY

The various anatomical and physiological changes in the senior population are to be kept in mind while planning the perioperative care of the patient to maximize patient safety and minimize poor outcomes in the elderly. There is an increased risk of postoperative pulmonary complications (PPCs) in older people[4] due to these changes. These alterations, summarized in the adjoining table **(Table 1)**, are essential in planning the perioperative care of the elderly cancer patient.

## GERIATRIC PHARMACOLOGY

- Alterations in the activity of the drug-metabolizing enzymes affect drug efficacy and toxicity in older people. **Tables 2 and 3** summarize the pharmacokinetic[5] and pharmacodynamic[6] drug considerations in older people.
  - Changes in hepatic blood flow, liver mass, or hepatic endothelium.
  - 30–50% ↓ clearance of drugs metabolized by the liver.
  - ↑ bioavailability of drugs (opioids, metoclopramide).
  - ↑ risk of dose-related adverse drug reactions (ADRs).
  - ↓ activation of prodrug/metabolites → ↓/delayed efficacy [angiotensin-converting enzyme inhibitors (ACEIs)].
  - No changes in drug microsomal enzyme activity.
- Phase 2 metabolism
  - Conjugation pathways remain relatively unchanged.
  - 30–35% ↓ in conjugation in patients taking an average of 5.2 prescription drugs/day.

## TABLE 1: Anatomical and physiological changes in the elderly.

| System | Changes |
|---|---|
| Respiratory | • *Increased alveolar-arterial (A-a) gradient due to:* Dysfunctional mucociliary transport system, connective tissue changes in the lung parenchyma causing reduced elasticity, reduced overall number of alveoli, and increase in alveolar duct size<br>• Impaired cough and swallow reflex leads to increased risk of aspiration<br>• Increased chances of hospitalization due to respiratory illness/infection, higher risk of respiratory failure, ARDS<br>• Reduced FEV and VC; increased risk of desaturation on apnea |
| Cardiovascular | • Attenuated parasympathetic responses and increased resting sympathetic tone<br>• Sinus node intrinsic rate and atrioventricular (AV) conduction slowing, resulting in bradycardia<br>• Valvular calcification, increased ventricular stiffness, diastolic dysfunction, and higher preload dependence<br>• Intra-arterial and venous wall changes causing vessel stiffness and fragility<br>• More vulnerable to the shifts in intravascular volume status; reduced cardiac index<br>• Increased incidence of heart failure, myocardial infarction, and cardiac arrythmias |
| Renal | • Reduced renal mass due to loss of renal cortex (>50 years); Decreased number of functioning glomeruli and ↑ size of the remaining glomeruli<br>• Reduced effective renal blood flow (up to 10% per decade)<br>• Reduced production and responsiveness of renin-angiotensin system<br>• Reduced ability to concentrate urine and potential risk for volume depletion<br>• More susceptible to injury or AKI from hypovolemia and nephrotoxins |
| Hepatic | • Reduced hepatic blood flow and function<br>• Decreased phase 1 (P450) enzyme reactions<br>• Increased drug levels/toxicity if dose adjustments not made |
| Brain/CNS | • Significant losses in gray and white matter volume<br>• Reduced cerebral blood flow<br>• Increased blood brain barrier permeability<br>• Increased risk of physical frailty and decline in cognitive function<br>• Decreased peripheral conduction velocity (demyelination)<br>• Reduced visual and auditory acuity, impaired vibration and position sense, and increased reaction time |
| Musculoskeletal | • Sarcopenia (exacerbated by inflammation, immobilization, endocrine stress responses, nutritional deficit, and impaired microcirculation)<br>• Proinflammatory mediators such as TNF alpha, IL-1, IL-6, GDF-15, illness-induced sodium channel dysfunction, and altered intracellular calcium homeostasis play role in muscle breakdown |

*Contd...*

*Contd...*

| System | Changes |
|---|---|
| | • Neuropathic changes include axonal degeneration, microvascular changes due to sepsis, and channelopathies and enhanced risk of ICU-associated weakness<br>• Osteoporosis leads to vertebral compression and hip fracture, increased chances of long bone fractures with trauma |
| Nutrition | • Increased chances of preexisting malnutrition and inadequate dietary intake, coupled with functional decline, sarcopenia, anemia, and poor wound healing<br>• Increased chances of infection |
| Immune system | • Immunosenescense due to: Increased level of proinflammatory cytokines at baseline and reduced antigenic response, chronic hyperstimulation of the immune system, risk of dysregulated systemic response to infection<br>• Enhanced risk of secondary and hospital acquired infections<br>• Changes in gut microbiome (by diet, lifestyle, medications, and overall health status) with an increase in proinflammatory bacteria associated with inflammatory dysregulation and immune dysfunction |
| Body composition | • Increased total body water: Increased initial plasma volumes for bolus doses<br>• Reduced lean body mass: Reduced volume of distribution of hydrophilic drugs |

(ARDS: acute respiratory distress syndrome; AKI: acute kidney injury; CNS: central nervous system; FEV: forced expiratory volume; IL: interleukin; GDF: growth differentiation factor; VC: vital capacity; TNF: tumor necrosis factor)

**TABLE 2:** Pharmacokinetic considerations in the elderly.

| System | Changes |
|---|---|
| Respiratory | • Increased alveolar-arterial (A-a) gradient due to: Dysfunctional mucociliary transport system, connective tissue changes in the lung parenchyma causing reduced elasticity, reduced overall number of alveoli and increase in alveolar duct size<br>• Impaired cough and swallow reflex leads to increased risk of aspiration<br>• Increased chances of hospitalization due to respiratory illness/infection, higher risk of respiratory failure, ARDS<br>• Reduced FEV and VC; increased risk of desaturation on apnea |
| Cardiovascular | • Attenuated parasympathetic responses and increased resting sympathetic tone<br>• Sinus node intrinsic rate and AV conduction slowing, resulting in bradycardia<br>• Valvular calcification, increased ventricular stiffness, diastolic dysfunction and higher preload dependence<br>• Intra-arterial and venous wall changes causing vessel stiffness and fragility<br>• More vulnerable to the shifts in intravascular volume status; reduced cardiac index |

*Contd...*

*Contd...*

| System | Changes |
|---|---|
| | • Increased incidence of heart failure, myocardial infarction and cardiac arrythmias |
| Renal | • Reduced renal mass due to loss of renal cortex (>50 years); decreased number of functioning glomeruli and ↑ size of the remaining glomeruli; Reduced effective renal blood flow (up to 10% per decade)<br>• Reduced production and responsiveness of renin-angiotensin system<br>• Reduced ability to concentrate urine and potential risk for volume depletion<br>• More susceptible to injury or AKI from hypovolemia and nephrotoxins |
| Hepatic | • Reduced hepatic blood flow and function<br>• Decreased phase 1 (P450) enzyme reactions<br>• Increased drug levels/toxicity if dose adjustments not made |
| Brain/CNS | • Significant losses in gray and white matter volume<br>• Reduced cerebral blood flow<br>• Increased blood brain barrier permeability<br>• Increased risk of physical frailty and decline in cognitive function<br>• Decreased peripheral conduction velocity (demyelination)<br>• Reduced visual and auditory acuity, impaired vibration and position sense and increased reaction time |
| Musculoskeletal | • Sarcopenia (exacerbated by inflammation, immobilization, endocrine stress responses, nutritional deficit, and impaired microcirculation)<br>• Proinflammatory mediators such as TNF alpha, IL-1, IL-6, GDF-15, illness-induced sodium channel dysfunction, and altered intracellular calcium homeostasis play role in muscle breakdown<br>• Neuropathic changes include axonal degeneration, microvascular changes due to sepsis, and channelopathies and enhanced risk of ICU-associated weakness<br>• Osteoporosis leads to vertebral compression and hip fracture, increased chances of long bone fractures with trauma |
| Nutrition | • Increased chances of preexisting malnutrition and inadequate dietary intake, coupled with functional decline, sarcopenia, anemia, and poor wound healing<br>• Increased chances of infection |
| Immune system | • Immunosenescense due to: Increased level of proinflammatory cytokines at baseline and reduced antigenic response, chronic hyperstimulation of the immune system, risk of dysregulated systemic response to infection<br>• Enhanced risk of secondary and hospital acquired infections<br>• Changes in gut microbiome (by diet, lifestyle, medications and overall health status) with an increase in proinflammatory bacteria associated with inflammatory dysregulation and immune dysfunction |
| Body Composition | • Increased total body water: increased initial plasma volumes for bolus doses<br>• Reduced lean body mass: Reduced volume of distribution of hydrophilic drugs |

(ARDS: acute respiratory distress syndrome; AKI: acute kidney injury; CNS: central nervous system; FEV: forced expiratory volume; IL: interleukin; GDF: growth differentiation factor; VC: vital capacity; TNF: tumor necrosis factor)

**TABLE 3:** Pharmacodynamic considerations in the elderly.

| System | Change | Clinical effect |
|---|---|---|
| Brain | • Brain atrophy<br>• ↓ catecholamines<br>• ↓ dopamine synthesis | • Forgetfulness, depression, Parkinsonism, insomnia, etc.<br>• ↑ sensitivity to sedation (opioids, anticonvulsants)<br>• Psychomotor impairment with CNS drugs |
| Endocrine | • Glucose intolerance<br>• ↓ BMR (vulnerable to stress) | • Dysglycemia risk |
| Cardiovascular | • ↓/altered homeostasis | • Need for hospitalization<br>• Risk of orthostatic hypotension<br>• ↑ risk of arrhythmias (digoxin) |
| Genitourinary | • BPH<br>• Vaginal/urethral mucosal atrophy | • ↑ residual urine and risk of infection<br>• Drug therapy<br>• ↓ diuretic effect of furosemide |

(CNS: central nervous system; BMR: basal metabolic rate; BPH: benign prostatic hyperplasia)

The latest American Geriatric Society (AGS) Beers criteria[7] for dose modification in elderly patients and potentially inappropriate medication use in the elderly need to be followed **(Table 4)**. Elderly patients are prone to adverse drug reactions due to unique physiological changes, polypharmacy, and age-related alterations in body composition and organ function. First introduced in 1991 and later updated in 2019 and 2023, the Beers criteria is classified into five categories.
1. Potentially inappropriate Medications.
2. Medications potentially inappropriate in patients with specific comorbidities or syndromes.
3. Medications to be used with caution.
4. Potentially inappropriate drug-drug interactions.
5. Medications with dosage adjustments based on renal function.

This criterion applies to adults 65 and older in all day-care, acute, and hospital settings, except those in hospice and end-of-life care settings.

## ■ PERIOPERATIVE CONCERNS IN THE GERIATRIC POPULATION

Accurate anesthesiology care is a prerequisite for optimal surgical outcomes in all patient groups, more so in the elderly population. The SIOG has formulated guidelines for elderly cancer patients. Their major perioperative concerns stem from the various physiological, anatomical, and pharmacological changes cited previously and the risks of different cancers and their therapies. In addition to the standard American Society of Anesthesiologists (ASA) and the New York Heart Association (NYHA) classification, the most common predictors of collective morbidities in older patients include preoperative transfusion, emergency surgery, weight loss, operative duration, and chronic obstructive pulmonary disease. The prime perioperative considerations[8] include the functional status of the elderly patient, cancer stage/metastases, extent/type of surgery planned along with anticipated complications, comorbid conditions

**TABLE 4:** American Geriatric Society (AGS)–Beers criteria drug dose modifications.

| Drug | GFR | Rationale | Recommendation | Quality | Evidence |
|---|---|---|---|---|---|
| Ciprofloxacin | <30 mL/min | ↑ risk of CNS effects (e.g., seizures, confusion) and tendon rupture | Dose ↓ when used to treat common infections | Moderate | Strong |
| Nitrofurantoin | <30 mL/min | Potential for pulmonary toxicity, hepatoxicity, and peripheral neuropathy, especially with long-term use | Avoid | Low | Strong |
| Cotrimoxazole | <30 mL/min | ↑ risk of worsening of kidney function and hyperkalemia; risk of hyperkalemia especially prominent with concurrent use of an ACE, ARB, or ARNI | • Reduce dosage if CrCl is 15–29 mL/min<br>• Avoid if CrCl <30 mL/min | Moderate | Strong |
| Enoxaparin | <30 mL/min | ↑ risk of bleeding | ↓ dose | Moderate | Strong |
| Fondaparinux | <30 mL/min | ↑ risk of bleeding | Avoid | Moderate | Strong |
| Dabigatran | <30 mL/min | Lack of evidence for efficacy and safety in individuals with a CrCl | Avoid when CrCl <30 mL/min. Dose adjustment when CrCl >30 mL/min in the presence of drug-drug interactions | Moderate | Strong |
| Rivaroxaban | <30 mL/min | Lack of efficacy or safety evidence in people with CrCl <15 mL/min | Avoid if CrCl <15 mL/min<br>↓ dose if CrCl is 15–50 mL/min following manufacturer dosing recommendations based on indication-specific dosing | Moderate | Strong |
| • Spironolactone (S)<br>• Triamterene (T) | <30 mL/min | Hyperkalemia with ST change<br>Hyponatremia with T | Avoid | Moderate | Strong |
| Baclofen | eGFR <60 mL/min/m² BSA | ↑ risk of encephalopathy in older adults with eGFR <60/chronic HD | • Avoid<br>• Use lowest possible dose when essential with close monitoring | Moderate | Strong |
| Levetiracetam | <80 | CNS adverse effects | ↓ dose | Moderate | Strong |
| Pregabalin and Gabapentin | <60 | CNS adverse effects | ↓ dose | Moderate | Strong |

(ACE: angiotensin converting enzyme; ARB: angiotensin receptor blocker; ARNI: angiotensin receptor-neprilysin inhibitor; BSA: body surface area; CNS: central nervous system; CrCl: creatinine clearance; GFR: glomerular filtration rate) with their level of optimization, nutritional status, pain management, postoperative critical care/intensive care unit (ICU) requirements, and palliative/end-of-life care decisions. With the advent of robotic surgery[9] for radical cancer resections, there have been positive results, given shorter ICU/hospital stays, reduced pain, and early return to preoperative status, though with newer challenges of patient safety for the perioperative care team. Promoting the application of prehabilitation enhances physical fitness and improves surgical outcomes in elderly cancer patients. Mortality indexes, such as the Schonberg or Lee indices,[10] which incorporate comorbid conditions, health status, functional status, and age, can help clinicians estimate life expectancy and guide cancer screening and treatment decisions. The type of malignancy also matters, in addition to age. Most geriatric patients who undergo breast cancer surgery have a lower incidence of complications as compared to patients who undergo CRS-HIPEC (cytoreductive surgery and hyperthermic intraperitoneal chemotherapy) and robotic-assisted laparoscopic prostatectomy, who develop more complications. The type of chemotherapy[11] administered also has a bearing. If succinylcholine is administered to a patient given cyclophosphamide, prolonged apnea can occur. Adriamycin or doxorubicin given for ovarian cancer can cause cardiac dysfunction and reduced ejection fraction [left ventricular ejection fraction (LVEF)], which can be deleterious during induction. Hence, it is preferable to use titrated doses of etomidate. In patients given bleomycin chemotherapy, it is preferable to keep lower inspired oxygen concentrations ($FiO_2$ ~33%), even during one-lung ventilation for lung cancer surgeries, due to the risk of oxygen toxicity, lung fibrosis, and risk of adult respiratory distress syndrome (ARDS).

## PREOPERATIVE ASSESSMENT AND RISK STRATIFICATION IN GERIATRIC ONCOLOGICAL PATIENTS

A thorough preoperative assessment of geriatric patients is beneficial in many ways, as it provides information about risk stratification and the presence of medical/nutritional problems requiring optimization, and it initiates postoperative planning regarding resource allocation and early rehabilitation. Return to intended oncologic therapy (RIOT)[12] is an important consideration to ensure the completeness of cancer treatment. As aging is a heterogeneous process, chronological age is less important than physiologic age in guiding surgical outcomes. Geriatric assessments involve multidisciplinary tools to assess the ability of the elderly patient to live their daily lives independently and evaluate physical and nutritional status, cognitive capacity, associated diseases, memory and psychological states, and access to social and financial support. Vital predictors in geriatric assessment regarding surgical outcomes in older patients with cancer include functional status, comorbidity, cognitive function, nutritional status, and depression. Preoperative risk stratification[13] can be done by slow gait speed (ability to walk 5 meters in >6 seconds) and cardiopulmonary exercise testing (CPET), a functional objective test in the elderly population. CPET measures estimated oxygen uptake at lactate threshold ($VO_2$ at LT) and peak exercise. Increased risk of perioperative mortality and morbidity following major surgery can be signaled by a $VO_2$ at LT <11 mL/Kg/min. Peak oxygen consumption and anaerobic threshold can also predict perioperative morbidity and mortality. CPET allows for decision-making regarding postoperative care and interventions to modify risk. Elderly patients with cancer have a higher risk of falling, which can cause a multitude of injuries like hip fractures. This can reduce the quality of life and survival. Early geriatric assessment can identify patients at risk of falls and prompt the implementation of measures to avoid falls, such as installing railings, starting physical and occupational therapy, and treating the underlying cause. The TUG or "timed up and go" evaluation is a screening test for the propensity to fall and also serves as a strong mortality indicator in the elderly.[14] Sarcopenia can be assessed by hand-grip dynamometry and gait speed walking (walking speed below 0.8 m/s in the 4 minutes walking test). Age-adjusted Charlson comorbidity index[15] can be used to identify higher-risk geriatric patients, and it is recommended that deep sedation be avoided in patients with greater scores. The American College of Surgeons National Surgical Quality Improvement Program/American Geriatric Society (ACSNSQIP/AGS)[16] advocates assessment using multiparametric frailty scales, as frailty strongly predicts adverse postoperative outcomes.

## ■ NUTRITIONAL ASSESSMENT

Malnutrition adversely affects body composition, physical function, and clinical outcomes. Nutritional assessment of older age group patients scheduled for oncosurgery includes diagnosis, prevention, and management of malnutrition. The diagnostic criteria[17] for malnutrition in geriatric oncology patients consist of the following:
- Significant weight loss (≥5% of premorbid weight) and/or low body mass index (BMI <22 kg/m$^2$);
- Hypoalbuminemia; and
- Significant and sustained reduction in food intake (<1,200 kcal/day in women, <1,500 kcal/day in men, or 22 and 25 kcal/kg/day, respectively).

Malnutrition in elderly cancer patients (MECP) is due to a multitude of factors, including progressive functional decline, medication effects, comorbid conditions, increased burden of symptoms such as anorexia/dysphagia/gastrointestinal dysmotility, psychosocial determinants, on-therapies like chemo/radiotherapy, and length of hospitalization. The most critical pathophysiologic mechanisms for the development of MECP include[18] starvation, sarcopenia, and cachexia. The chronic inflammatory and metabolic stress responses to cancer produce the vicious cycle of fat-muscle wasting, anorexia, fatigue, anemia, and hypoalbuminemia, resulting in anorexia-cachexia syndrome. Morley and Krenzle proposed a pneumonic "meals on wheels"[19] for treatable causes of MECP (M: medication side effects; E: emotional problems; A: anorexia; L: late-life paranoia; S: swallowing disorders; O: oral factors; N: nosocomial infections; W: wandering and other dementia-related behaviors; H: hyper/hypothyroidism, hyperparathyroidism, hypoadrenalism; E: enteric problems; L: low salt/low-cholesterol diets; S: smell/taste abnormalities). Nutritional assessment in older patients with cancer can be done by anthropometry (weight, BMI, skinfold, mid-arm and mid-calf circumferences), biochemistry [serum prealbumin/albumin, C-reactive protein (CRP), leptin, interleukin (IL)-6, interferon-γ, and tumor necrosis factor alpha (TNF-α)], functional (handgrip dynamometry and gait speed), body composition [bioelectrical impedance analysis, dual X-ray absorptiometry, computed tomography (CT)/magnetic resonance imaging (MRI)], and tests for energy metabolism as well as food intake. The standardized screening tools[20] for MECP include malnutrition universal screening tool (MUST), malnutrition screening tool

(MST), short nutritional assessment questionnaire (SNAQ), nutritional risk screening (NRS), mini nutritional assessment (MNA), nutrition risk index (NRI), subjective global assessment (SGA), and patient-generated subjective global assessment (PG-SGA). Hand grip dynamometer[21] is a quick, inexpensive, portable, and reliable tool to assess muscle strength, with values adjusted for age and gender. Perioperative nutritional therapy can be helpful in moderate to severe malnutrition if given for 7–14 days preoperatively, especially in patients who cannot ingest or absorb nutrients for a long time (e.g., oral cancer and free flap surgery patients). The risk-benefit ratio of the possibility of delaying onco-surgery for improving nutrition must be evaluated against the risk of cancer progression. Omega-3 fatty acid supplementation[22] may stabilize weight in cancer patients on oral diets experiencing progressive, unintentional weight loss. Immunonutrition with enteral feeds with arginine, nucleic acids, and essential fatty acids may benefit malnourished patients.

## ▪ PERIOPERATIVE MANAGEMENT

Perioperative management of geriatric cancer patients is more complex and labor-intensive than that of the general population. An electively performed cancer surgery is more successful than that performed in an emergency. Understanding the physiological, anatomical, nutritional, functional, and pharmacological characteristics/changes in elderly patients is paramount in anesthetic management. These patients' main focus of recovery is maintaining function and independence. On average, elderly patients take 3 months to reattain preoperative levels of activities of daily living and about 6 months for independent activities of daily living.[23] They must be handled gently as their skin is fragile and are prone to falls, injuries/bruising, and hypothermia. A thick layer of cotton padding must be wrapped around the upper arm beneath the blood pressure cuff, in exposed areas, and at pressure points. Additional time for preoxygenation must be given in older people to prevent induction hypoxia. Invasive monitoring may be instituted in the presence of comorbid illness for accurate fluid therapy, blood gas monitoring, cardiac output measurements, and administration of drug infusions. Transesophageal echocardiography is an effective evaluation tool for cardiac function and detecting diastolic dysfunction in older people. Care must be taken regarding perioperative positioning, judicious fluid therapy, and strict procedural asepsis. All inhalational agents' minimum alveolar concentration (MAC) declines with advancing age (30% lower for 80-year-old patients).[24] The MAC is reduced by 6% per decade of increasing age. They also need lesser amounts of intravenous (IV) induction agents. BIS monitoring is recommended for these patients. Thiopental sleep-dose requirements decrease linearly with age, with increased sensitivity to thiopental due to a decrease in central volume of distribution. Elderly patients are more sensitive to the soothing and hemodynamic effects of propofol. The bolus dose of propofol is reduced by 20% and the infusion dose by 30%. There is enhanced sensitivity to etomidate due to pharmacokinetic changes in older people. The induction-awakening times are prolonged, mandating careful dose titration and avoiding hemodynamic instability. The opioid doses (fentanyl, alfentanil, and remifentanil) required to achieve a given level of electroencephalogram (EEG) depression are reduced by 50% from 20 to 89 years of age.[25] Regarding remifentanil, the central volume and its clearance are decreased in elderly patients, resulting in higher plasma concentrations. To achieve the same effect, the bolus doses of remifentanil are halved, and the infusion rates are reduced to one-third of the adult dosage in the elderly population. There is a nearly 50% reduction in the bolus doses of morphine, fentanyl, and remifentanil in older patients. Dose requirements of muscle relaxants and anticholinergic drugs are unaffected by age. Nevertheless, recovery is prolonged due to changes in pharmacokinetics. Generalized muscle atrophy with senile motor neuron degeneration predisposes elderly patients to the exaggerated effects of muscle relaxants and muscle weakness. The sensitivity to the sedative effects of benzodiazepines (midazolam) is higher in geriatric patients due to pharmacodynamic changes within the gamma butyric acid type receptors.[26] Shorter-acting midazolam is preferred over diazepam. As per research, choosing total intravenous anesthesia (TIVA) over inhaled anesthetics may decrease postoperative delirium (POD) risk. As BIS correlates with the depth of sedation, independent of the patient's age, BIS-guided[27] anesthesia in the elderly can mitigate the risks of TIVA and reduce the anesthetic doses, with faster emergence and positive patient outcomes. It is advisable to use BIS-guided anesthesia maintenance, with BIS levels kept between 50 and 60. With advancing age, both central and peripheral nervous systems are affected, resulting in prolonged duration of neural blockade, increased epidural/spinal anesthesia level, and greater incidence of hemodynamic instability. Due to enhanced sympathetic tone in elderly patients, anesthetic agents with sympathomimetic properties are poorly tolerated in those with cardiovascular disorders. In addition, there are interactions between anesthetic agents and cytotoxic agents. There can be prolonged apnea after succinylcholine in patients who have received cyclophosphamide. Azathioprine can reduce the potency of curare as compared to the potentiation of neuromuscular blockade by alkylating agents. Pulmonary toxicity and ARDS can occur when excessive oxygen is administered in patients who have received bleomycin therapy. Several geriatric syndromes may affect older patients, resulting in prolonged hospital stays and attendant complications. In anesthetic management, it is preferable to avoid long-acting benzodiazepines preoperatively and clear fluids can be given up to 2 hours before surgery. Adequate analgesia must be ensured with IV fentanyl or remifentanil and epidural or nerve block anesthesia, wherever possible. There is evidence that intraoperative dexmedetomidine prevents the emergence of delirium. As per meta-analysis by Yang W et al.,[28] it reduces postoperative cognitive dysfunction (POCD) at day seven due to neuroprotective, analgesic, and anti-inflammatory effects. Maintaining vital parameters within 20% of the baseline must ensure hemodynamic stability during the perioperative period. Avoid intraoperative hypotension (systolic blood pressure (SBP) <80 mm Hg and mean arterial pressure (MAP) <65 mm Hg) and maintain normoxia, normothermia, normovolemia, and normocarbia.

## PAIN RELIEF AND POSTOPERATIVE CARE IN GERIATRIC ONCOLOGICAL PATIENTS

Enhanced recovery after surgery (EARS) protocol must be utilized in all these patients. Postoperative nausea vomiting (PONV) requires prophylaxis in these patients, especially if the Apfel score >2. Refractory PONV may require multimodal PONV prophylaxis[29] with droperidol-dexamethasone before anesthesia induction, on danseur before reversal of anesthesia, and fosaprepitant or amisulpride as rescue drugs. Some of these cancer patients may be on opioids, and to reduce opioid-related PONV, alternative analgesics can be substituted, like IV lidocaine (1.5 mg/kg followed by 2 mg/kg) until discharge from surgical ICU or magnesium sulfate (40 mg/kg over 10 minutes). The primary postoperative concern is the prevention and management of delirium, as the perioperative period poses several risk factors for its development in elderly patients. Apart from advancing age, the level of patient education and evidence of preexisting cerebrospinal-vascular disease are strong predictors of perioperative delirium.[30] Early provision of reading glasses, hearing aids, and dentures, and making the patient aware of the time-place-person and daylight exposure can make a positive outcome. Neuroleptics like haloperidol 0.5–1 mg may be administered with strict electrocardiogram (ECG) (QTc interval) monitoring for POD. Early mobilization, early enteral nutrition, and early removal of drains and catheters are also beneficial in these elderly patients. Both prehabilitation and rehabilitation can be helpful in this regard. Another consideration is the prevention and management of POCD[31] in the elderly population, which is characterized by progressive deterioration from baseline in cognitive neuropsychological functioning lasting for months to years and occurs due to micro-emboli, neuroinflammation, neuronal death, and cholinergic dysfunction. POCD leads to a higher risk of death at 1-year postsurgery due to cardiopulmonary complications such as pneumonia, deep vein thrombosis (DVT), and stroke.

Pain is often undertreated in older people due to underestimation of their sensitivity to pain and the fear of side effects. They have reduced pain tolerance, with significant interpatient variability in older people. There is a shift in balance within the autonomic nervous system (ANS)[32] toward sympathetic tone predominance. This leads to limited stress adaptability, reduced basal parasympathetic nervous system activity, decreased baroreflex sensitivity, and weakened homeostatic functions. There is a decrease in the dose of analgesic drugs to prevent the risk of increased plasma drug accumulation and accumulation of active metabolites. Patient-controlled analgesia (PCA) and epidural analgesia are more effective in elderly patients as compared to conventional opioid regimens. The opioid requirements are reduced in older people due to age-related pharmacokinetic and pharmacodynamic changes. The addition of IV lidocaine[33] can significantly reduce postoperative pain intensity and opioid consumption, along with shortened hospital stays in elderly patients. The most standard treatment of cancer pain is oral analgesics as per the World Health Organization (WHO's) three-step analgesic ladder.[34] Acetaminophen is the first-line agent with analgesic-antipyretic (central action) but no anti-inflammatory activity. IV paracetamol 1 g is used frequently for pain relief. Nonsteroidal anti-inflammatory drugs (NSAIDs) act peripherally, demonstrate ceiling effects and varying adverse effects, and have no habit-forming potential. Opioids are the mainstay of cancer pain management. Moderate cancer pain can be treated with step 2 opioids such as codeine, tramadol, and propoxyphene. Dextropropoxyphene is preferably avoided in geriatric cancer patients due to the accumulation of its toxic metabolite (norpropoxyphene) and prolonged half-life. Moderate to severe cancer pain requires more potent opioids such as morphine, oxycodone, hydromorphone, methadone, and transdermal drugs, with the concept of "start slow and go slow". When cancer pain does not respond to escalating doses of an opioid, switching over to an alternative opioid with a proper conversion ratio in equianalgesic doses can help. Adjuvant analgesics[35] can be added for treating chronic cancer pain, including antidepressants, anticonvulsants, corticosteroids, bisphosphonates, and sedatives. Gabapentin is particularly useful for radiotherapy and chemotherapy-related neuropathic pain in older people. There is evidence that placement of a thoracic epidural catheter can improve left ventricular function and increase myocardial oxygen availability, which is beneficial in those with ischemic heart disease. Per surgical requirements, ultrasound-guided nerve blocks can be given during the perioperative period, which helps reduce stress response, prevent DVT, and early rehabilitation.

## ■ GERIATRIC ONCOLOGY IN INDIA

The number of older patients with cancer is exponentially increasing in India. In contrast to Japan, where the age cutoff for the senior population is 75 years, in India, an older person is defined as anyone 60 years or older (as per the National Program for Health Care of the Elderly, Government of India). Nearly 8.6% of the Indian population (around 103 million) is elderly. By 2050, 21.2 % of the world's population will be aged 60 years, and the most significant numbers reside in the developing world.[36] There is a pressing need for research into the prevention of cancer and the planning of treatment and care for the elders. As compared with the significant causes of death among the elderly, cancer incidence and mortality have not, in general, declined, indicating that primary prevention (especially cessation of tobacco smoking) is the most valuable approach to decreasing mortality. A practical and comprehensive "Geriatric Model of Care" needs to be envisaged and followed for the elderly patients in our country for better outcomes. "Comprehensive Geriatric Assessment" or CGA model[37] proposed by the perioperative management of elderly patients (PriME). Recommendations for older people can be followed, comprising physical, functional, psychological, and social considerations. In those exhibiting TUG test result duration >20 seconds (propensity to falls), a CGA evaluation is recommended in elderly patients. There is an urgent need for multidisciplinary geriatric oncology services for elderly cancer patients in India. In addition to geriatric assessment, one must evaluate chemotherapy-toxicity risk,[38] patient and caregiver expectations, nononcological life expectancy, and overall quality of life.

## ■ CONCLUSION

Many cancers in older people are diagnosed at a later stage, as early cancer symptoms can be mistaken for other conditions or minor illnesses associated with old age. As a result, cancer treatment often starts late, which increases the complexity of treatment and the likelihood of severe side effects and reduces the chances of a successful treatment outcome. Geriatric perioperative care of the onco-surgical patients is quite challenging for the anesthesiologists and requires a multidisciplinary approach for a positive outcome. Preoperative assessment must be meticulous with the optimization of comorbid illnesses and nutritional therapy for MECP. Evaluation of various geriatric syndromes such as constipation, insomnia, urinary incontinence, lower urinary tract infections, osteoporosis, pressure sores, and visual and auditory impairment, along with oral/dental health evaluation, must be done. With advancements in surgical techniques and novel anticancer therapies, anesthesiologists must be geared toward newer challenges in perioperative care of geriatric cancer patients. Robotic cancer surgeries are frequently performed in elderly patients, which require special precautions regarding positioning, fluid therapy, muscle relaxation, and the care of tubes and lines. Adequate analgesia, palliative therapy, and end-of-life care must be integrated into perioperative care of elderly onco-surgical patients. The focus must be on prehabilitation, optimization of associated diseases, and prevention and management of complications such as hemodynamic instability, malnutrition, delirium, cognitive decline, frailty, thromboembolism, chronic pain, and cardiopulmonary events.

## REFERENCES

1. Wildiers H, Heeren P, Puts M, Topinkova E, Janssen-Heijnen ML, Extermann M, et al. International Society of Geriatric Oncology consensus on geriatric assessment in older patients with cancer. J Clin Oncol. 2014;32(24):2595-603.
2. Koolhaas W, van der Klink JJ, Groothoff JW, Brouwer S. Towards a sustainable healthy working life: associations between chronological age, functional age, and work outcomes. Eur J Public Health. 2012;22(3):424-9.
3. Cinar D, Tas D. Cancer in the elderly. North Clin Istanb. 2015;2(1):73-80.
4. Yang LQ, Zhu L, Shi X, Miao CH, Yuan HB, Liu ZQ, et al. POLMA-EP investigators. Postoperative pulmonary complications in older patients undergoing elective surgery with a supraglottic airway device or tracheal intubation. Anaesthesia. 2023;78(8):953-62.
5. Mukker JK, Singh RSP, Derendorf H. Pharmacokinetic and Pharmacodynamic Considerations in Elderly Population. In: Stegemann S (Ed). Developing Drug Products in an Aging Society. AAPS Advances in the Pharmaceutical Sciences Series, Volume 26. New York: Springer, Cham; 2016. pp. 139-51.
6. Bowie MW, Slattum PW. Pharmacodynamics in older adults: A review. Am J Geriatr Pharmacother. 2007;5(3):263-303.
7. American Geriatrics Society 2012 Beers Criteria Update Expert Panel. American Geriatrics Society updated Beers Criteria for potentially inappropriate medication use in older adults. J Am Geriatr Soc. 2012;60(4):616-31.
8. Aceto P, Incalzi RA, Bettelli G, Carron M, Chiumiento F, Corcione A, et al.; Società Italiana di Anestesia Analgesia Rianimazione e Terapia Intensiva (SIAARTI), Società Italiana di Gerontologia e Geriatria (SIGG), Società Italiana di Chirurgia (SIC), Società Italiana di Chirurgia Geriatrica (SICG) and Associazione Italiana di Psicogeriatria (AIP). Perioperative management of elderly PATIENTS (PriME): Recommendations from an Italian intersociety consensus. Aging Clin Exp Res. 2020;32(9):1647-73.
9. Ceccarelli G, Andolfi E, Biancafarina A, Rocca A, Amato M, Milone M, et al. Robot-assisted surgery in elderly and very elderly population: our experience in oncologic and general surgery with literature review. Aging Clin Exp Res. 2017;29(Suppl 1):55-63.
10. Lee SJ, Lindquist K, Segal MR, Covinsky KE. Development and validation of a prognostic index for 4-year mortality in older adults. JAMA. 2006;295(7):801-8.
11. Allan N, Siller C, Breen A. Anaesthetic implications of chemotherapy. Continuing Education in Anaesthesia Critical Care & Pain. 2012;12(2):52-6.
12. Aloia TA, Zimmitti G, Conrad C, Gottumukkala V, Kopetz S, Vauthey JN. Return to intended oncologic treatment (RIOT): a novel metric for evaluating the quality of oncosurgical therapy for malignancy. J Surg Oncol. 2014;110(2):107-14.
13. Ramesh HS, Boase T, Audisio RA. Risk assessment for cancer surgery in elderly patients. Clin Interv Aging. 2006;1(3):221-7.
14. Cruz-Jentoft AJ, Bahat G, Bauer J, Boirie Y, Bruyère O, Cederholm T, et al. Writing Group for the European Working Group on Sarcopenia in Older People 2 (EWGSOP2), and the

Extended Group for EWGSOP2, Sarcopenia: revised European consensus on definition and diagnosis. Age Ageing. 2019;48(1):16-31.
15. Zhou S, Zhang XH, Zhang Y, Gong G, Yang X, Wan WH. The age-adjusted Charlson comorbidity index predicts prognosis in elderly cancer patients. Cancer Manag Res. 2022;14:1683-91.
16. Jones DM, Song X, Rockwood K. Operationalizing a frailty index from a standardized comprehensive geriatric assessment. J Am Geriatr Soc. 2004;52(11):1929-33.
17. Mislang AR, Di Donato S, Hubbard J, Krishna L, Mottino G, Bozzetti F, et al. Nutritional management of older adults with gastrointestinal cancers: an International Society of Geriatric Oncology (SIOG) review paper. J Geriatr Onco. 2018;9(4):382-92.
18. Zhang Q, Qian L, Liu T, Ding JS, Zhang Z, Song MM, et al; Investigation on nutrition status and its clinical outcome of common cancers (INSCOC) group. Prevalence and prognostic value of malnutrition among elderly cancer patients using three scoring systems. Front Nutr. 2021;8:738550.
19. Stanga Z. Basics in clinical nutrition: Nutrition in the elderly. e-SPEN, the European e-Journal of Clinical Nutrition and Metabolism. 2009;4(6):e289-99.
20. Harris D, Haboubi N. Malnutrition screening in the elderly population. J R Soc Med. 2005;98(9):411-4.
21. Wiraguna A, Setiati S. Correlation of hand grip strength with quality of life in elderly patients. J Phys Conf Ser. 2018;1073:042033.
22. Molfino A, Gioia G, Rossi Fanelli F, Muscaritoli M. The role for dietary omega-3 fatty acids supplementation in older adults. Nutrients. 2014;6(10):4058-73.
23. Montroni I, Ugolini G, Saur NM, Rostoft S, Spinelli A, Van Leeuwen BL, et al. SIOG Surgical Task Force/ESSO GOSAFE Study Group. Quality of life in older adults after major cancer surgery: The GOSAFE International Study. J Natl Cancer Inst. 2022;114(7):969-78.
24. Cooter M, Ni K, Thomas J, Gupta DK, Hopkins TJ, Miller TE, et al. Age-dependent decrease in minimum alveolar concentration of inhaled anaesthetics: a systematic search of published studies and meta-regression analysis. Br J Anaesth. 2020;124(1):e4-7.
25. Borsheski R, Johnson QL. Pain management in the geriatric population. Mo Med. 2014;111(6):508-11.
26. Lei VJ, Navathe AS, Seki SM, Neuman MD. Perioperative benzodiazepine administration among older surgical patients. Br J Anaesth. 2021;127(2):E69-71.
27. Yang Y, Song C, Song C, Li C. Comparison of bispectral index-guided individualized anesthesia with standard general anesthesia on inadequate emergence and postoperative delirium in elderly patients undergoing esophagectomy: a retrospective study at a single center. Med Sci Monit. 2020;26:e925314.
28. Yang X, Huang X, Li M, Jiang Y, Zhang H. Identification of individuals at risk for postoperative cognitive dysfunction (POCD). Ther Adv Neurol Disord. 2022;15: 17562864221114356.
29. Huang L, Zhang T, Wang K, Chang B, Fu D, Chen X, et al. Postoperative multimodal analgesia strategy for enhanced recovery after surgery in elderly colorectal cancer patients. Pain Ther. 2024;4:745-66.
30. Korc-Grodzicki B, Root JC, Alici Y. Prevention of post-operative delirium in older patients with cancer undergoing surgery. J Geriatr Oncol. 2015;6(1):60-9.
31. Plas M, Rotteveel E, Izaks GJ, Spikman JM, van der Wal-Huisman H, B. van Etten B, et al. Cognitive decline after major oncological surgery in the elderly. Eur J Cancer. 2017;86: 394-402.
32. Giunta S, Xia S, Pelliccioni G, Olivieri F. Autonomic nervous system imbalance during aging contributes to impair endogenous anti-inflammaging strategies. GeroScience. 2024;46(1):113-27.

33. Zhu Y, Wang F, Yang L, Zhu T. Intravenous lidocaine infusion reduce post-operative pain and length of hospital in elderly patients undergoing surgery: Meta-analysis of randomized controlled trials. Surg Innov. 2022;29(5):632-45.
34. Rao A, Cohen HJ. Symptom management in the elderly cancer patient: Fatigue, pain, and depression. JNCI Monographs. J Natl Cancer Inst Monogr. 2004;(32):150-7.
35. Portenoy RK. A practical approach to using adjuvant analgesics in older adults. J Am Geriatr Soc. 2020;68(4):691-8.
36. Noronha V, Rao AR, Ramaswamy A, Kumar A, Pillai A, Dhekale R, et al. The current status of geriatric oncology in India. Ecancermedicalscience. 2023;17:1595.
37. Extermann M, Aapro M, Bernabei R, Cohen HJ, Droz JP, Lichtman S, et al. Use of comprehensive geriatric assessment in older cancer patients: Recommendations from the task force on CGA of the International Society of Geriatric Oncology (SIOG) Crit Rev Oncol Hematol. 2005;55(3):241-52.
38. Extermann M, Boler I, Reich RR, Lyman GH, Brown RH, DeFelice J, et al. Predicting the risk of chemotherapy toxicity in older patients: the chemotherapy risk assessment scale for high-age patients (CRASH) score. Cancer. 2012;118(13):3377-86.

# CHAPTER 14

# Perioperative POCUS

*Massimiliano Meineri*

## ABSTRACT

Perioperative point-of-care ultrasound (POCUS) consists of using ultrasound (US) at the bedside to answer qualitative questions during the perioperative period. We defined the perioperative period from preoperative patient assessment to immediate postoperative care. Several POCUS modalities have been described in this clinical situation, but their use was usually first described in other settings. They include cardiac, lung, diaphragm, airway, and gastric US. Although their utility and potential impact in clinical practice seems apparent, there is still scattered evidence on their use in perioperative settings, especially regarding their effect on patients' outcomes. Training in POCUS has been well-defined, and some national and international guidelines are available. Quality control remains a challenge, mainly due to the lack of storage.

**Keywords:** Ultrasound; Perioperative; Point-of-care

## KEY POINTS

- Point-of-care ultrasound (POCUS) finds its natural setting in perioperative care. The need to answer critical binary questions, especially in emergencies, makes it a valuable tool to be added to the anesthesia armamentarium.
- Focused cardiac ultrasound (FCU) consists of obtaining five views to qualitatively assess ventricular function, pericardial effusion, and gross valvular abnormalities. It is indicated before induction to optimize hemodynamics and in case of intraoperative hemodynamic instability. Focused transesophageal echocardiography constitutes an excellent alternative with a higher image quality.
- Lung ultrasound (LUS) has been proven more specific and sensitive than chest X-ray in detecting pneumothorax and pleural effusion. In the preoperative settings, it can determine the presence of lung edema and identify patients at risk of postoperative pulmonary complications.
- Gastric ultrasound (GUS) can accurately identify and quantify gastric content, allowing better fasting assessment. However, it has yet to be integrated into current guidelines.
- Airway and diaphragm ultrasound provides accurate location of the cricothyroid membrane, detects esophageal intubation, and quantifies diaphragmatic contraction and strength. A reduced diaphragmatic contractility correlates to an increased incidence of postoperative pulmonary complications.

## ■ INTRODUCTION

Point-of-care ultrasound (POCUS) involves using ultrasound (US) to answer binary questions at the bedside that can be integrated immediately into the patient's management. The information provided is usually not obtainable or very difficult to obtain through standard physical examination, such as the presence of pericardiac effusion, pneumothorax, and abdominal free fluid.

The POCUS has grown enormously in the past few years due to the increased availability of US machines, the growth of knowledge, and the scientific validation of established and new applications.

Ultrasound-guided line insertion[1] and regional blocks have been the first clinical applications of US and are now a standard of care. Similarly, intraoperative transesophageal echocardiography (TEE)[2] is also a very well-established practice in the hands of cardiac anesthesiologists that contributed to the increased number of available US machines in the perioperative setting. Hand-held systems have become wireless, with multiple probes and high image quality, but their cost is high. However, it has decreased in the last few years and remains a burden for individual practitioners.

In a fast-paced, digital, and very "visual" world, POCUS was warmly received in the perioperative setting, and its use is enthusiastically encouraged by many editorials. Navigating among the multiple POCUS applications, the scientific evidence supporting them, and the lack of national and international guidelines remains a big challenge for most practitioners.

In this review, we define the perioperative setting as the care of patients by the anesthesiologist from preoperative assessment to the recovery room after surgery.

This narrative review will discuss which POCUS applications offer helpful clinical tools in the perioperative setting, what questions can be answered, and what evidence supports their use. We will also discuss the challenges involved in POCUS training and current available guidelines.

## ■ FOCUSED CARDIAC ULTRASOUND

Focused cardiac ultrasound (FCU) entails the application of a limited number of transthoracic echocardiography (TTE) views without the use of Doppler and without any measurements to answer (A) the following questions (Q):
*Q1:* Is the left ventricular function?
*A:* Normal or abnormal.
*Q2:* Is the right ventricular function?
*A:* Normal or abnormal.
*Q3:* Is there pericardial effusion?
*A:* Yes or no.
*Q4:* What is the volume status?
*A:* Full or empty.

The FCU is the first noncardiologist application of echocardiography that the American Society of Echocardiography (ASE) supported.[3]

The more recent international evidence-based recommendations[4] added the following question:
*Q5:* Is there gross valvular abnormality of the mitral and aortic valve?
*A:* Yes or no.

Focused echocardiography performed at the bedside by anesthesiologists has been successfully applied to preoperative assessment, allowing new diagnoses and excluding suspected ones, thus resulting in extra or less invasive monitoring.[5] Despite its apparent benefits, the impact on patient outcomes must be investigated further.[6,7] Various schemes for a simplified TTE exam have been described in this setting with significant variability of questions, from the six basic FCU questions to the detection of pulmonary hypertension.[8]

Assessment of volume status before induction of anesthesia using FCU for emergent procedures has shown to be effective in avoiding postinduction hypotension.[9] In this setting, detecting cardiac pathologies may also favorably impact the choice of anesthetic technique and monitoring undergoing emergency surgery.[6] Intraoperative use of FCU is often impractical due to sterile draping and patient position; however, its use has been well described and provides an effective tool to identify the cause of hemodynamic instability.[10] FCU has been widely integrated into resuscitation for cardiac arrest.[11] Typically, only the subcostal view can be used and only during the 10 seconds of pulse check. A dedicated resuscitation team member should be in charge of performing the scan.[11] Under no circumstances should FCU delay cardiac compressions and resuscitative efforts. In this context, FCU can answer the following question:

*Q6:* Is there any coordinated cardiac contraction?
*A:* Yes or no.

Evidence of cardiac contraction in the absence of a palpable pulse is common and defines pseudo-pulseless electric activity, which prompts further resuscitation. On the contrary, the lack of cardiac contraction (cardiac standstill) questions the effectiveness of any additional efforts.[12]

The FCU may play an essential role in the perioperative setting, but it has yet to be studied explicitly in the recovery room after surgery. However, many "intraoperative" and "perioperative" studies included the immediate postoperative period.[7]

Nevertheless, FCU finds its application in the perioperative care of cardiac surgical patients despite the technical challenges due to fresh surgical wounds and drainages, which are also in the hands of critical care nurses.[13]

## FOCUSED INTRAOPERATIVE TRANSESOPHAGEAL ECHOCARDIOGRAPHY

Intraoperative transesophageal echocardiography by cardiac anesthetists is established during cardiac surgery and is regulated by national certification, training pathways, and accreditation. The increased availability of TEE equipment and trained personnel allowed the spread of intraoperative TEE outside of cardiac surgical procedures. A limited TEE exam (basic TEE) is described to answer binary questions on the causes of hemodynamic instability and intraoperative complications such as air embolism in this setting. TEE remains a natural alternative to TTE in patients intubated with difficult imaging windows.

"Rescue" TEE is indicated to manage intraoperative hemodynamic instability.[14]

A further simplified TEE protocol, like FCU, has been described in the emergency setting.[15] They include only five views without measurements and use of Doppler to answer Q1 to Q6 and further:

*Q7:* Is there any aortic dissection?
*A:* Yes or no.

Focused TEE has been deemed feasible for emergency physicians after minimal training.[16] It has also gained popularity in its application during cardiopulmonary resuscitation.[17,18] TEE can be performed continuously without discontinuing chest compression and reliably provides good-quality images. It is also beneficial in guiding extracorporeal membrane oxygenator implantation.[19] Furthermore, single-used, single-plane TEE probes, allowing minimal views, have been reported to be reliable tools for continuous postoperative hemodynamic monitoring in cardiac surgical patients.[20,21]

## ■ LUNG ULTRASOUND

Lung ultrasound (LUS) relies on the interpretation of artifacts and has been proven more accurate than clinical examination in determining the cause of respiratory failure in the emergency department.[22] It can be performed with any US probe, although lower-frequency ones (phased and curved arrays) are required to assess deeper structures such as the costophrenic angle.

Several imaging algorithms have been proposed, including a variable number of views. However, depending on the patient's position, the highest point on the chest has to be assessed to exclude the presence of pleural air and the deepest to exclude fluid.

The LUS can reliably answer the following questions:
*Q8:* Is the lung ventilated?
*A:* Yes or no.
*Q9:* Is there a pneumothorax?
*A:* Yes or no.
*Q10:* Is there pleural effusion?
*A:* Yes or no.
*Q11:* Is there pulmonary edema?
*A:* Yes or no.

Current guidelines suggest that LUS can detect pneumothorax with greater sensitivity and specificity than chest X-ray in trauma patients by demonstrating the lack of pleural sliding and pulsatility.[23] The same applies to pleural effusion. The presence of multiple bilateral B lines suggests lung edema.

This feature of LUS has been used in the preoperative assessment of surgical patients and to stratify the risk of postoperative complications by indirectly identifying underlying heart failure.[24,25] The number of B lines correlates with the amount of interstitial lung fluid and has been used to guide fluid management in thoracic surgical patients.[26]

After the central line insertion and nerve blocks are performed, the same linear probe can rule out the presence of pneumothorax when lung sliding is present. LUS further allows the detection of lung ventilation and confirms endotracheal intubation and one-lung ventilation.[27,28] Intraoperatively, LUS has been used to optimize ventilation to avoid atelectasis, which seems to impact postoperative respiratory complications.[29]

The LUS lends itself perfectly to intraoperative use in case of hypoxia; however, its use as an intraoperative tool has yet to be widely studied.[30] Conversely, TEE may also provide continuous lung assessment without interfering with surgery.[31]

In immediate postoperative care, LUS has proven helpful in assessing atelectasis; however, its potential obvious application in managing postoperative hypoxia has yet to be studied explicitly in the recovery room.[24,32]

## ■ DIAPHRAGMATIC ULTRASOUND

Diaphragmatic US (DUS) evaluates the diaphragm's muscular part at the lateral costophrenic angle level. In this location, the diaphragmatic muscle fibers run craniocaudally parallel to the skin and can be imaged using a linear array probe.

The DUS answers the following question:
*Q12:* Does the diaphragm contract?
*A:* Yes or no.

The DUS has been successfully used intraoperatively to detect diaphragmatic palsy after regional anesthesia.[33] The percent of diaphragmatic muscle thickening (thickening fraction) at the zone of apposition to the chest wall correlates to diaphragmatic contraction strength. This parameter has been used preoperatively as a surrogate of lung function.[34] In cardiac surgical patients, a value of <38% was reported to correlate to an increased risk of postoperative pulmonary complications.[35]

## ■ AIRWAY ULTRASOUND

Airway ultrasound (AUS) primarily allows precise localization of the cricothyroid membrane and not just simple palpation.[36] In the intensive care unit setting, AUS is also used to define the ideal point of percutaneous tracheostomy.[37] Preinduction identification of cricothyroid membrane may benefit patients with predicted difficult intubation in which the airway may have to be emergently secured with a cricothyroidotomy. Its application has been proven successful in obese and pregnant patients.[38] AUS also has the potential to identify other features of difficult intubation, such as distance from skin to airway structures such as epiglottis and hyoid bone.[39]

It answers the following questions:
*Q13:* Where is the cricothyroid membrane located?
*A:* Precise location.
*Q14:* Is the tube in the trachea?
*A:* Yes or no.

The AUS has also been used to assess difficult airways with scattered weak evidence; nevertheless, it allows measurement of tracheal diameter, which guides the choice of single- and double-lumen tubes.[40]

The AUS was proven very sensitive in the emergency medicine setting to detect the dynamic sliding of the endotracheal tube on the anterior tracheal wall or esophageal intubation before ventilation, thus avoiding the risks of unnecessary gastric insufflation. It could be used in addition to or as a replacement for auscultation.[41]

## ■ GASTRIC ULTRASOUND

Gastric ultrasound (GUS) assesses the gastric antrum to detect the presence of gastric content and define its type and amount.[42]

It answers the following questions:
*Q15:* Is the stomach empty?
*A:* Yes or no
*Q16:* What type of gastric content is there?
*A:* Fluid or solids.
*Q17:* How much gastric fluid is there?
*A:* Amount in mL.

The GUS was developed to assess fasting and aspiration risk.[43] The quantification of gastric fluid is precise[44] and reliable; however, GUS still needs to be integrated into the current fasting guidelines. GUS can also accurately assess the risk of aspiration before tracheal extubation in the intensive care unit.[45] GUS is essential in identifying delayed gastric emptying and residual gastric content.[46]

## ■ TRAINING

Training in POCUS has been extensively described and includes four essential components: (1) Indication, (2) image acquisition, (3) image interpretation, and (4) clinical decision-making.[47] Hands-on teaching is a critical training component and can be complemented and enhanced using simulators, although surface US can be comfortably performed on healthy volunteers. Integration of POCUS teaching into residency curricula remains scattered around the world.[48,49] Supervised training remains a big challenge because it requires a significant time commitment as well as the availability of experts.

## ■ CERTIFICATION AND QUALITY CONTROL

The ASE has established a certification through the National Board of Echocardiography for POCUS for intensive care physicians,[50] but there is still no specific certification in perioperative medicine. Many national societies have established training pathways that remain a suggestion to practice but have yet to be made mandatory.[51] The German Society of Anesthesia requires the completion of hybrid courses (online and hands-on) as well as the creation of a portfolio.[52] Although most guidelines suggest establishing a quality control system, it is seldom implemented due to time constraints, the lack of stored video loops, and available experts for review.

## ■ CONCLUSION

The POCUS is ideal for the perioperative setting as a valuable tool to answer critical binary questions. Unfortunately, there is no specific evidence for the perioperative application of many of the POCUS modalities, especially regarding their impact on patient outcomes.

Given the availability of US systems and the growing body of literature on perioperative use, POCUS should be integrated into the training program of anesthesia residents to become a standard tool in the anesthetist's armamentarium. The need for quality control should be addressed with more accessible and cheaper image storage solutions and, eventually, virtual external audits. The latter could be part of center-specific POCUS certification.

## ■ REFERENCES

1. American Society of Anesthesiologists Task Force on Central Venous Access; Rupp SM, Apfelbaum JL, Blitt C, Caplan RA, Connis RT, Domino KB, et al. Practice guidelines for central venous access: a report by the American Society of Anesthesiologists Task Force on Central Venous Access. Anesthesiology. 2012;116(3):539-73.
2. Hahn RT, Abraham T, Adams MS, Bruce CJ, Glas KE, Lang RM, et al. Guidelines for performing a comprehensive transesophageal echocardiographic examination: recommendations from the American Society of Echocardiography and the Society of Cardiovascular Anesthesiologists. J Am Soc Echocardiogr. 2013;26(9):921-64.

3. Spencer KT, Kimura BJ, Korcarz CE, Pellikka PA, Rahko PS, Siegel RJ. Focused cardiac ultrasound: recommendations from the American Society of Echocardiography. J Am Soc Echocardiogr. 2013;26(6):567-81.
4. Via G, Hussain A, Wells M, Reardon R, ElBarbary M, Noble VE, et al. International evidence-based recommendations for focused cardiac ultrasound. J Am Soc Echocardiogr. 2014;27(7):683.e1-e33.
5. Cowie CJ, Strachan R. Ultrasound preferred as the immediate preoperative investigation before three-pin rigid fixation. Childs Nerv Syst. 2011;27(9):1365-6.
6. Canty DJ, Heiberg J, Yang Y, Royse AG, Margale S, Nanjappa N, et al. Pilot multi-centre randomised trial of the impact of pre-operative focused cardiac ultrasound on mortality and morbidity in patients having surgery for femoral neck fractures (ECHONOF-2 pilot). Anaesthesia. 2018;73(4):428-37.
7. Cowie B. Focused transthoracic echocardiography predicts perioperative cardiovascular morbidity. J Cardiothorac Vasc Anesth. 2012;26(6):989-93.
8. Mahmood F, Matyal R, Skubas N, Montealegre-Gallegos M, Swaminathan M, Denault A, et al. Perioperative Ultrasound Training in Anesthesiology: A Call to Action. Anesth Analg. 2016;122(6):1794-804.
9. Dana E, Dana HK, De Castro C, Bueno Rey L, Li Q, Tomlinson G, et al. Inferior vena cava ultrasound to predict hypotension after general anesthesia induction: a systematic review and meta-analysis of observational studies. Can J Anaesth. 2024;71(8):1078-91.
10. Navas-Blanco JR, Louro J, Reynolds J, Epstein RH, Dudaryk R. Intraoperative focused cardiac ultrasound for assessment of hypotension: a systematic review. Anesth Analg. 2021;133(4):852-9.
11. Breitkreutz R, Walcher F, Seeger FH. ALS conformed use of echocardiography or ultrasound in resuscitation management. Resuscitation. 2008;77(2):270-2.
12. Breitkreutz R, Price S, Steiger HV, Seeger FH, Ilper H, Ackermann H, et al. Focused echocardiographic evaluation in life support and peri-resuscitation of emergency patients: a prospective trial. Resuscitation. 2010;81(11):1527-33.
13. Laastad Sorensen M, Oterhals K, Ponitz V, Morken IM. Point-of-care examinations using handheld ultrasound devices performed by intensive care nurses in a cardiac intensive care unit. Eur J Cardiovasc Nurs. 2023;22(5):482-8.
14. Reeves ST, Finley AC, Skubas NJ, Swaminathan M, Whitley WS, Glas KE, et al. Basic perioperative transesophageal echocardiography examination: a consensus statement of the American Society of Echocardiography and the Society of Cardiovascular Anesthesiologists. J Am Soc Echocardiogr. 2013;26(5):443-56.
15. Arntfield R, Pace J, McLeod S, Granton J, Hegazy A, Lingard L. Focused transesophageal echocardiography for emergency physicians-description and results from simulation training of a structured four-view examination. Crit Ultrasound J. 2015;7(1):27.
16. Arntfield R, Pace J, Hewak M, Thompson D. Focused transesophageal echocardiography by emergency physicians is feasible and clinically influential: observational results from a novel ultrasound program. J Emerg Med. 2016;50(2):286-94.
17. Prager R, Ainsworth C, Arntfield R. Critical care transesophageal echocardiography for the resuscitation of shock: an important diagnostic skill for the modern intensivist. Chest. 2023;163(2):268-9.
18. Prager R, Walser E, Balta KY, Anton Nikouline MD, Leeper WR, Vogt K, et al. Resuscitative transesophageal echocardiography during the acute resuscitation of trauma: a retrospective observational study. J Crit Care. 2024;79:154426.
19. Nicoara A, Skubas N, Ad N, Finley A, Hahn RT, Mahmood F, et al. Guidelines for the use of transesophageal echocardiography to assist with surgical decision-making in the operating room: a surgery-based approach: from the American Society of Echocardiography in collaboration with the Society of Cardiovascular Anesthesiologists and the Society of Thoracic Surgeons. J Am Soc Echocardiogr. 2020;33(6):692-734.

20. Hlaing M, He J, Haglund N, Takayama H, Flynn BC. Impact of a Monoplane Hemodynamic TEE (hTEE) Monitoring Device on Decision Making in a Heterogeneous Hemodynamically Unstable Intensive Care Unit Population: A Prospective, Observational Study. J Cardiothorac Vasc Anesth. 2018;32(3):1308-13.
21. Treskatsch S, Balzer F, Knebel F, Habicher M, Braun JP, Kastrup M, et al. Feasibility and influence of hTEE monitoring on postoperative management in cardiac surgery patients. Int J Cardiovasc Imaging. 2015;31(7):1327-35.
22. Lichtenstein D. Lung ultrasound in acute respiratory failure an introduction to the BLUE-protocol. Minerva Anestesiol. 2009;75(5):313-7.
23. Volpicelli G, Elbarbary M, Blaivas M, Lichtenstein DA, Mathis G, Kirkpatrick AW, et al. International evidence-based recommendations for point-of-care lung ultrasound. Intensive Care Med. 2012;38(4):577-91.
24. Xie C, Sun K, You Y, Ming Y, Yu X, Yu L, et al. Feasibility and efficacy of lung ultrasound to investigate pulmonary complications in patients who developed postoperative Hypoxaemia-a prospective study. BMC Anesthesiol. 2020;20(1):220.
25. Gillmann HJ, Dieding J, Schrimpf C, Janssen H, Sahlmann B, Rustum S, et al. Prospective evaluation of preoperative lung ultrasound for prediction of perioperative outcome and myocardial injury in adult patients undergoing vascular surgery (LUPPO study). Minerva Anestesiol. 2020;86(11):1151-60.
26. Assaad S, Kratzert WB, Perrino AC, Jr. Extravascular lung water monitoring for thoracic and lung transplant surgeries. Curr Opin Anaesthesiol. 2019;32(1):29-38.
27. Yang FM, Ma BZ, Liu Y, Sun Q, Li N, Feng SY, et al. Lung ultrasound for detecting tracheal and mainstem intubation: a systematic review and meta-analysis. Ultrasound Med Biol. 2022;48(1):3-9.
28. Kanavitoon S, Raksamani K, Troy MP, Suphathamwit A, Thongcharoen P, Suksompong S, et al. Lung ultrasound is non-inferior to bronchoscopy for confirmation of double-lumen endotracheal tube positioning: a randomized controlled noninferiority study. BMC Anesthesiol. 2022;22(1):168.
29. Tonelotto B, Pereira SM, Tucci MR, Vaz DF, Vieira JE, Malbouisson LM, et al. Intraoperative pulmonary hyperdistension estimated by transthoracic lung ultrasound: A pilot study. Anaesth Crit Care Pain Med. 2020;39(6):825-31.
30. Diaz-Gomez JL, Renew JR, Ratzlaff RA, Ramakrishna H, Torp K, Via G. Can lung ultrasound be the first-line tool for evaluation of intraoperative hypoxemia? Anesth Analg. 2018;126(6):2146-7.
31. Cavayas YA, Girard M, Desjardins G, Denault AY. Transesophageal lung ultrasonography: a novel technique for investigating hypoxemia. Can J Anaesth. 2016;63(11):1266-76.
32. Wu L, Yang Y, Yin Y, Yang L, Sun X, Zhang J. Lung ultrasound for evaluating perioperative atelectasis and aeration in the post-anesthesia care unit. J Clin Monit Comput. 2023;37(5):1295-302.
33. Da Conceicao D, Perlas A, Giron Arango L, Wild K, Li Q, Huszti E, et al. Validation of a novel point-of-care ultrasound method to assess diaphragmatic excursion. Reg Anesth Pain Med. 2023;rapm-2023:104983.
34. Qian Z, Yang M, Li L, Chen Y. Ultrasound assessment of diaphragmatic dysfunction as a predictor of weaning outcome from mechanical ventilation: a systematic review and meta-analysis. BMJ Open. 2018;8(9):e021189.
35. Cavayas YA, Eljaiek R, Rodrigue E, Lamarche Y, Girard M, Wang HT, et al. Preoperative Diaphragm Function Is Associated With Postoperative Pulmonary Complications After Cardiac Surgery. Crit Care Med. 2019;47(12):e966-e74.
36. Siddiqui N, Yu E, Boulis S, You-Ten KE. Ultrasound Is superior to palpation in identifying the cricothyroid membrane in subjects with poorly defined neck landmarks: A randomized clinical trial. Anesthesiology. 2018;129(6):1132-9.

37. Lin J, Bellinger R, Shedd A, Wolfshohl J, Walker J, Healy J, et al. Point-of-care ultrasound in airway evaluation and management: A comprehensive review. Diagnostics (Basel). 2023;13(9):1541.
38. You-Ten KE, Desai D, Postonogova T, Siddiqui N. Accuracy of conventional digital palpation and ultrasound of the cricothyroid membrane in obese women in labour. Anaesthesia. 2015;70(11):1230-4.
39. Carsetti A, Sorbello M, Adrario E, Donati A, Falcetta S. Airway ultrasound as predictor of difficult direct laryngoscopy: a systematic review and meta-analysis. Anesth Analg. 2022;134(4):740-50.
40. Ahn JH, Park JH, Kim MS, Kang HC, Kim IS. Point of care airway ultrasound to select tracheal tube and determine insertion depth in cleft repair surgery. Sci Rep. 2021;11(1):4743.
41. Hossein-Nejad H, Mehrjerdi MS, Abdollahi A, Loesche MA, Schulwolf S, Ghadipasha M, et al. Ultrasound for intubation confirmation: a randomized controlled study among emergency medicine residents. Ultrasound Med Biol. 2021;47(2):230-5.
42. Van de Putte P, Perlas A. Ultrasound assessment of gastric content and volume. Br J Anaesth. 2014;113(1):12-22.
43. Kruisselbrink R, Arzola C, Jackson T, Okrainec A, Chan V, Perlas A. Ultrasound assessment of gastric volume in severely obese individuals: a validation study. Br J Anaesth. 2017;118(1):77-82.
44. Kruisselbrink R, Arzola C, Endersby R, Tse C, Chan V, Perlas A. Intra- and interrater reliability of ultrasound assessment of gastric volume. Anesthesiology. 2014;121(1):46-51.
45. O'Donoghue SD, Pincus JM, Pang GKF, Roach RE, Anstey CM, Perlas A, et al. Impact of fasting on the gastric volume of critically ill patients before extubation: a prospective observational study using gastric ultrasound. BJA Open. 2022;3:100023.
46. Arzola C, Perlas A, Siddiqui NT, Downey K, Ye XY, Carvalho JCA. Gastric ultrasound in the third trimester of pregnancy: a randomised controlled trial to develop a predictive model of volume assessment. Anaesthesia. 2018;73(3):295-303.
47. Perlas A, Van de Putte P, Van Houwe P, Chan VW. I-AIM framework for point-of-care gastric ultrasound. Br J Anaesth. 2016;116(1):7-11.
48. Sanders JA, Navas-Blanco JR, Yeldo NS, Han X, Guruswamy J, Williams DV. Incorporating Perioperative Point-of-Care Ultrasound as Part of the Anesthesia Residency Curriculum. J Cardiothorac Vasc Anesth. 2019;33(9):2414-8.
49. Mok D, Schwarz SKW, Rondi K. Point-of-care ultrasonography in Canadian anesthesiology residency programs: a national survey of program directors. Can J Anaesth. 2017;64(10):1023-36.
50. Kirkpatrick JN, Grimm R, Johri AM, Kimura BJ, Kort S, Labovitz AJ, et al. Recommendations for echocardiography laboratories participating in cardiac point of care cardiac ultrasound (POCUS) and critical care echocardiography training: Report from the American Society of Echocardiography. J Am Soc Echocardiogr. 2020;33(4):409-22.e4.
51. Meineri M, Arellano R, Bryson G, Arzola C, Chen R, Collins P, et al. Canadian recommendations for training and performance in basic perioperative point-of-care ultrasound: recommendations from a consensus of Canadian anesthesiology academic centres. Can J Anaesth. 2021;68(3):376-86.
52. Greim C-A, Weber SU, Göpfert M, Ender J, Schwemmer U, Seidel R, et al. Anästhesiefokussierte sonographie (AFS). Anästh Intensivmed. 2020;(61):532-52.

# CHAPTER 15

# Fluid Stewardship in the Critically Ill

*Nishant Kumar, Anshu Gupta, Maitree Pandey*

## ABSTRACT

Fluids are drugs that are often prescribed injudiciously and can cause harm rather than benefit, leading to increased morbidity and mortality, especially in the critically ill. In most institutes, fluid prescription is based on individual physicians' discretion. This chapter describes the goals of fluid stewardship, including the 5 Ps, and discusses how these goals can be achieved utilizing the 7 Ds. The need for a multidisciplinary team is highlighted, and its components are discussed. The strengthening of a fluid stewardship program with the help of education, training, documentation, auditing, reviewing, and its impact on cost-effectiveness is emphasized. Current problems in developing an excellent fluid stewardship program are also discussed.

**Keywords:** Fluid stewardship; Fluid overload; Fluid responsiveness; Fluid tolerance

## KEY POINTS

- Fluids are drugs often prescribed indiscriminately, leading to an increase in morbidity and mortality of critically ill patients.
- Fluid stewardship results in individualized, appropriate fluid therapy, early detection of inappropriate fluid prescription and helps in preventing complications.
- The 5 Ps (patient, prescriber, prescription, preparation, and pharmacist) are essential in setting goals for fluid stewardship, and the 7 Ds (definition, diagnosis, drug, dose, duration, de-escalation, and documentation) are critical to achieving them.
- A multidisciplinary team approach, focusing on education, training, auditing, and reviewing helps achieve the desired outcome.

## ■ INTRODUCTION

Fluids are drugs. Unfortunately, they are prescribed indiscriminately and have the potential to cause harm and increase morbidity and even mortality, especially in the critically ill, who hang between a delicate balance of when, what, how much fluids to administer, and when to stop.

The initial phase of critical illness usually requires the administration of a large bolus of fluid, followed by a period of maintenance, stabilization, and de-escalation. Therefore, the correct prescription of fluid requires a deep understanding of the underlying pathophysiology, associated comorbidities of the patient, and associated fluid dynamics and kinetics about the former.

The importance of fluid therapy must be considered. The jury still needs to be made clear about the ideal fluid to be used during the different phases of illness and which dose to use. Despite the guidelines by the United Kingdom's National Institute for Health and Care Excellence (NICE)[1] and other efforts such as the British Consensus Guidelines on Intravenous Fluid Therapy for Adult Surgical Patients (GIFTASUP),[2] the Perioperative Quality Initiative (POQI),[3] and International Fluid Academy (IFA) guidance,[4,5] prescription of fluids is based mainly on individual treating physician's discretion, leading to inappropriate therapy with consequent potential impact on disease outcome and healthcare costs. Reasons cited include lack of consistent training and education.[4] If efforts are made to focus on education, recordkeeping, and auditing, adherence to guidelines and outcomes may be improved. Development of such guidelines depends on extensive data analysis and constant evaluation and re-evaluation, which can be fostered by adopting the principles of fluid stewardship, not unlike antimicrobial stewardship, to prevent injudicious use and misprescription, with an eye on health and economic outcome.

## ■ FLUID STEWARDSHIP

*Fluid stewardship* is defined as a series of coordinated interventions for judicious intravenous (IV) fluid administration, with a primary goal of limiting the harmful effects of inappropriate fluid prescription and fluid overload or accumulation and optimizing the clinical outcomes.[6]

### Purpose

Fluid stewardship serves three primary purposes:
1. Individualized, appropriate therapy in terms of choice of therapy, dose, duration, and appropriate withdrawal.[7]
2. Early detection and prevention of inappropriate fluid prescription to prevent associated complications.[8]
3. Implementation of preventive quality improvement measures, leading to economic benefit.[9]

### Goals

Although defined primarily for preventing hypervolemia, fluid stewardship, in the broadest terms, refers to under- and overprescribing fluids. While hypervolemia is more common, it does not imply that fluid restriction or hypovolemia is without adverse effects, as restrictive fluid therapy entails early and prudent administration of vasoactive drugs with their inherent adverse effects and potential for systemic harm, such as acute kidney injury and subsequent requirement of renal replacement therapy as concluded by the RELIEF (Restrictive versus Liberal Fluid Therapy for Major Abdominal Surgery) trial.[10] The primary goal of fluid stewardship covers the first two aims and may be defined as optimizing clinical outcomes and minimizing the harmful effects of fluid administration.[7]

The secondary goal stems from the third goal, reducing healthcare costs through awareness, research, education, training, and quality assurance exercises by establishing fluid stewardship teams.[6]

The aforementioned goals, in turn, depend on the 5 Ps, and it is essential to consider each one.[11,12]
1. *Patient*: Fluid is ordered as per the clinical condition and requirement of the patient.

2. Prescriber: Physician or intensivist who decides fluid administration
3. Prescription: Written orders that specify the type of fluid, rate (dose), and duration of therapy
4. Preparation: Individualized fluid with additions or deletions
5. Pharmacist: Crosschecks for any inconsistencies

Therefore, the prescriber can design adequate and accurate fluid therapy with the patient's underlying condition in mind. He can deliver the detailed written prescription to the pharmacist for the individual fluid to be prepared, with the resuscitative goals and the addition and/or deletion of any of the components, such as electrolytes, for maintenance and replacement. The prescription should be made keeping in mind the 7 Ds:[7,12]

1. Definitions
2. Diagnosis
3. Drug
4. Dose
5. Duration
6. De-escalation
7. Documentation at discharge

## Definitions

The inconsistencies in the literature regarding various terminologies and definitions of fluid therapy lead to confusion and make it difficult to standardize regimens for comparison and measure the impact of habits and practices. Some of the common terminologies used are restrictive vs. liberal fluid therapy, hypovolemia, hypervolemia, maintenance fluids, resuscitation fluids, and goal-directed therapy, which should be considered in perspective to the patient rather than absolute terms, e.g., hypervolemia and hypovolemia are defined as ±10% of net fluid balance.

## Diagnosis

This refers to the patient's underlying condition, which decides the type of fluid, and the patient's volume status, which helps determine the amount of fluid to be administered.

Patients in shock often require rapid administration of fluids, mainly crystalloids, whereas the consensus on the type and amount of fluid for maintenance is lacking as it is best judged by the volume status of the patient and is based on the dynamic rather than static hemodynamic parameters **(Table 1)**.[13]

## Drug

Fluids, like drugs, are available in various formulations. The four basic categories are crystalloids, balanced crystalloids, colloids, and balanced colloids. The prefix balanced refers to the composition as close to plasma as possible regarding osmolality and electrolyte concentrations.

Critical considerations for choosing a particular fluid include composition and suitability for the indication of fluid therapy while keeping in mind the contraindications and intended and nonintentional side effects that this therapy might cause.

to achieve objective dynamic hemodynamic parameters, as described in **Table 1**. The fluid balance during this stage is positive.

Optimization: This refers to the phase when the fluid deficit has been corrected (objective dynamic target concerning fluids has been achieved), but the hemodynamics remain unstable. Fluids in this phase are administered with constant assessment of the fluid status. This phase aims to optimize perfusion to the tissues rather than pressure goals to maintain oxygenation to prevent and limit organ damage. Markers of microcirculation may be helpful to guide the therapy, but lactate, prolonged capillary refill time, and mottling score, unfortunately, rely on microcirculation as well.

Stabilization: This phase starts with the patient achieving stable hemodynamics. The aim is to maintain and return the fluid and electrolyte levels to the physiological baseline by replacing ongoing losses and providing organ support. The target in this phase shifts to zero or slightly negative fluid balance. Administration of starches in this phase has shown a harmful effect, thus undermining their use.

Evacuation (De-escalation): This is the final phase that aims to remove any excess fluid accumulated by using diuretics or ultrafiltration unless the patient themselves does not digress, often taken as a sign of recovery.

## Duration

Before a fluid is prescribed, the ordering physician must ask the basic four questions of fluid therapy:

### Q1: When to start IV fluids?
This aims to guide the prescription on whether fluids are required, how to determine whether fluids are required, or if some other intervention would be more beneficial. It should also be answered whether fluid administration would not further deteriorate the patient's clinical condition.

### Q2: When to stop IV fluids?
This should be answered to prevent either hypovolemia or hypervolemia and should be guided by objective measurements of fluid responsiveness and tolerance.

### Q3: When to start fluid removal?
This pertains to active fluid removal from the body using diuretics or renal replacement therapy with ultrafiltration and aims to prevent complications due to hypervolemia.

### Q4: When to stop fluid removal?
This aims to avoid hypoperfusion once the patient is stabilized.

These four questions include the above steps as well as monitoring, assessment for fluid requirement (responsiveness and tolerance), and help in maintaining an average cumulative fluid balance of 2-5-5% at day 7.[12]

Fluid responsiveness is an objective increase in cardiac output ≥10% in response to a fluid bolus. This has been used as a marker for the need for more fluids, but fluid responsiveness may not constantly improve tissue oxygenation despite causing an increase in pressure. It may, in fact, harm tissue perfusion due to venous congestion.[19]

This has led to the origin of a better term called fluid tolerance, which refers to the degree to which a patient can tolerate the administration of fluids without causing

**TABLE 1:** Dynamic hemodynamic parameters.

| Assessment measure | Cut off value | Limitations |
|---|---|---|
| PLR | • 10% increase in CO<br>• 10% increase in PPV | • Requires CO measurement<br>• Severe hypovolemia<br>• IAP ≥16 mm Hg |
| Fluid challenge | 15% increase in CO | • Requires CO measurement<br>• Volume overload |
| SVV | >12% | • Spontaneous breathing<br>• Arrhythmias<br>• Increased IAP<br>• Low tidal volume/compliance<br>• Right ventricular failure |
| PPV | >12% | Same as above— |
| IVC collapsibility | 12% change in vessel diameter | • Spontaneous breathing<br>• Increased IAP<br>• Low tidal volume/compliance |
| End expiratory occlusion test[14] | 5% increase in CO | • Low tidal volume<br>• Should tolerate 15 seconds apnea |
| $EtCO_2$[15] | $\Delta EtCO_2 \geq 5\%$ with PLR | • Spontaneous breathing |
| Tidal volume challenge[16] | • 3.5% increase in PPV<br>• 2.5% increase in SVV | • Only for ARDS patients |

(ARDS: acute respiratory distress syndrome; CO: cardiac output; $EtCO_2$: end-tidal carbon dioxide; IAP: intra-abdominal pressure; IVC: inferior vena cava; PLR: passive leg raise; PPV: pulse pressure variation; SVV: stroke volume variation)

## Dose

*"All things are poison, and nothing is without poison; the dosage alone makes it so a thing is not a poison".* Paracelsus's statement holds for fluids as well.

The daily essential requirement of fluid and electrolyte requirements for a healthy person is described as: Water: 1 mL/kg/h, Glucose: 1–1.5 g/kg/day, Sodium: 1–1.5 mmol/kg/day, Potassium: 1 mmol/kg/day, and Chlorine 1 mmol/kg/day.[12]

However, the patients admitted to the intensive care unit (ICU), apart from the underlying disease, are homeostatically challenged, with a disturbed electrolyte milieu of the plasma, which requires significant adjustments to the requirements above.

Apart from this, the phases of fluid therapy should also be considered in patients with shock. These phases can be described as salvage, optimization, stabilization, and de-escalation, acronymized as SOSD,[17] which by preference was changed to ROSE: Resuscitation, Optimization, Stabilization, and Evacuation.[18]

*Resuscitation (Salvage):* This refers to the initial rapid administration of fluid (usually 3–4 mL/kg over 10–15 minutes, repeated as necessary) to correct hemodynamic shock and maintain adequate pulse pressure. This stage should be guided by advanced hemodynamic monitors, and appropriate therapy fluid, vasopressors, or both should be initiated, personalized to the patient's requirements rather than fixed amounts. This has been referred to as early goal-directed therapy organ dysfunction and indicates the herald of fluid overload and the need for fluid limitation or removal.[19]

## De-escalation

De-escalation and deresuscitation are the terms often used interchangeably. While deresuscitation is defined as active fluid removal in patients with fluid overload using diuretics or ultrafiltration, de-escalation refers to limiting the amount and/or rate of fluids being administered.[20]

De-escalation should begin soon after resuscitation goals have been met, and further fluid may impact organ function. Resuscitative fluids account for only 6% of the total, whereas the bulk comprises nutrition (33%), drug administration (fluid creep; 33%), maintenance (25%), and the remaining 3% by blood and blood products.[20]

De-escalation should stop once the goals are met or the under-administration compromises organ function.[20] The entire phase is dynamic, and defining actual timelines would need to be more concise.

## Documentation

Documentation provides detailed instructions, prescriptions, and records for comparison, audit, and research purposes. It should include not only the 5 Ps but also the 6 Ds with a detailed discharge plan.

Thus, the genesis of appropriate fluid prescription may be summarized as in **Figure 1**.

These changes cannot be adopted by the prescriber alone. It is the duty of the entire healthcare team involved in the care of the critically ill patient to be involved. Also, when it comes to the institution, constant evaluation, feedback, re-evaluation, and revisiting are required before guidelines can be formed or modified. The fluid stewardship team can best handle this task.

## ■ FLUID STEWARDSHIP TEAM

Since cohesive guidelines for fluid administration are lacking, the practices vary widely. A recent survey of practices worldwide revealed the absence of

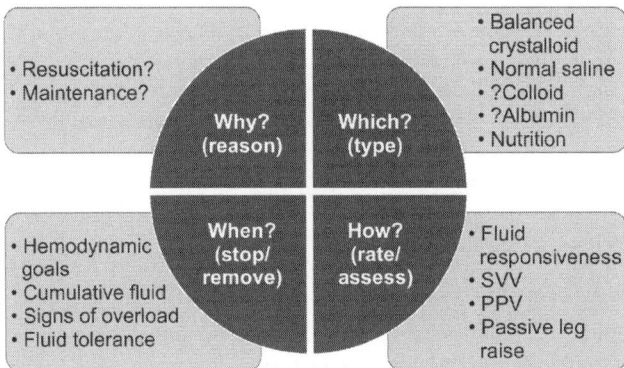

**Fig. 1:** Appropriate fluid prescription. (PPV: pulse pressure variation; SVV: stroke volume variation)

hospital-based guidelines in three-fourths of the respondent hospitals, and only 6.5% of the respondents performed above average on the knowledge score regarding the administration of fluids.[21]

It is a must to have fluid stewardship teams to achieve the aims and goals of fluid administration, provide personalized fluid therapy, education, training, and skill sets, and gather data for audits, research, guideline framing, and clinical practice improvement.

The fluid stewardship team should consist of:[12]
- Emergency physician
- Intensivist
- Treating specialty physician (nephrologist/cardiologist)
- Anesthesiologist
- Pharmacist
- Nurse
- Member of quality assurance team

The responsibilities of the team include:[12,22]
- Safe prescription
- Adherence to guidelines
- Recognize and manage complications
- Liaison with team members
- Education and training
- Defining key performing indices
- Feedback on practice and adherence
- Data collection
- Audits
- Collaboration and research
- Change in practice and continuous improvement in outcomes

## Knowledge Gaps

The fluid stewardship teams are formed to usher in personalized fluid treatment. However, the initial stumbling blocks may be:
- Lack of standardization of guidelines and best practices
- Lack of consensus on metrics/measurement of the impact of fluid stewardship
- Standardized education and training
- Integration of fluid stewardship program with clinical work and its implementation
- Standardized data collection
- Study the economic considerations concerning the resources utilized and actual cost savings for the patient
- Collaboration with like-minded teams across institutes to reduce bias and generate evidence-based strategies to optimize fluid management practices and improve patient outcomes.[22]

## Stepwise Approach to set up a Fluid Stewardship Program[12,22]

Once the concept of fluid stewardship is understood and ready to be adopted, the following steps may help in establishing the team:
- Identification of leads
- Agreement across clinical departments

- Support from the organization
- Local institutional guidelines built on evidence-based medicine
- Education of prescribers, nurses, and audit teams
- Collection of data and interpretation
- Review of prescriptions and documentation
- Calculate the economic impact concerning resource utilization and patient outcome
- Analysis, revisiting, and reformulating guidelines as required

## Indicators of Good Compliance

Even if the stewardship program is implemented, its impact must be studied and assessed for appropriate use and patient outcomes. The following metrics may be helpful:[12]

- Total quantity of fluids purchased
- Type of fluids purchased
- Timing of administration
- Rate of administration
- Duration of administration
- Factors contributing to hypervolemia
- Patient outcome

## Strategies for Improving Education and Training

Awareness, education, and training are needed to change healthcare professionals' mindsets. Hard facts and medicine should not be countered by "my way or the highway". Healthcare professionals must recognize that the ultimate goal of fluid therapy is to "restore and maintain tissue fluid, electrolyte homeostasis, and central euvolemia".

The educational programs may be designed with the goals of:[22]

- Improving and expanding training
- Involving professionals across specialties, including nurses
- Evidence-based medicine and guidelines
- Resources to disseminate knowledge

## Best Practices for Fluid Stewardship

To summarize, the process of administration of fluids may be based on the following questions:[22]

- Are fluids required? And if so, are they beneficial?
- What is the indication of fluid (resuscitation, maintenance, redistribution, or creep)?
- Which fluid is to be used?
- How much fluid (dose, rate, duration, route)?
- When to stop fluids?
- When to de-escalate?
- When and if to de-resuscitate?
- When should fluid removal (to prevent hypovolemia) be stopped?

## Areas of Future Research

We still have a long way to go about fluid therapy, especially in the critically ill, as they are on the brink and require a delicate balance of drug, dose, duration, and electrolyte homeostasis. Guidelines are needed to standardize the type of fluids (crystalloid vs. colloids, saline vs. balanced, etc.), amount of fluids required (restrictive vs. liberal therapy), clinical assessment of hemodynamic status (maintenance of pressures vs. oxygen delivery), evaluation of fluid status (responsiveness, tolerance), and associated outcomes in terms of morbidity, mortality, and costs.

Focus is also required to identify indicators and monitoring strategies to evaluate stewardship programs. Interventions must be agreed upon to promote and provide educational activities and training with maximal impact. It is imperative to establish standardized protocols for data collection and analysis, use of electronic health records, programs, and software for fluid calculation and management, to facilitate benchmarking, quality improvement, and research in fluid stewardship. The role of simulation and software such as Situational Awareness and Preparedness for Public Health Incidences and Reasoning Engines (SAPPHIRE) and nomograms needs to be studied in detail and validated for generalized use.[12,22]

## ■ CONCLUSION

Additional evidence and research are required to develop robust guidelines for the optimal prescription of fluids and prevent their misuse and consequent harm. Establishing fluid stewardship teams in the hospital may be the first step in educating, training, and regulating fluid prescriptions. Other steps include auditing the available data with the help of emerging technologies and seamlessly integrating recent advances into existing guidelines to improve patient outcomes.

## ■ REFERENCES

1. National Institute for Health and Care Excellence (NICE). (2013). Intravenous fluid therapy in adults in hospital: clinical guideline CG174. Available from: https://www.nice.org.uk/guidance/cg174/resources/intravenous-fluid-therapy-in-adults-in-hospital-pdf-35109752233669 [Last accessed July, 2024].
2. Powell-Tuck J, Gosling P, Lobo D, et al. (2018). British consensus guidelines on intravenous fluid therapy for adult surgical patients. Available from: https://www.bapen.org.uk/resources-and-education/education-and-guidance/bapen-principles-of-good-nutritional-practice/giftasup. [Last accessed July, 2024].
3. Martin GS, Kaufman DA, Marik PE, Shapiro NI, Levett DZH, Whittle J, et al. Perioperative Quality Initiative (POQI) consensus statement on fundamental concepts in perioperative fluid management: fluid responsiveness and venous capacitance. Perioper Med (Lond). 2020;9:12.
4. McDougall M, Guthrie B, Doyle A, Timmins A, Bateson M, Ridley E, et al. Introducing NICE guidelines for intravenous fluid therapy into a district general hospital. BMJ Open Qual. 2022;11(1):e001636.
5. Silversides JA, Perner A, Malbrain MLNG. Liberal versus restrictive fluid therapy in critically ill patients. Intensive Care Med. 2019;45(10):1440-2.
6. Malbrain M, Rice TW, Mythen M, Wuyts S. It is time for improved fluid stewardship. ICU Manage Pract. 2018;18(3):158-62.
7. Malbrain MLNG, Van Regenmortel N, Saugel B, De Tavernier B, Van Gaal PJ, Joannes-Boyau O, et al. Principles of fluid management and stewardship in septic shock: It is

time to consider the four D's and the four phases of fluid therapy. Ann Intensive Care. 2018;8(1):66.
8. Bates DW, Cullen DJ, Laird N, Petersen LA, Small SD, Servi D, et al. Incidence of adverse drug events and potential adverse drug events. Implications for prevention. ADE Prevention Study Group. JAMA. 1995;274(1):29-34.
9. Etchells E, Koo M, Daneman N, McDonald A, Baker M, Matlow A, et al. Comparative economic analyses of patient safety improvement strategies in acute care: a systematic review. BMJ Qual Saf. 2012;21(6):448-56.
10. Myles PS, Bellomo R, Corcoran T, Forbes A, Peyton P, Story D, et al. Australian and New Zealand College of Anaesthetists Clinical Trials Network and the Australian and New Zealand Intensive Care Society Clinical Trials Group. Restrictive versus Liberal Fluid Therapy for Major Abdominal Surgery. N Engl J Med. 2018;378(24):2263-74.
11. Malbrain MLNG, Langer T, Annane D, Gattinoni L Elbers P, Hahn RG, et al. Intravenous fluid therapy in the perioperative and critical care setting: Executive summary of the International Fluid Academy (IFA). Ann Intensive Care. 2020;10:64.
12. Wong A, Wilkinson J, Nasa P, Malbrain MLNG. Introduction to fluid stewardship. In: Malbrain MLNG, Wong A, Nasa P, Ghosh S (Eds). Rational Use of Intravenous Fluids in Critically Ill Patients, 1st edition. Cham, Switzerland: Springer Nature; 2024. p. 545-66.
13. Carr JR, Hawkins AW, Newsome AS, Smith SE, Clemmens AB, Bland CM, et al. Fluid stewardship of maintenance intravenous fluids. J Pharm Pract. 2022;35(5):769-82.
14. Gavelli F, Shi R, Teboul JL, Azzolina D, Monnet X. The end-expiratory occlusion test for detecting preload responsiveness: a systematic review and meta-analysis. Ann Intensive Care. 2020;10(1):65.
15. Toupin F, Clairoux A, Deschamps A, Lebon JS, Lamarche Y, Lambert J, et al. Assessment of fluid responsiveness with end-tidal carbon dioxide using a simplified passive leg raising maneuver: a prospective observational study. Can J Anaesth. 2016;63(9):1033-41.
16. Myatra S, Monnet X, Teboul JL. Use 'tidal volume challenge' to improve the reliability of pulse pressure variation. Crit Care. 2017;21:60.
17. Hoste EA, Maitland K, Brudney CS, Mehta R, Vincent JL, Yates D, et al. Four phases of intravenous fluid therapy: a conceptual model. Br J Anaesth. 2014;113(5):740-7.
18. Malbrain ML, Marik PE, Witters I, Cordemans C, Kirkpatrick AW, Roberts DJ, et al. Fluid overload, de-resuscitation, and outcomes in critically ill or injured patients: a systematic review with suggestions for clinical practice. Anaesthesiol Intensive Ther. 2014;46:361-80.
19. Kattan E, Castro R, Miralles-Aguiar F, Hernandez G. The emerging concept of fluid tolerance: A position paper. J Crit Care. 2022;71:154070.
20. Malbrain MLNG, Martin G, Ostermann M. Everything you need to know about deresuscitation. Intensive Care Med. 2022;48(12):1781-6.
21. Nasa P, Wise R, Elbers PWG, Wong A, Dabrowski W, Regenmortel NV, et al. Intravenous fluid therapy in perioperative and critical care setting-Knowledge test and practice: an international cross-sectional survey. J Crit Care. 2022;71:154122.
22. Malbrain MLNG, Caironi P, Hahn RG, Llau JV, McDougall M, Patrao L, et al. Multidisciplinary expert panel report on fluid stewardship: perspectives and practice. Ann Crit Care. 2023;13:89.

# CHAPTER 16

# Noninvasive Ventilation in Critical Care

*Matthew Camilleri, Giles Coverdale, Mathew Patteril*

## ABSTRACT

Noninvasive ventilation (NIV) is a mainstay of intensive care unit (ICU) care, and it has various forms and patient interfaces. Current modalities of NIV include continuous positive airway pressure (CPAP), bilevel positive airway pressure (BiPAP), and high-flow nasal oxygen (HFNO). Positive airway pressure (PAP) has various effects on the physiology of the respiratory and cardiac systems. This chapter explores the wide range of indications for NIV, including current trends in use, evidence, and international guidelines relating to its application. Well-established indications include exacerbations of chronic obstructive pulmonary disease (COPD), interstitial lung disease (ILD), pulmonary edema, restrictive lung disease, and obesity hypoventilation syndrome (OHS) with or without obstructive sleep apnea (OSA). More controversial but increasingly relevant indications include pneumonia and acute respiratory distress syndrome (ARDS), as well as acute exacerbations of asthma. Indicators of NIV treatment failure and the appropriate use of NIV as a ceiling of treatment will also be discussed, along with how NIV may be used around intubation and liberation from invasive ventilation.

**Keywords:** Noninvasive ventilation; Intensive care unit; High flow nasal oxygenation; Respiratory failure

## KEY POINTS

- Most modern ventilators can perform continuous positive airway pressure (CPAP) and bilevel positive airway pressure (BiPAP) functions with various patient interfaces. High-flow nasal oxygen (HFNO) is a simple air oxygen blender with humidification but can deliver high flows and fraction of inspired oxygen ($FiO_2$) to match peak inspiratory flows.
- The benefits of noninvasive ventilation (NIV) on the pulmonary system may include recruiting lung units to improve ventilation/perfusion (V/Q) matching, splinting airways to prevent collapse, and improving breathing work. There are potential benefits on the left ventricle with systolic dysfunction, but it should be used with caution in preload-dependent states and patients with right ventricular (RV) dysfunction.
- NIV's use in the management of pneumonia, acute respiratory distress syndrome (ARDS), and acute asthma exacerbations remains controversial, with no clear evidence base or guidelines. Nevertheless, NIV is increasingly employed to manage these conditions in the intensive care unit (ICU) initially.

*Contd...*

*Contd...*

- CPAP is an established and evidenced therapy for pulmonary edema that benefits respiratory and cardiac physiology.
- BiPAP is an established treatment for hypercapnic respiratory failure due to COPD, interstitial lung disease (ILD), restrictive lung disease, and obesity hypoventilation syndrome (OHS). It has a sound evidence base and is recommended by international guidelines.
- Monitoring response to NIV is critical to ensuring prompt escalation where appropriate. Lack of improvement in physiological parameters after an initial period of optimal treatment suggests treatment failure.
- There is currently no good evidence regarding the superiority of mask ventilation, NIV, or HFNO for preoxygenation in critically ill patients before intubation.
- NIV has evidence of the benefit of improving the success of weaning high-risk patients from mechanical ventilation. Still, evidence suggests it should not be used as a late rescue of patients deteriorating following tracheal extubation.

## ■ INTRODUCTION

Noninvasive ventilation (NIV) delivers respiratory support by positive-pressure oxygen or air without requiring tracheal intubation or supraglottic airway device insertion.

The NIV can be categorized as delivering continuous positive airway pressure (CPAP) or bilevel positive airway pressure (BiPAP). More recently, high-flow nasal oxygen (HFNO) therapy has been classified as a form of NIV. Many devices can deliver oxygen flow rates exceeding 60 L/min with positive end-expiratory pressure (PEEP).

The NIV, in all its forms, is commonplace in critical care. It is used to prevent the need for tracheal intubation in patients with respiratory failure, reduce the risk of oxygen desaturation during intubation attempts, improve the success rate of liberation from invasive mechanical ventilation (IMV), and as a rescue for patients who deteriorate postextubation. Being less invasive than tracheal intubation and IMV, it may also be used as a ceiling of treatment or destination therapy for patients with advanced frailty or severe chronic respiratory disease who may not be suitable for more advanced organ support.

## ■ NONINVASIVE VENTILATION EQUIPMENT

High-flow nasal oxygen devices consist of an oxygen flowmeter with an air/oxygen blender, a gas analyzer, a heating system, a sterile water tank for humidification, and oxygen tubing connected to wide-bore nasal prongs.[1] HFNO devices typically deliver gas flow rates of up to 60 L/min with 95–100% relative humidity at body temperature. Therefore, they can provide fraction of inspired oxygen ($FiO_2$) of nearly 1.0 by matching the peak inspiratory flow rates in spontaneously breathing critically ill patients. The high flow rates delivered nasally produce a variable CPAP effect of 3.2–7.4 $cmH_2O$, particularly when closed mouth breathing, improving ventilation/perfusion (V/Q) matching, and reducing atelectasis. Humidification functions improve comfort and promote secretion clearance.

The CPAP and BiPAP can be delivered as NIV by most modern ventilators. Many bespoke NIV machines are designed for spontaneously breathing patients without tracheal intubation. Various tight-fitting facemasks, nasal masks, and hoods are available, and they can include heat and moisture exchangers (HMEs) or active humidification systems in the circuits. Simple devices deliver a fixed CPAP throughout the respiratory cycle. In contrast, more advanced equipment usually has variable PEEP settings (often up to 15 cmH$_2$O) with pressure support (PS) functions set separately to provide BiPAP and augment a patient's tidal volume. The PS functions synchronize with a patient's innate ventilation by detecting a pressure or flow change in the circuit with a spontaneous breath and delivering PS. Some advanced NIV machines also provide a set backup breathing rate to avoid apnoea.[2] Like HFNO equipment, advanced NIV systems can provide high O$_2$ flow rates to match a patient's peak inspiratory flow and deliver near to 100% oxygen if required.

## PHYSIOLOGICAL EFFECTS OF NONINVASIVE VENTILATION

### Noninvasive Ventilation and Respiratory Mechanics

Applying positive pressure to the lungs and airways affects respiratory mechanics and function. At its most basic, CPAP, unlike other oxygen delivery devices, is a closed-circuit device that can deliver high flows and high FiO$_2$ to correct hypoxemia in respiratory failure. CPAP generates continuous increases in airway pressures and PEEP.

Creating a negative intrapleural pressure is the process of inspiration performed by the respiratory muscles, with the diaphragm being the most important. Compliance represents the change in lung volume from a resultant change in transpulmonary pressure. Compliance can be reduced in various pathophysiological processes that may increase the work of breathing by increasing the required pressure to increase lung volume. Positive airway pressure (PAP) can reduce the work of breathing through various mechanism.[3] PEEP can elevate resting alveolar pressure, preventing alveolar collapse and optimizing the point on the compliance curve at which inspiration is initiated, reducing the negative intrapleural pressure the respiratory muscles are required to generate. PEEP increases mean airway pressure, potentially recruiting under ventilated lung units, increasing the surface area available for gas exchange,[4] and reducing shunt. PEEP may also splint open airways to reduce resistance and improve flow, increasing mean airway pressure and relieving obstructed airways, and increasing CO$_2$ elimination through increased alveolar ventilation. Higher alveolar pressures will reduce fluid extravasation in pulmonary oedema[5] through changes in starling forces.

Inspiratory positive airway pressure (IPAP) augments a patient's inspiratory effort to increase transpulmonary pressure and reduce the work of breathing. IPAP will augment tidal volumes, thus improving ventilation and reducing CO$_2$. PEEP and IPAP facilitate more uniform overall ventilation, improving V/Q mismatch.

### Noninvasive Ventilation and Cardiac Function

Positive airway pressure has various complex interactions with cardiac function, with ventricular transmural pressure a key determinant of effective filling and emptying of the heart.[6] Increases in intrathoracic pressure reduce venous return during systole, thus reducing right ventricular (RV) and left ventricular (LV) venous return, which is helpful in an overloaded heart.[6] PAP during systole will reduce the transmural pressure required for each cardiac contraction and decrease afterload. Increased intrathoracic pressure throughout the cardiac cycle may reduce heart rate due to higher parasympathetic tone.[6] All these elements are helpful in LV systolic dysfunction; however, in patients with diastolic dysfunction with higher filling pressure requirements, a fall in venous return may be detrimental, reducing filling and precipitating hypotension.[7]

Interactions of PAP with the RV are even more complex due to the highly variable effect on pulmonary vascular resistance. PEEP's impact on the RV will reduce venous return as described earlier but may decrease or increase the RV's afterload, depending on the effect on pulmonary vascular resistance. In some patients, changes in lung volume relative to functional residual capacity may maximize pulmonary arterial flow by reducing hypoxic vasoconstriction, thus recruiting alveolar units, potentially leading to a reduction in pulmonary arterial pressure, and reduced afterload.[7] However, increased intrathoracic pressure through PEEP and even higher IPAP pressure may also increase RV afterload due to high intrathoracic pressures, myocardial work, and oxygen demand in a failing ventricle. NIV with high intrathoracic pressures must be considered with caution in patients with pulmonary hypertension or RV failure.

## ■ NONINVASIVE VENTILATION TO PREVENT INTUBATION

### Noninvasive Ventilation in Pneumonia and Acute Respiratory Distress Syndrome

The use of CPAP in pneumonia and acute respiratory distress syndrome (ARDS) due to causes other than coronavirus disease-2019 (COVID-19) remains a controversial subject without clear guidelines or definitive evidence of benefit.[8] There has been an increasing trend in the use of tracheal intubation in patients without other indications for IMV. This practice was accelerated during the recent COVID-19 pandemic. CPAP and HFNO were increasingly utilized to avoid the risks of prolonged mechanical ventilation, and critical care units were overwhelmed by the high numbers of patients. Studies such as RECOVERY-RS showed that NIV was safe and effective in providing respiratory support to patients with COVID-19 and may improve the risk of a combined endpoint of death or the need for mechanical ventilation compared to standard oxygen therapy,[9] primarily due to a reduction in the need for intubation. The benefit of HFNO, or when HFNO could be used as an alternative to CPAP, for these patients needed to be clarified.[10] HFNO and CPAP both became established as reasonable strategies as first-line respiratory support for hypoxemic respiratory failure due to COVID-19.

There is difficulty in generalizing the studies on COVID-19 to the broader population of mixed etiology hypoxemic respiratory failure, where the benefits of reducing the need for tracheal intubation are less clear. As in COVID-19 patients, there is a legitimate concern that delaying intubation and IMV for long trials of NIV could contribute to patient self-induced lung injury (p-SILI) and worse outcomes. In non-COVID-19 type 1 respiratory failure, there is some evidence that NIV can reduce the need for tracheal intubation, but there is no apparent effect on mortality.[11] The European Respiratory Society (ERS) has recently issued guidance recommending HFNO as first-line for hypoxemic respiratory failure based on a possible reduction in intensive care unit (ICU) stay compared to CPAP. This recommendation came with a low level of certainty,[12] and they acknowledge that the choice of CPAP or HFNO may be patient-specific.

The increasing trend in CPAP or HFNO as the first line for acute hypoxemic respiratory failure is despite no clear evidence for a mortality benefit or harm associated with this strategy. There are no clear international guidelines to dictate which patients are suitable or when treatment has failed and should be escalated to IMV.

## Continuous Positive Airway Pressure in Pulmonary Edema

Continuous positive airway pressure with or without PS (BiPAP) has been established as a safe, effective treatment alongside medical therapy for acute decompensated cardiac failure with pulmonary edema. It is recommended by the European Society of Cardiology (ESC)[13] for patients with signs of respiratory distress (respiratory rate >25 breaths/min or arterial saturations <90% despite oxygen therapy). CPAP may also improve cardiac output and LV dynamics by reducing LV afterload and wall tension in LV dysfunction. However, caution is required in hypotensive, hypovolemic, or preload-dependent patients and patients with RV dysfunction. In these patients, the rise in intrathoracic pressure can precipitate worsening hypotension.

Although individual studies have failed to show a benefit in applying CPAP to patients with acute decompensated cardiac failure, meta-analyses have shown significantly improved hospital mortality and reduced intubation rates.[14] NIV is now well established as an adjunct to medical therapy and highly recommended for suitable patients in acute cardiogenic pulmonary edema.

## Noninvasive Ventilation in Chronic Obstructive Pulmonary Disease

The use of NIV, in the form of BiPAP, is widespread in critical care for the treatment of acute hypercapnic chronic obstructive pulmonary disease (COPD) exacerbations with acidemia (pH <7.35) and dyspnea despite optimal medical therapy. This is supported by numerous international guidelines, including the 2017 ERS/American Thoracic Society (ATS)[8] clinical practice guidelines for the use of NIV in acute respiratory failure, and the UK National Institute of Health and Care Excellence (NICE) 2019 COPD guidelines.[15]

Available evidence strongly supports the use of NIV in acute exacerbations of COPD with respiratory acidosis and a pH of 7.25-7.35. There is an improvement in survival in these patients, an improvement in subjective dyspnea, and a reduction in the need for emergency intubation. Evidence is less clear for patients with hypercapnic respiratory failure and a pH <7.25. They may be safely trialed with NIV as an alternative to immediate tracheal intubation if there are no other contraindications (for example, respiratory arrest, bradycardia, hypotension, delirium, and agitation) and they are closely monitored. There has been no significant difference in mortality demonstrated for these patients with severe hypercapnic respiratory failure, but some may avoid intubation and have a reduced length of ICU stay. Overall, there is no recommended lower limit to pH below which NIV is inadvisable; however, the likelihood of treatment failure and the requirement for emergent intubation increases with worsening pH.

Although few studies investigated the use of NIV when the pH is normal (>7.35), the available evidence does not show any benefit, and there may be a worsening in agitation and compliance with treatment. It is, therefore, not recommended for this cohort.

## Noninvasive Ventilation in Asthma

The use of NIV in acute asthma exacerbations remains controversial. It is rarely used in adult populations but is more commonplace in pediatrics. In theory, NIV in acute asthma exacerbations may offload respiratory muscles and improve gas exchange. NIV may reduce the risk of gas trapping by splinting open airways, improving diameter and gas exchange, and potentially decreasing fatigue.[16]

There are increasing numbers of small studies supporting the use of NIV in acute exacerbations of asthma, but their quality is variable. A Cochrane review from 2012 with five randomized controlled trials (RCTs) and 203 patients concluded that there needed to be more evidence to support NIV use in acute asthma exacerbations.[17] Despite this, NIV use in asthma has increased in popularity. Overall, there may be an improvement in the failure rate of NIV based on careful patient selection.[16] Evidence in pediatric populations is also limited, but a meta-analysis of 10 small RCTs demonstrated positive effects on gas exchange and length of stay.[17]

Current guidelines from the British Thoracic Society (BTS) and Intensive Care Society (ICS) on managing hypercapnic respiratory failure[18] do not recommend using NIV in acute asthma. This is not surprising as patients meeting the criteria for hypercapnic respiratory failure are likely to be categorized in the life-threatening spectrum and may be past the point at which NIV is a suitable treatment. The BTS guidelines for the management of asthma agree regarding the use of NIV, suggesting that any patient with hypercapnia would require intubation rather than NIV and reiterating that there is a lack of evidence for NIV in acute asthma and that it should only be considered in an ICU or equivalent setting.[19]

## Noninvasive Ventilation in Obesity Hypoventilation Syndrome and Obstructive Sleep Apnea

Obesity hypoventilation syndrome (OHS) is defined as a combination of sleep-disordered breathing and daytime hypercapnia during wakefulness in individuals with body mass index (BMI) >30 kg/m$^2$.[20] The interaction of OHS and the spectrum of sleep-disordered breathing, including obstructive sleep apnea (OSA), leads to multiple phenotypes with potentially different optimal management approaches.[12] OHS has multisystem effects but is mainly associated with RV dysfunction. CPAP is the primary modality for the management of OHS, both acutely and chronically. Combined BTS/ICS guidelines on hypercapnic respiratory failure[19] recommend the initiation of NIV based on the same criteria as for COPD. It also further recommends it in patients with OHS without acidosis to correct elevated daytime partial pressure of carbon dioxide ($PCO_2$). The treatment of choice for patients with severe OSA is to be managed on CPAP, with BiPAP for those who have failed CPAP, or for OHS with mild OSA or sleep disorder breathing of a nonobstructive nature.[20]

## Noninvasive Ventilation in Interstitial and Restrictive Lung Disease

Invasive ventilation was previously the mainstay of management of interstitial lung disease (ILD) with acute respiratory failure, often with poor outcomes. NIV has increasingly become an alternative therapy, especially in inpatient groups where invasive ventilation is not advisable due to the severity of the disease.[21] While there are no current guidelines for the use of NIV in ILD, some recent small studies support its use[21,22] for acute hypoxic and hypercapnic respiratory failure, initiated as early as possible to avoid IMV.

Restrictive lung disease also represents a heterogeneous group of disorders ranging from neuromuscular disorders to chest wall deformity. NIV is indicated in hypercapnic respiratory failure and is an established arm of treatment both in the acute and domiciliary setting, with much of the evidence for its effectiveness coming from long-term use.[23] Current guidelines[18] recommend early trialing in unwell patients with hypercapnia even before acidosis develops. They also recommend mandatory ventilation modes due to the higher risk of patients being unable to trigger supportive modes. Lastly, they state NIV should not be persevered with in deteriorating patients that are appropriate for IMV.

## Noninvasive Ventilation Failure/Decision to Intubate

Failure of NIV in acute respiratory failure is a possibility for every patient commencing therapy. The endpoint of failure is escalation to IMV or death, hopefully with appropriate advanced care planning. Predictors of patients at high risk of failure have not been agreed. Possible predictors of NIV failure include previous history of NIV failure, high initial heart rate, high initial respiratory rate, low initial pH ($<7.25$) at 1-2 hours and 4-6 hours, high $PCO_2$ at 1-2 hours and 4-6 hours and low initial sodium level.[16] However, attempting a list of indicators may be overly simplistic as different pathologies and patient factors will respond variably.[24] Certainly, agitation/tolerance of therapy, high secretion loads, and anatomical or technical issues with the NIV interface are also possible causes of failure. BTS/ICS guidelines[18] suggest that NIV in hypercapnic acute respiratory failure caused by obstructive or restrictive disease processes, including obesity, should be considered failing if there is no pH or $PCO_2$ level improvement with a trial on optimal settings despite ruling out equipment problems.[25]

## Noninvasive Ventilation as a Destination Therapy/Ceiling of Treatment

Multidisciplinary advanced care planning is integral to managing patients with severe comorbidities. The use of NIV as a treatment ceiling for those in whom mechanical ventilation would not be suitable has increased over recent years, with an estimated 20% of patients in critical care having NIV as a ceiling of therapy.[24] This raises an interesting question about the use of essential care resources with the ability to provide NIV in the ward. Another trend noted is that ward-based units are increasingly admitting patients outside of their inclusion parameters, and this is suspected to be due to pressure on providing NIV as a ceiling of care therapy.[26] Outcomes relating to using NIV as a ceiling of care are variable, and correct patient selection for those that will genuinely benefit is crucial.[27] NIV is suitable as a palliative therapy[18] to improve dyspnea and continuation of NIV for patient comfort and preference should be agreed upon if indicated, with all clinicians who manage NIV having training in end-of-life care.

# NONINVASIVE VENTILATION AND HIGH-FLOW NASAL OXYGEN PREVENT DESATURATION DURING INTUBATION

Preoxygenation is an essential precursor to endotracheal intubation in elective and emergency settings. Denitrogenating the lungs with oxygen gives an extended apneic period in which intubation can be undertaken without desaturation and hypoxemia.

Positive airway pressure via CPAP or BiPAP should improve gas exchange, reduce the effort of breathing, and reduce atelectasis, all elements that may improve preoxygenation. However, there is a significant increase in patient discomfort from a tight mask interface. HFNO is significantly more comfortable and provides high $FiO_2$, PAP of up to 0.7 $cmH_2O$ per 10 $L.min^{-1}$ flow rate, pharyngeal dead-space "washout", and improved respiratory mechanics.[28] HFNO has been used in treating respiratory failure for many years within critical care and emergency department settings and has also been used for preoxygenation of hypoxemic patients needing intubation for invasive ventilation before HFNO adoption for use in anaesthesia.[28]

In critically ill patients with hypoxemic respiratory failure, the benefits of NIV are less clear. NIV may not be superior when compared to usual mask preoxygenation;[29] similarly, a large RCT also found no significant difference in hypoxemic episodes between NIV and HFNO for preoxygenation of patients with severe respiratory failure, but on an individual patient basis, there were no episodes of desaturation in the HFNO group, unlike the NIV group.[30] The lack of a clear superiority over the various techniques is manifest in the current guidance with mask ventilation using CPAP, the primary modality recommended for intubation of critically ill patients, but with allowances for both HFNO and NIV as methods for preoxygenation.[31]

# NONINVASIVE VENTILATION FOLLOWING TRACHEAL EXTUBATION

## Tracheal Extubation onto Noninvasive Ventilation (Prophylactic)

Noninvasive ventilation has an established role in reducing the risk of respiratory failure following the tracheal extubation of high-risk patients and in the early tracheal extubation of patients with type 2 respiratory failure and COPD exacerbations. The ERS recommended it for both these indications in their 2017 guidelines,[8] albeit supported by low levels of evidence.

Since these guidelines, a systematic review of 32 randomized studies (5,063 patients)[32] has confirmed an improvement in postextubation respiratory failure with NIV (no difference in the overall population was found between HFNO and CPAP/BiPAP). The review found an odds ratio for respiratory failure requiring reintubation of 0.60 [confidence interval (CI) 0.43–0.84]. In subgroup analysis, only high-risk patients benefitted from NIV, while there was no significant improvement in those perceived to be at low risk of extubation failure. As well as improving the risk of reintubation, NIV improved ICU length of stay and hospital mortality (seen with mask-based NIV only, not HFNO).

Early tracheal extubation onto NIV for patients failing a spontaneous breathing trial (SBT) has mixed results depending on the patient population. Studies investigating all-comers intubated and ventilated with respiratory failure and weaning difficulty, such as BREATHE published in 2018,[33] did not demonstrate benefit in overall time to liberation from ventilatory support when comparing early tracheal extubation onto NIV and a protocolized weaning regime with ongoing invasive ventilation. There is the potential for harm in unselected patients associated with increased reintubation rates. However, there may be benefits in considering early tracheal extubation directly onto NIV in carefully selected patients. A mortality benefit and a reduction in ventilator-associated pneumonia were found for patients in a 2012 Cochrane review of 16 small studies, mainly in patients with hypercapnic respiratory failure, where the effect was particularly pronounced in patients with pre-existing COPD.[34]

There is good evidence of the benefit of applying NIV (mask-based or HFNO) prophylactically to patients at high risk of respiratory failure following tracheal extubation. The benefit has not been demonstrated in lower-risk patients and is likely to cause increased discomfort. Early tracheal extubation onto NIV for patients failing standard weaning or a SBT is not generally recommended, except in selected patients with COPD and hypercapnic respiratory failure.[8]

## Rescue Noninvasive Ventilation for Respiratory Failure Following Tracheal Extubation

Studies assessing the use of NIV (including HFNO) as an emergency treatment for postextubation respiratory failure do not show benefits in an overall population, either for reintubation rates or mortality. It may be associated with harm if reintubation is delayed in those that eventually require it.[8] One multicenter randomized trial, published in 2004,[35] showed an increased risk of mortality for patients with postextubation respiratory failure who were given NIV rather than standard therapy, apart from those with COPD. It is generally recommended that reintubation should not be delayed for a trial of NIV if indications of extubation failure develop and patients are suitable for reescalation of therapy.[36]

## ■ CONCLUSION

Noninvasive ventilation is recommended by international guidelines, with a strong evidence base, as an adjunct to medical therapy in acute pulmonary edema with respiratory distress and COPD exacerbations or obesity hypoventilation syndrome with hypercapnic respiratory failure and acidosis. The use of NIV for hypoxemic respiratory failure of other etiologies can be considered in appropriately monitored environments if intubation is not significantly delayed in those that are suitable but deteriorating despite therapy. The use of NIV in acute asthma exacerbations remains a controversial area and is not generally recommended. NIV, particularly HFNO, is frequently used in a general critical care population to increase the apnea time during intubation, prevent oxygenation desaturation during intubation attempts, and initiate IMV.

There is good evidence that patients at high risk of respiratory deterioration benefit from tracheal extubation onto immediate NIV, with improved reintubation rates and reduced hospital mortality. However, it is not generally recommended to delay re-establishing IMV for a trial of NIV in those that have already developed respiratory failure postextubation, except in selected cases treating type 2 respiratory failure in patients with COPD. Generally, patients failing standard weaning techniques should not be extubated early onto NIV. However, it may be considered in those with COPD exacerbations and isolated hypercapnic respiratory failure who are otherwise suitable.

Noninvasive ventilation has an established role in treating respiratory failure in critical care due to various causes. If used wisely, it is a crucial tool that can improve patient outcomes and reduce the need for IMV.

## REFERENCES

1. Ashraf-Kashani N, Kumar R. High-flow nasal oxygen therapy. BJA Education. 2017;17(2):57-62.
2. Bauchmuller K, Glossop AJ. Non-invasive ventilation in the perioperative period. BJA Education. 2016;16(9):299-304.
3. Gong Y, Sankari A. Noninvasive Ventilation. Treasure Island (FL): StatPearls Publishing; 2022.
4. British Thoracic Society Standards of Care Committee. Non-invasive ventilation in acute respiratory failure. Thorax. 2002;57(3):192-211.
5. Carbonara P, Nava S. Noninvasive mechanical ventilation. Clin Respir Med. 2012:431-6.
6. Agarwal R, Aggarwal AN, Gupta D, Jindal SK. Non-invasive ventilation in acute cardiogenic pulmonary edema. Postgrad Med J. 2005;81(960):637-43.
7. Pengo MF, Bonafini S, Fava C, Steier J. Cardiorespiratory interaction with continuous positive airway pressure. J Thorac Dis. 2018;10(Suppl 1):S57.
8. Rochwerg B, Brochard L, Elliott MW, Hess D, Hill NS, Nava S, et al. Official ERS/ATS clinical practice guidelines: noninvasive ventilation for acute respiratory failure. Eur Respir J. 2017;50(2):1602426.
9. Perkins GD, Ji C, Connolly BA, Couper K, Lall R, Baillie JK, et al. Effect of noninvasive respiratory strategies on intubation or mortality among patients with acute hypoxemic respiratory failure and COVID-19: the RECOVERY-RS randomized clinical trial. JAMA. 2022;327(6):546-58.
10. Zampieri FG, Ferreira JC. Defining optimal respiratory support for patients with COVID-19. JAMA. 2022;327(6):531-3.
11. Aswanetmanee P, Limsuwat C, Maneechotesuwan K, Wongsurakiat P. Noninvasive ventilation in patients with acute hypoxemic respiratory failure: a systematic review and meta-analysis of randomized controlled trials. Sci Rep. 2023;13(1):8283.
12. Oczkowski S, Ergan B, Bos L, Chatwin M, Ferrer M, Gregoretti C, et al. ERS clinical practice guidelines: high-flow nasal cannula in acute respiratory failure. Eur Respir J. 2022;59(4):2101574.
13. McDonagh TA, Metra M, Adamo M, Gardner RS, Baumbach A, Böhm M, et al. 2021 ESC Guidelines for the diagnosis and treatment of acute and chronic heart failure: Developed by the Task Force for the diagnosis and treatment of acute and chronic heart failure of the European Society of Cardiology (ESC) With the special contribution of the Heart Failure Association (HFA) of the ESC. Eur Heart J. 2021;42(36):3599-726.
14. Berbenetz N, Wang Y, Brown J, Godfrey C, Ahmad M, Vital FM, et al. Non-invasive positive pressure ventilation (CPAP or bilevel NPPV) for cardiogenic pulmonary oedema. Cochrane Database Syst Rev. 2019;4(4):CD005351.
15. National Institute for Health and Care Excellence. Chronic Obstructive Pulmonary Disease in Over 16s: Diagnosis and Management. London: National Institute for Health and Care Excellence (NICE); 2019.
16. Manglani R, Landaeta M, Maldonado M, Hoge G, Basir R, Menon V. The use of non-invasive ventilation in asthma exacerbation–a two year retrospective analysis of outcomes. J Community Hosp Intern Med Perspect. 2021;11(5):727-32.
17. Lim WJ, Akram RM, Carson KV, Mysore S, Labiszewski NA, Wedzicha JA, et al. Non-invasive positive pressure ventilation for treatment of respiratory failure due to severe acute exacerbations of asthma. Cochrane Database Syst Rev. 2012;12:CD004360.
18. Dai J, Wang L, Wang F, Wang L, Wen Q. Noninvasive positive-pressure ventilation for children with acute asthma: a meta-analysis of randomized controlled trials. Front Pediatr. 2023;11:1167506.
19. Davidson AC, Banham S, Elliott M, Kennedy D, Gelder C, Glossop A, et al. BTS/ICS guideline for the ventilatory management of acute hypercapnic respiratory failure in adults. Thorax. 2016;71(Suppl 2):ii1-35.

20. British Thoracic Society. SIGN 158: British Guideline on the Management of Asthma London: British Thoracic Society; 2019.
21. Masa JF, Pépin JL, Borel JC, Mokhlesi B, Murphy PB, Sánchez-Quiroga MÁ. Obesity hypoventilation syndrome. Eur Respir Rev. 2019;28(151):180097.
22. Ahmed NB, Abou Zeid AA, Elhasab MA, Elwafa GS. Noninvasive ventilation in acute exacerbation of interstitial lung diseases. Egypt J Chest Dis Tuberc. 2023;72(1):99-104.
23. Soltaninejad F, Samim A, Salmasi M, Schöbel C, Penzel T, Feizi A, et al. Non Invasive Ventilation's Effectiveness (NIV) in Patients with Interstitial Lung Disease and Hypercapnic Respiratory Failure. Tanaffos. 2022;21(3):302.
24. Dwarakanath A, Elliott M. Noninvasive ventilation in the management of acute hypercapnic respiratory failure. Breathe. 2013;9:338-48.
25. Ozyilmaz E, Ugurlu AO, Nava S. Timing of noninvasive ventilation failure: causes, risk factors, and potential remedies. BMC Pulm Med. 2014;14:19.
26. Azoulay É, Kouatchet A, Jaber S, Lambert J, Meziani F, Schmidt M, et al. Noninvasive mechanical ventilation in patients having declined tracheal intubation. Intens Care Med. 2013;39:292-301.
27. Livesey A, Antoine-Pitterson P, Oakes A, Chakraborty B, Mukherjee R. Ward-based Non-invasive ventilation (NIV) as Ceiling of Care in Acute Hypercapnic Respiratory Failure (AHRF). Eur Respir J. 2018;52(suppl 62):PA2356.
28. Innocenti F, Giordano L, Gualtieri S, Gandini A, Taurino L, Nesa M, et al. Prediction of mortality with the use of noninvasive ventilation for acute respiratory failure. Respir Care. 2020;65(12):1847-56.
29. Sud A, Patel A. THRIVE: five years on and into the COVID-19 era. Br J Anaesth. 2021;126(4):768-73.
30. Baillard C, Prat G, Jung B, Futier E, Lefrant JY, Vincent F, et al. Effect of preoxygenation using non-invasive ventilation before intubation on subsequent organ failures in hypoxaemic patients: a randomised clinical trial. Br J Anaesth. 2018;120(2):361-7.
31. Frat JP, Ricard JD, Quenot JP, Pichon N, Demoule A, Forel JM, et al. Non-invasive ventilation versus high-flow nasal cannula oxygen therapy with apnoeic oxygenation for preoxygenation before intubation of patients with acute hypoxaemic respiratory failure: a randomised, multicentre, open-label trial. Lancet Respir Med. 2019;7(4):303-12.
32. Higgs A, McGrath BA, Goddard C, Rangasami J, Suntharalingam G, Gale R, et al. Guidelines for the management of tracheal intubation in critically ill adults. Br J Anaesth. 2018;120(2):323-52.
33. Boscolo A, Pettenuzzo T, Sella N, Zatta M, Salvagno M, Tassone M, et al. Noninvasive respiratory support after extubation: a systematic review and network meta-analysis. Eur Respir Rev. 2023;32(168):220196.
34. Perkins GD, Mistry D, Gates S, Gao F, Snelson C, Hart N, et al. Effect of protocolized weaning with early extubation to noninvasive ventilation vs invasive weaning on time to liberation from mechanical ventilation among patients with respiratory failure: the breathe randomized clinical trial. JAMA. 2018;320(18):1881-8.
35. Burns KE, Meade MO, Premji A, Adhikari NK. Noninvasive positive-pressure ventilation as a weaning strategy for intubated adults with respiratory failure. Cochrane Database Syst Rev. 2013;2013(12):CD004127.
36. Esteban A, Frutos-Vivar F, Ferguson ND, Arabi Y, Apezteguía C, González M, et al. Noninvasive positive-pressure ventilation for respiratory failure after extubation. N Engl J Med. 2004;350(24):2452-60.

# CHAPTER 17

# Point-of-care Ultrasound in Critical Care

*Vijayalaxmi Bellana, Nageswar Bandla*

## ABSTRACT

Point-of-care ultrasound (POCUS) is a critical tool in modern medical practice, providing real-time diagnostic imaging at the bedside. This chapter explores the fundamentals of ultrasound physics, knobology, sonoanatomy, and practical applications in vascular access, lung, cardiac, and renal ultrasound. We emphasize enhancing clinical skills and improving patient outcomes through the proficient use of POCUS.

**Keywords:** POCUS; Ultrasound physics; Knobology; Sonoanatomy; Vascular access; Lung ultrasound; Cardiac ultrasound; Fluid responsiveness; Renal ultrasound

## KEY POINTS

- POCUS provides immediate diagnostic imaging and enhances clinical decision-making.
- An understanding of ultrasound physics and knobology is essential for optimal image acquisition.
- Proficiency in sonoanatomy allows an accurate interpretation of ultrasound images.
- POCUS is invaluable in guiding vascular access, assessing lung pathology, evaluating cardiac function, and diagnosing renal conditions. It is becoming increasingly popular among intensive care physicians in other areas, such as transcranial ultrasound, orbital ultrasound, and airway ultrasound.

## ■ INTRODUCTION

Point-of-care ultrasound (POCUS) has revolutionized bedside diagnostic capabilities, allowing clinicians to make prompt and accurate decisions. This chapter provides a comprehensive overview of POCUS, including the physics behind ultrasound, the operation of ultrasound machines (knobology), and the anatomical landmarks (sonoanatomy) necessary for accurate imaging. Additionally, it covers the applications of POCUS in vascular access and lung, cardiac, and renal assessments.

## ■ ULTRASOUND PHYSICS

Understanding the principles of ultrasound physics is fundamental to effectively utilizing POCUS. Ultrasound uses high-frequency sound waves to produce images of internal structures.

These sound waves are transmitted into the body, where they are reflected off tissues with varying densities, creating an image based on the echoes received by the transducer **(Figs. 1 and 2)**.[1,2]

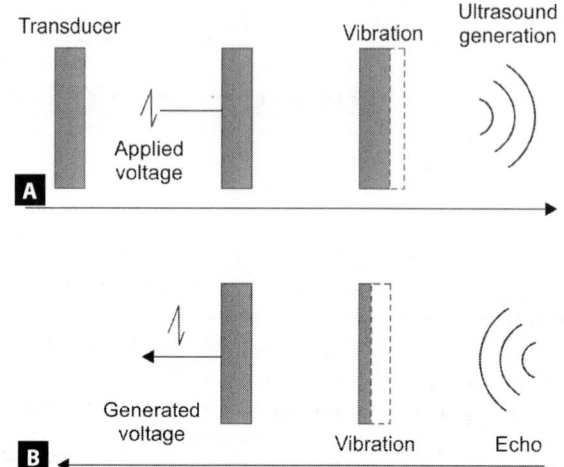

**Figs. 1A and B:** Sound waves reflected off tissues create an echo, which is received by the transducer.[1,2]

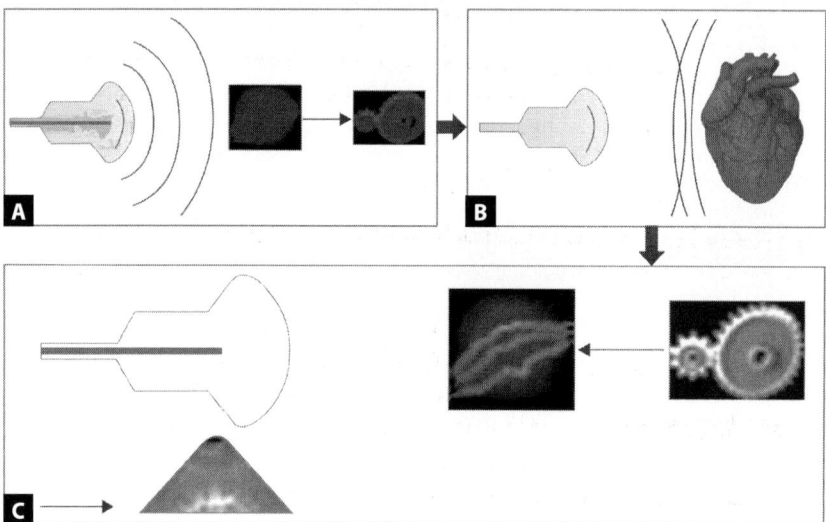

**Figs. 2A to C:** The piezoelectric effect converts kinetic or mechanical energy into electrical energy. This effect is used in ultrasound transducers to receive sound waves. (A) Electric energy is converted into sound waves; (B) Sound waves are reflected by body tissue based on the tissue density; and (C) Reflected sound waves are converted back to electric energy to generate an image.

## Sound Wave Properties

- *Frequency:* Higher frequencies provide better resolution but less penetration, which is suitable for superficial structures.[3]
- *Wavelength:* The distance between successive wave peaks, inversely related to frequency.[4]
- Velocity is the speed at which sound travels through different tissues, averaging 1,540 m/s in soft tissue.[5]

## Image Formation
- *Reflection:* Occurs at tissue boundaries with differing acoustic impedances.[6]
- *Refraction:* Bending of sound waves at interfaces, affecting image quality[7]
- *Attenuation:* Reduction in sound wave intensity due to absorption, scattering, and reflection.[8]

## Probes
The footprint is the part of the probe that contacts the patient's skin. The probes range from the largest (curvilinear) to the smallest (phased array). The standard probes in use are shown in **Figures 3A to C.**[4]
- *Linear probe (5–15 MHz):* It is best for imaging soft tissues, musculoskeletal areas, pediatrics, eyes, trachea, thyroid, chest, most procedures, deep vein thrombosis (DVT), appendicitis, and testicular examinations. It offers high resolution for structures <8 cm deep.
- *Curvilinear probe (2–5 MHz):* It is suitable for abdominal examinations (gallbladder and liver), extended focused assessment with sonography in trauma (eFAST), renal, aorta, inferior vena cava (IVC), bladder, bowel, and obstetrics/gynecology. Its large footprint provides excellent lateral resolution but could be more effective between ribs.
- *Phased array probe (1–5 MHz):* It is ideal for cardiac, abdominal, eFAST, renal, bladder, bowel, and IVC imaging. Its small footprint makes it perfect for cardiac examinations and scanning between ribs.

## Artifacts
- Due to reflection, refraction, and scatter as ultrasound waves pass through various media **(Figs. 4A to C)**.[9]

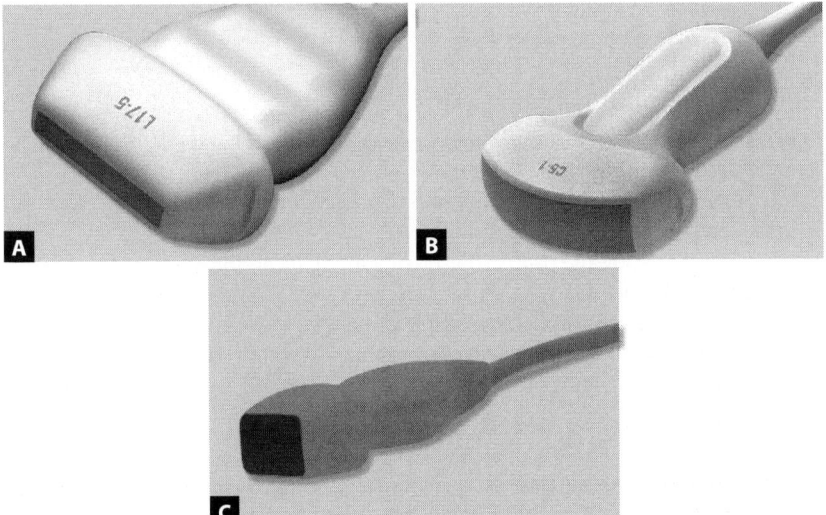

**Figs. 3A to C:** Commonly used ultrasound probes. (A) Linear probe; (B) Curvilinear probe; and (C) Phased array probe.

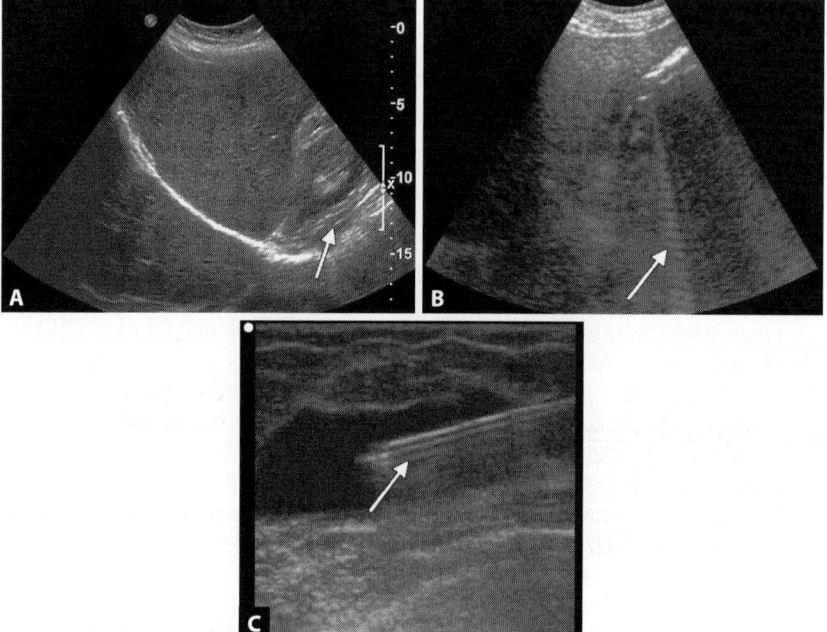

**Figs. 4A to C:** Artifacts that can be seen during an ultrasound. (A) Reverberation seen as a mirror image; (B) Comet tail artifact; and (C) Reflection artifact.

- *Types:*
    - Reverberation
    - Comet-tail
    - Reflection
    - Attenuation artifact
    - Acoustic enhancement

## Fundamental Ultrasound Movements

Effective probe handling and movement are vital to obtaining the best images. The four primary movements are:
1. *Slide:* Moving the entire probe to find a better imaging window[10]
2. *Rock:* Tilting the probe along its long axis[11]
3. *Tilt (Fan):* Moving the probe side-to-side along its short axis to capture cross-sectional images[12]
4. *Rotate:* Turning the probe clockwise or counterclockwise along its central axis.[13]

In addition, compression involves pressing down with the probe to compress tissues and improve image clarity.[14]

## Basic Ultrasound Modes

Familiarity with ultrasound modes is essential for effective scanning. The modes are:
- *B-mode (brightness mode):* It is the default mode for most ultrasound machines, providing two-dimensional grayscale images.[15]

- *Color Doppler mode:* This mode visualizes blood flow with color coding (red for flow toward the probe, blue for flow away), which is remembered by the mnemonic BART (blue away, red towards).[16]
- *Power Doppler mode:* This mode is more sensitive than color Doppler and detects low blood flow with a single color (usually yellow).[17]
- *Pulse wave (PW) Doppler:* This mode measures blood flow velocity in a specific area.[18]
- *Continuous wave (CW) Doppler:* This mode measures high-velocity blood flow and is typically used in cardiac assessments.[19]
- *Tissue Doppler imaging (TDI):* This mode is used to assess myocardial movement velocity to evaluate diastolic function.[20]

## Steps for Optimal Imaging

*Select the correct probe:* Use the appropriate probe based on the specific application.[21]
- *Adjust depth:* Set the depth to visualize the target structure adequately without excess[22]
- *Modify gain:* Adjust the overall gain to control the image brightness[23]
- *Choose application presets:* Select the correct preset for the probe and application, which automatically adjusts the frequency, depth, and gain.[24]

## KNOBOLOGY

Knobology refers to the understanding and manipulation of the various controls on an ultrasound machine to optimize image quality.

### Basic Controls

- *Gain:* Adjusts the brightness of the image.[25]
- *Depth:* Controls the field of view, allowing visualization of structures at different depths.
- *Focus:* Enhances the resolution at a particular depth.
- *Mode:* Different modes, such as B-mode (brightness), M-mode (motion), and Doppler, are used to assess blood flow.

## SONOANATOMY

Sonoanatomy involves the identification of anatomical structures using ultrasound.

### Vascular Structures

- *Arteries:* Appear as round, pulsatile structures with thicker walls
- *Veins:* Compressible, thinner-walled structures

### Lung

- *Pleura:* The sliding motion of the pleura is a crucial indicator of normal lung function[1]
- *A-lines and B-lines:* Artifacts indicating different lung pathologies.[3]

### Heart

- *Chambers and valves:* Visualization of the cardiac chambers, valves, and contractility
- *Pericardium:* Assessment for effusion

## Kidneys

- *Cortex and medulla:* Differentiation of renal parenchyma
- *Pelvis:* Identification of hydronephrosis

## ■ VASCULAR ACCESS

The POCUS is invaluable for guiding vascular access, enhancing success rates, and reducing complications. Ultrasound's real-time imaging capability allows for precise needle placement, minimizing the risk of complications such as arterial puncture, hematoma, and pneumothorax.

## Central Venous Access

Central venous access is critical in many clinical settings, including intensive care units, emergency departments, and operating rooms. Ultrasound guidance significantly improves the success rate and safety of central venous catheterization.

### *Internal Jugular Vein*

- *Preferred site:* The internal jugular vein (IJV) is commonly used for central venous access due to its superficial location and easy visualization with ultrasound.
- *Visualization:* The IJV can be visualized in transverse (short axis) and longitudinal (long axis) planes. In the transverse plane, the vein appears as a compressible, anechoic (dark) structure lateral to the carotid artery. In the longitudinal plane, the vein appears as a long, tubular structure, and the needle can be seen entering the vein in real time **(Figs. 5 and 6)**. The vein can also be visualized by following the course of the needle tip with the transducer (needle tip dynamic needle tip positioning) **(Fig. 7)**.

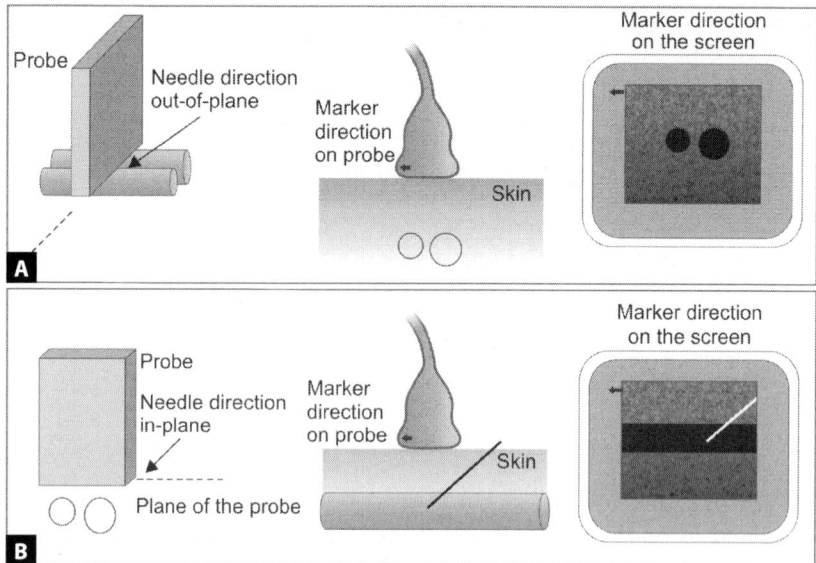

**Figs. 5A and B:** Ultrasound visualization—(A) Out-of-plane; (B) In-plane.

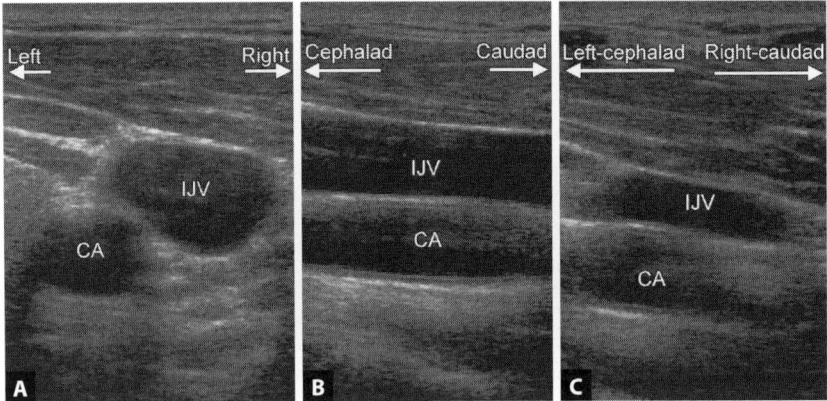

**Figs. 6A to C:** Out-of-plane and in-plane ultrasound cannulation and the view in an oblique axis. (A) Short axis; (B) Long axis; and (C) Oblique axis. (CA: carotid artery; IJV: internal jugular vein)

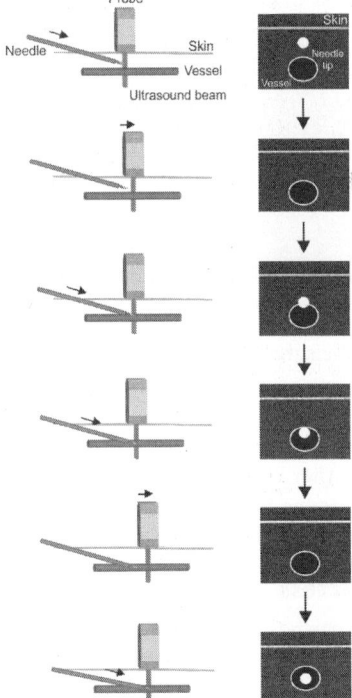

**Fig. 7:** Dynamic needle tip positioning in out-of-plane technique.

## Subclavian Vein

The subclavian vein is located beneath the clavicle and can be more challenging due to its deep location and proximity to the lung apex. However, ultrasound guidance can improve the success rate and reduce complications. **Figures 8A and B** show

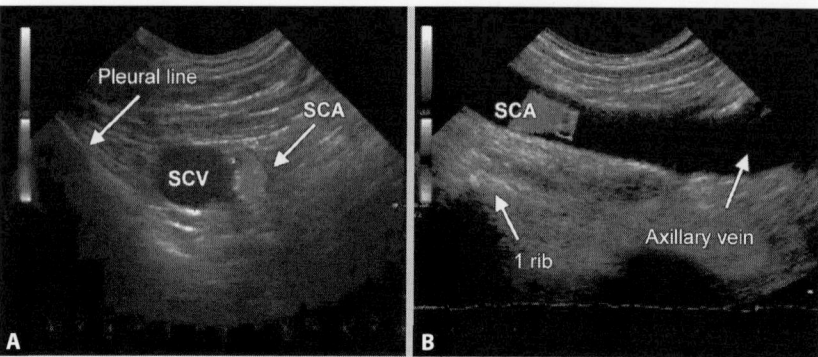

**Figs. 8A and B:** Subclavian vein cannulation. (SCA: subclavian artery; SCV: subclavian vein)

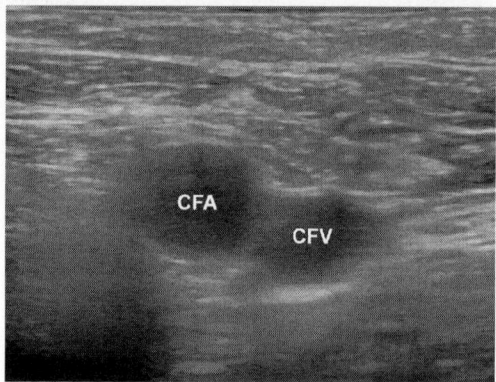

**Fig. 9:** Femoral vein cannulation. (CFA: common femoral artery; CFV: common femoral vein)

the ultrasound views of the subclavian artery and subclavian vein on both the short and long axes.

## Femoral Vein

The femoral vein is another central venous access alternative, particularly in emergencies. It is medial to the femoral artery in the groin region and can be easily visualized with ultrasound **(Fig. 9)**.

## Peripheral Venous Access

Peripheral venous access can be challenging in patients with difficult IV access due to obesity, chronic illness, or frequent hospitalizations. POCUS can facilitate peripheral IV placement by identifying suitable veins that are not easily palpable or visible.

### Difficult IV Access

*Visualization:* Ultrasound can identify deep or small veins, increasing the success rate of cannulation. The veins can be visualized in transverse and longitudinal planes, similar to central venous access. Real-time imaging allows for precise needle guidance, reducing the need for multiple attempts and minimizing patient discomfort.

## LUNG ULTRASOUND

Lung ultrasound is crucial in diagnosing various pulmonary conditions. It is a noninvasive, bedside tool that provides immediate information about lung pathology.[6] Lung ultrasound can diagnose acute respiratory failure **(Flowchart 1)**.

### Pneumothorax

Pneumothorax is the presence of air in the pleural space, which can lead to lung collapse. Early detection and management are critical.

#### Indicators of Pneumothorax

- *Absent lung sliding:* The absence of lung sliding is a key sonographic sign of pneumothorax. Usually, the visceral and parietal pleura glide smoothly against each other during respiration, creating a sliding motion on ultrasound. The absence of this motion suggests that the pleural layers are separated by air, indicating pneumothorax.[2]
- *Absence of normal lung motion or barcode sign:* The barcode sign (also known as the stratosphere sign) is another indicator of pneumothorax. On M-mode

**Flowchart 1:** The BLUE protocol to diagnose acute respiratory failure using lung ultrasound.

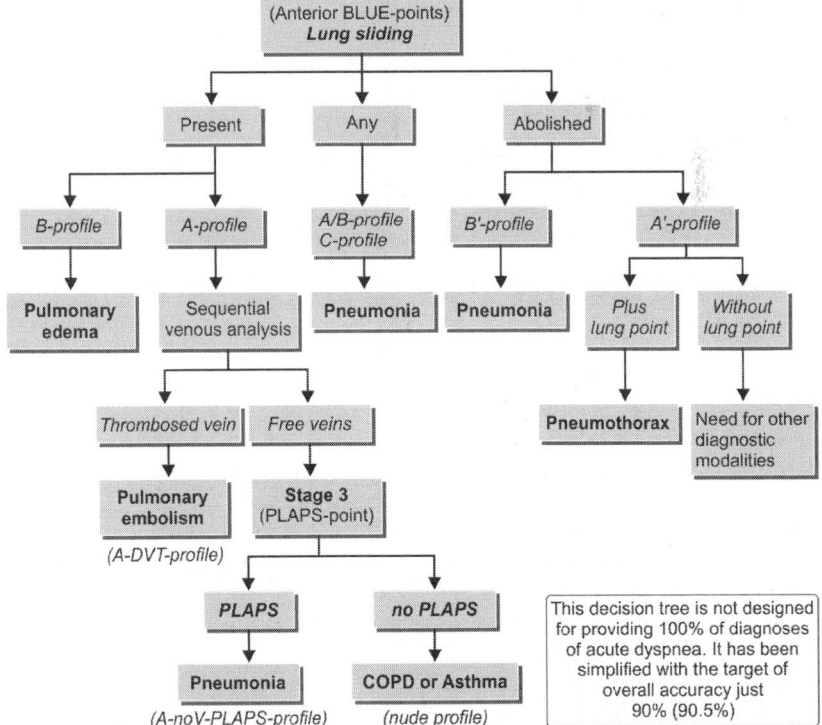

(BLUE: Bedside Lung Ultrasound in Emergency; PLAPS: posterolateral alveolar and/or pleural syndrome)
(*Source:* Adapted from Lichtenstein and Meziere with permission of chest).

ultrasound, normal lung sliding produces a characteristic seashore sign with a granular pattern below the pleural line. In pneumothorax, this pattern is replaced by horizontal lines resembling a barcode, indicating the absence of normal lung motion **(Fig. 10)**.[2]

## Pleural Effusion

Pleural effusion is the accumulation of fluid in the pleural space. Lung ultrasound is highly sensitive in detecting even small pleural effusions.[2]

### Anechoic Fluid Collection

Pleural effusion appears as an anechoic (dark) fluid collection in the dependent areas of the thorax **(Fig. 11)**. Due to gravity, the fluid accumulates in the lowest parts of the pleural cavity, making it easily identifiable with ultrasound. The diaphragm and liver or spleen can serve as landmarks to distinguish pleural effusion from other intrathoracic pathologies.[2]

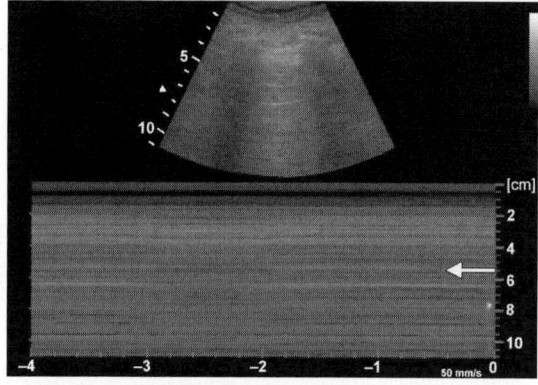

**Fig. 10:** The barcode or stratosphere sign on lung ultrasound.

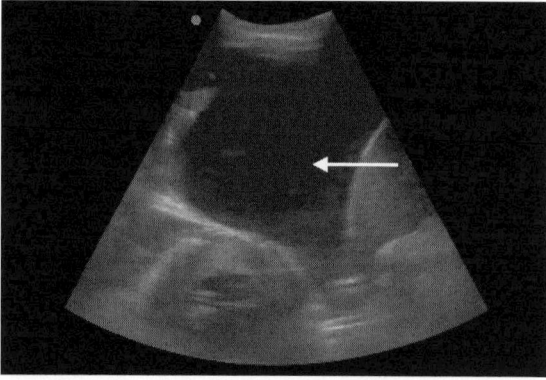

**Fig. 11:** Large pleural effusion.

## Pulmonary Edema

- Cardiogenic pulmonary edema is when increased pressure in the heart's left ventricle increases pressure in the left atrium.
- This elevated pressure in the left atrium, in turn, causes increased pressure in the pulmonary veins and, ultimately, in the pulmonary capillaries.
- The development of cardiogenic pulmonary edema is often associated with cardiac dysfunction, such as heart failure or left ventricular dysfunction.[9]

B-lines are ultrasound artifacts that appear as vertical lines in the image **(Figs. 12A to C)**.

- B-lines start at the pleural line and go to the bottom of the image, breaking up horizontal lines.
- When there are many close together, they merge into one line.
- They are caused by ultrasound energy bouncing off fluid-filled areas surrounded by air in the lungs.

## Diaphragm

*Assessment for diaphragmatic movement:* Ultrasound can also assess diaphragmatic movement, which is crucial in patients with pleural effusion. Reduced or absent diaphragmatic movement may indicate diaphragmatic paralysis or severe effusion, necessitating further intervention **(Figs. 13A and B)**.

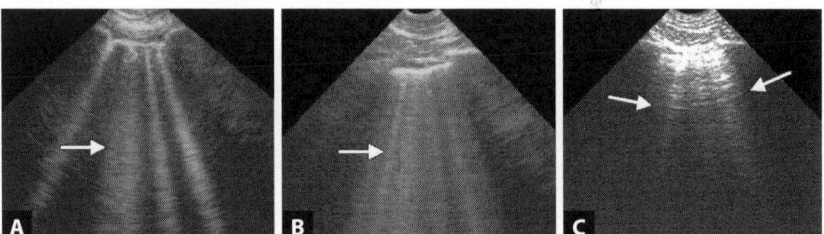

**Figs. 12A to C:** Pulmonary edema. Arrows indicate B-lines.

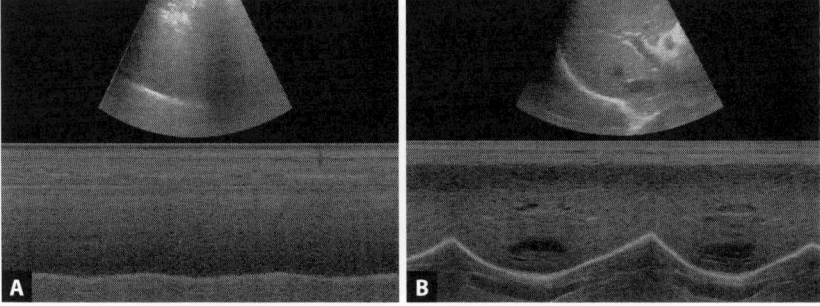

**Figs. 13A and B:** Diaphragmatic movement on ultrasound.
(A) Paralyzed diaphragm; (B) Normal diaphragm.

## ■ CARDIAC ULTRASOUND

Cardiac POCUS enables rapid cardiac function and hemodynamics assessment, providing crucial information for managing various cardiac conditions. It is instrumental in emergency and critical care settings.

### Left Ventricular Function

Assessment of left ventricular function is a fundamental component of cardiac ultrasound, aiding in diagnosing and managing heart failure, myocardial infarction, and other cardiac pathologies.

### Ejection Fraction

Ejection fraction (EF) measures the percentage of blood the left ventricle ejects with each contraction. It is a crucial indicator of cardiac function.

### Estimation Using Visual Assessment or Simpson's Method

The EF can be estimated visually by experienced clinicians or calculated more precisely using Simpson's method. This method involves tracing the endocardial borders in the apical four-chamber and two-chamber views to calculate the ventricular volumes at end-diastole and end-systole, as seen in **Figure 14**. A dilated left ventricle with a low EF can also be seen in the ultrasound, as seen in **Figure 15**.

### Wall Motion Abnormalities

*Indicators of ischemia or infarction:* Wall motion abnormalities are detected by observing the contraction patterns of the left ventricular walls. Hypokinesis (reduced movement), akinesis (absence of movement), and dyskinesis (paradoxical movement) can indicate areas of ischemia or infarction. These abnormalities are often segmental and correspond to the territory supplied by a specific coronary artery.

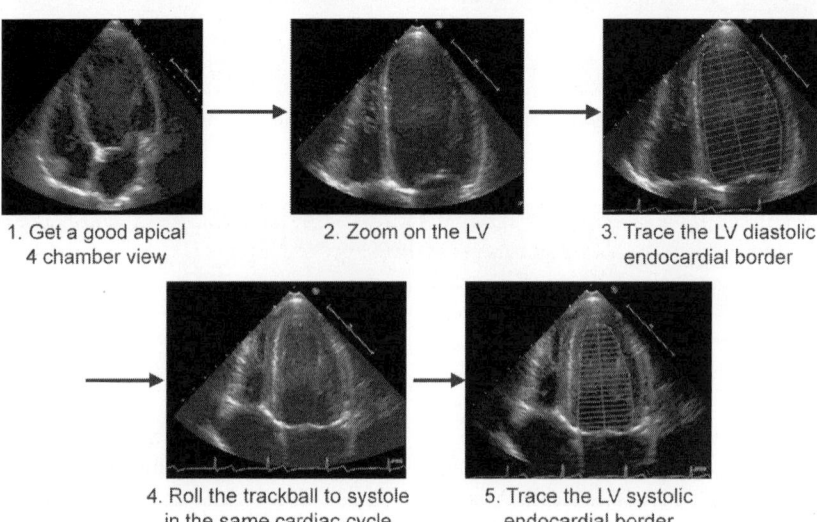

1. Get a good apical 4 chamber view
2. Zoom on the LV
3. Trace the LV diastolic endocardial border
4. Roll the trackball to systole in the same cardiac cycle
5. Trace the LV systolic endocardial border

**Fig. 14:** Estimating the ejection fraction using the Simpson's method.

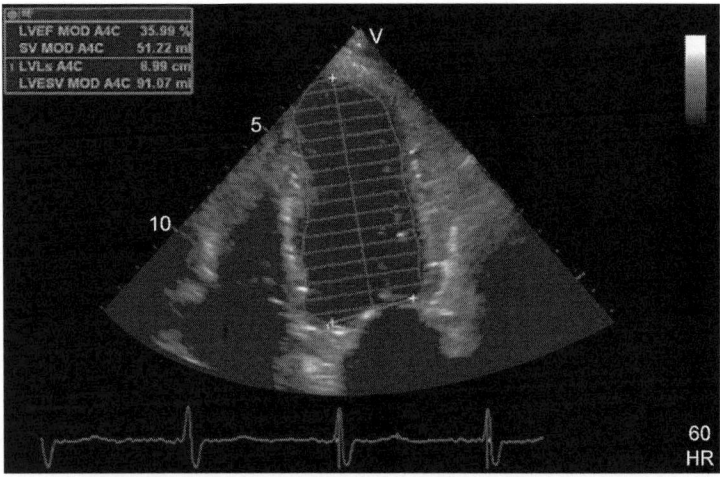

**Fig. 15:** A dilated left ventricle with a low ejection fraction.

*Pericardial effusion:* It refers to fluid accumulation in the pericardial sac surrounding the heart, which can lead to cardiac tamponade, a life-threatening condition. Anechoic space surrounds the heart, indicating effusion. On ultrasound, pericardial effusion appears as an anechoic (dark) space surrounding the heart **(Figs. 16A to E)**. The amount of fluid can vary from small, clinically insignificant effusions to large, compressive ones.

## Tamponade Physiology

### Assessment for Hemodynamic Compromise

Cardiac tamponade occurs when the pressure from the pericardial effusion compresses the heart, impairing its ability to fill and pump effectively. Ultrasound signs of tamponade include right atrial and right ventricular diastolic collapse, dilated IVC without respiratory variation, and exaggerated respiratory variation in transvalvular Doppler flow.

## Right Ventricle

Enlargement of the right ventricle is determined by the ratio of the right ventricle end-diastolic area (RVEDA) with the left ventricle end-diastolic area (LVEDA) **(Fig. 17)**.
- No dilatation—RVEDA/LVEDA <0.6
- Moderate dilatation—RVEDA/LVEDA 0.6–1.0
- Severe dilatation—RVEDA/LVEDA >1.0

## ■ ASSESSMENT OF VOLUME STATUS

*Volume status assessment* is crucial in managing acutely unwell patients. It determines whether they will respond to fluids and how much fluid should be administered. Techniques such as IVC and left ventricular outflow tract velocity time integral (LVOT VTI) assessments guide this assessment, offering real-time data to guide clinical decisions.

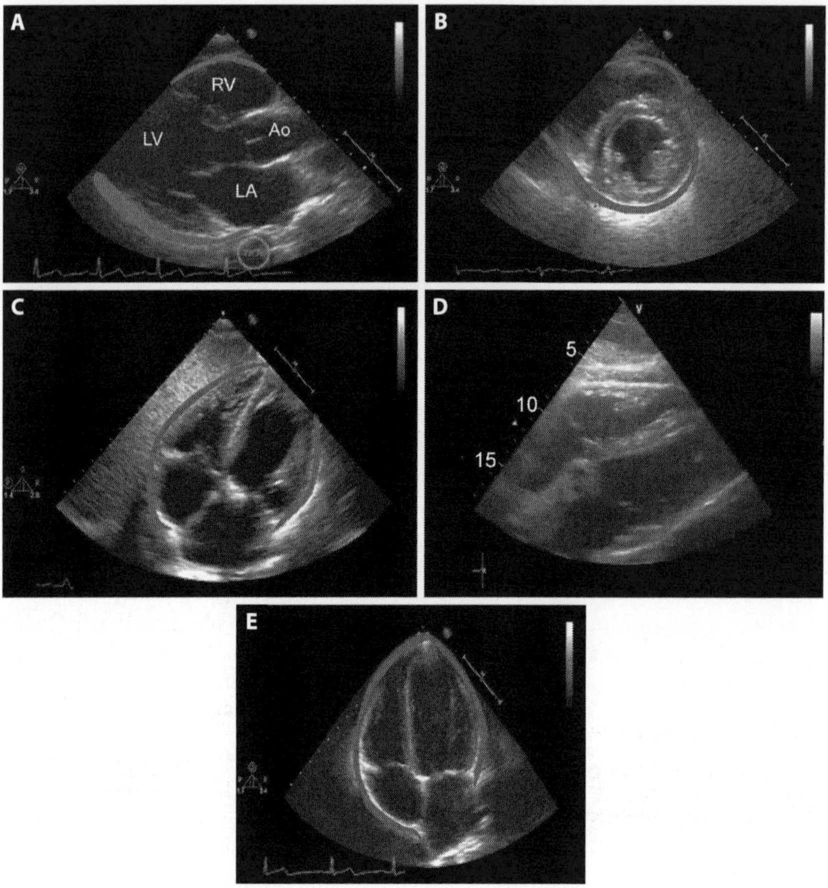

**Figs. 16A to E:** Pericardial effusion around the heart chambers.

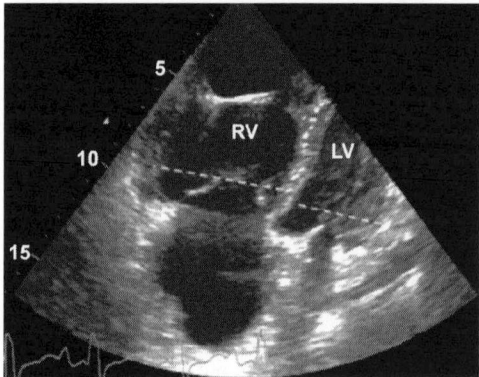

**Fig. 17:** Severely dilated right ventricle with RVEDA/LVEDA >1.0. (LVEDA: left ventricle end-diastolic area; RVEDA: right ventricle end-diastolic area)

## Inferior Vena Cava

### Inferior Vena Cava Assessment

The IVC's size and collapsibility during respiration help estimate right atrial pressure and fluid responsiveness. A collapsing, flat IVC suggests fluid responsiveness **(Figs. 18A and B)**.[10]

### Inferior Vena Cava Collapsibility Index

In spontaneously breathing patients, near total collapsibility indicates fluid responsiveness **(Fig. 19 and Table 1)**.[10]

### Inferior Vena Cava Distensibility Index

In mechanically ventilated patients, the IVC distends during inspiration **(Fig. 20)**.[10] The distensibility index can be used to assess fluid responsiveness. **Table 2** shows the formulas for calculating the collapse and distensibility indices.

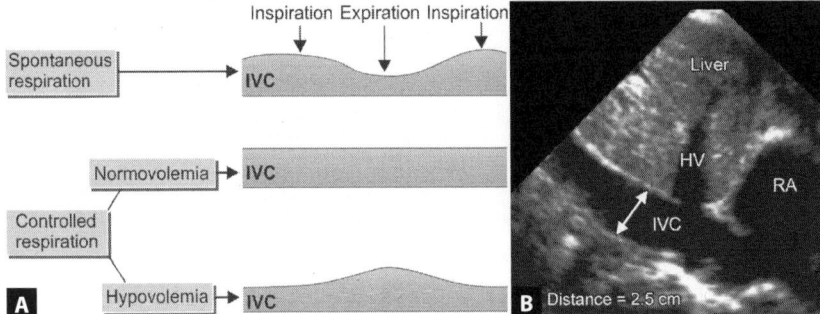

**Figs. 18A and B:** (A) The diameter of the inferior vena cava (IVC) in spontaneous respiration varies with the phase of respiration. During controlled ventilation, it collapses during inspiration in hypovolemic patients but not in normovolemic patients. (B) Measuring the IVC.

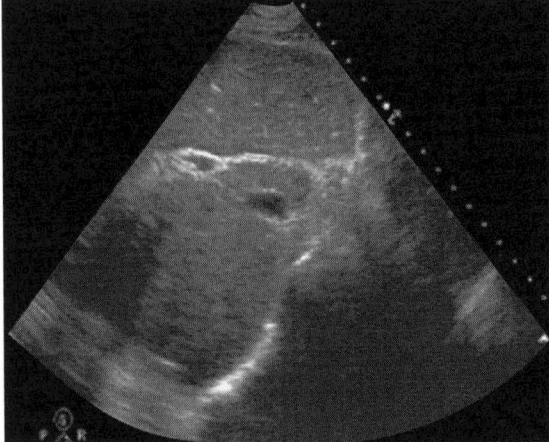

**Fig. 19:** In a spontaneously breathing patient, collapsed IVC is suggestive of fluid responsiveness.

**TABLE 1:** Relationship between the right atrial pressures, IVC diameter, and IVC collapsibility in spontaneously breathing patients.

| Mean right atrial pressure (mm Hg) | Inferior vena cava diameter (cm) | Inferior vena cava inspiratory collapse (%) |
|---|---|---|
| 0–5 | <20 | >50 |
| 5–10 | <20 | <50 |
| 10–15 | >20 | <50 |
| >15 | >25 | No inspiratory collapse |

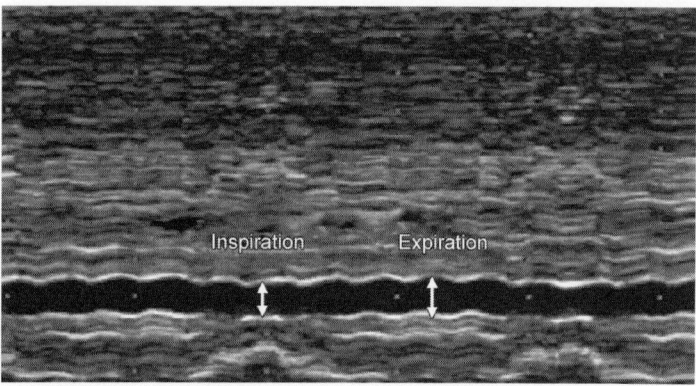

**Fig. 20:** IVC in mechanically ventilated patients. Distensibility index >12–18% indicates fluid responsiveness.

**TABLE 2:** Collapsibility and distensibility indices (CI and DI).

| Collapsibility index (spontaneous breathing) | Distensibility index (mechanical breathing) |
|---|---|
| CI = (Dmax − Dmin)/Dmax × 100% | DI = (Dmax − Dmin)/Dmin × 100% |

## Left Ventricular Outflow Tract Velocity Time Integral Variation

*LVOT VTI:* Stroke volume can be measured with pulsed wave (PW) Doppler at the LVOT. Variation in LVOT VTI (**Fig. 21**),[10] especially a rise in VTI with passive leg raise, indicates fluid responsiveness (**Figs. 22A and B**).

## Tracheal Ultrasound

The sonoanatomy of the upper airway is shown in **Figures 23 to 25**.

## Applications in Airway Management

### Confirmation of Endotracheal Tube Placement

- *Importance:* Ensures that the endotracheal tube (ETT) is correctly positioned in the trachea rather than the esophagus.[13]
- *Method:* Visualizing the ETT within the trachea using ultrasound immediately confirms correct placement (**Figs. 26A and B**).[13]

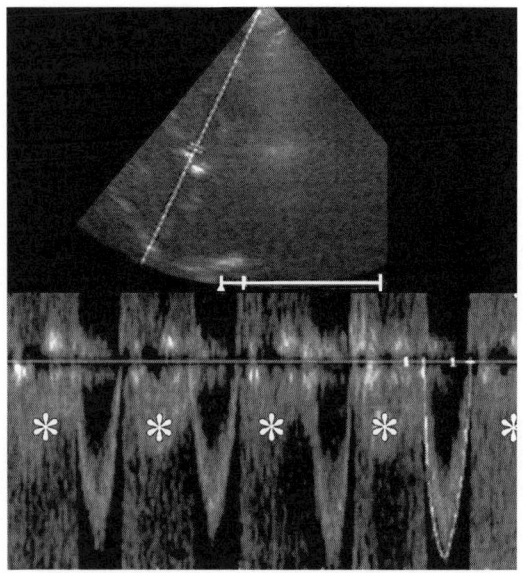

**Fig. 21:** The ratio of LVOT velocity time integral and peak systolic variability for fluid responsiveness.

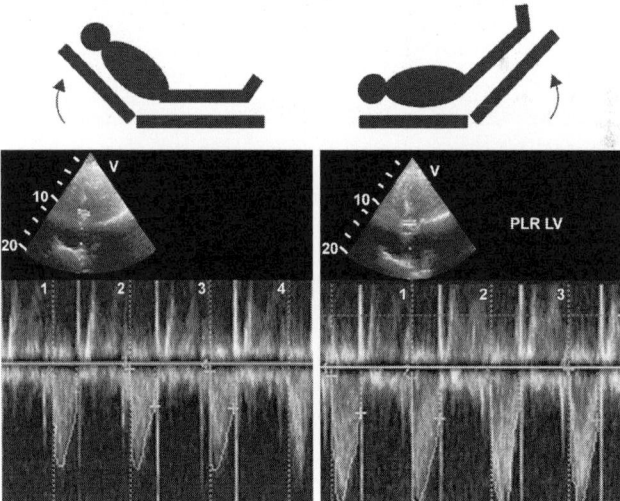

**Figs. 22A and B:** Passive leg raise test in spontaneously breathing patients for fluid responsiveness.

- *Advantages:* It is instrumental in noisy environments or patients where traditional methods such as auscultation and capnography might be less effective.[13]

## Percutaneous Tracheostomy

Ultrasound offers anatomical guidance for percutaneous dilatational tracheostomy (PDT) **(Fig. 27)**. It helps clinicians to determine the correct tracheostomy tube size

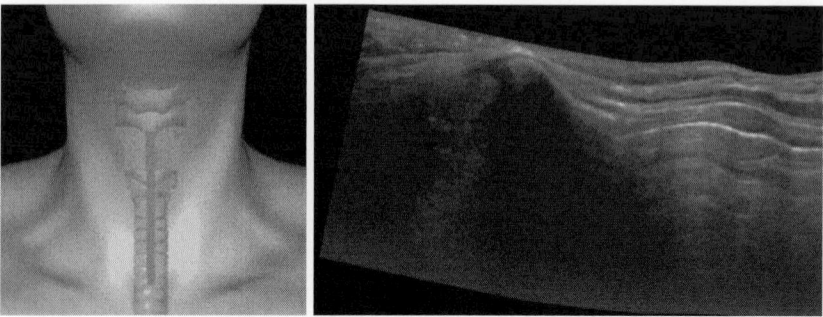

**Fig. 23:** Tracheal sonoanatomy in transverse section.

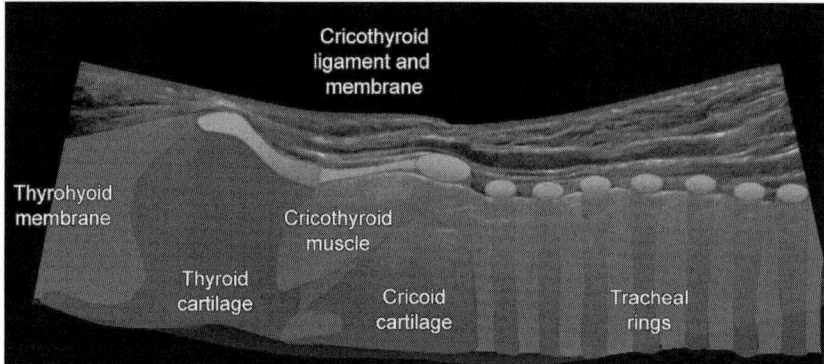

**Fig. 24:** Tracheal anatomy showing laryngeal and tracheal cartilages.

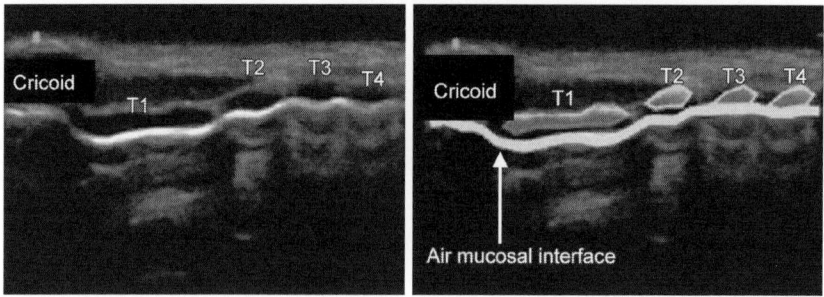

**Fig. 25:** Cricoid cartilage and tracheal cartilage longitudinal plane.

and length, avoid structures in the front of the neck, and prevent injuries to the back wall of the trachea.[13.]

Using ultrasound before the procedure enhances the safety of PDT. Research indicates that about 25% of patients needed their PDT puncture site adjusted based on ultrasound findings.

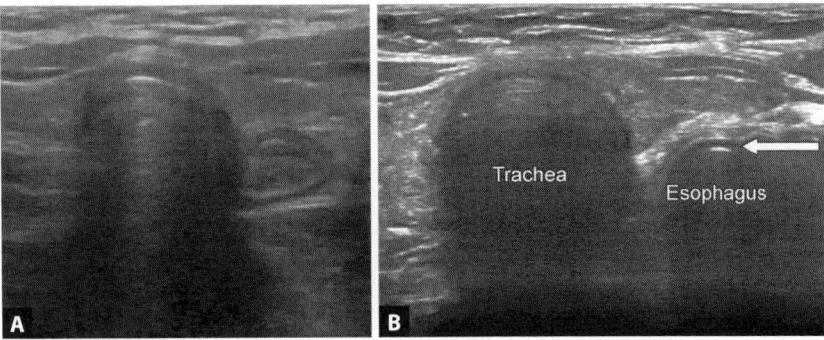

**Figs. 26A and B:** (A) Transverse view of an endotracheal tube in the trachea (esophagus is seen collapsed); (B) Transverse view of an endotracheal tube in the esophagus (seen as a "double tract" sign).

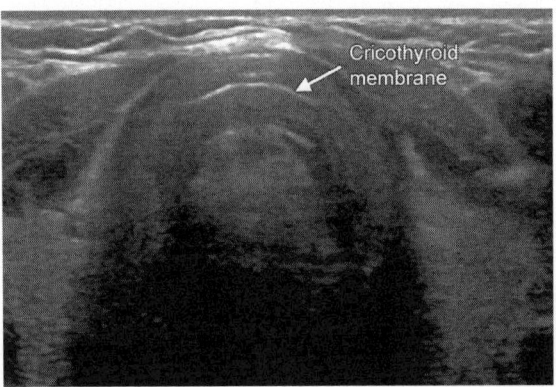

**Fig. 27:** The cricothyroid membrane in the transverse plane.

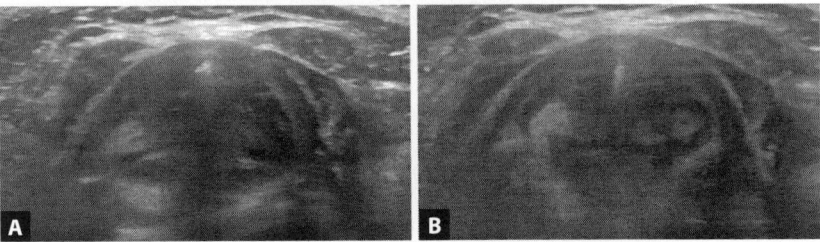

**Figs. 28A and B:** (A) Vocal cord function depicting vocal cord abduction and (B) vocal cord adduction.

## Evaluation of Vocal Cord Function (Figs. 28A and B)

### Function Assessment
- *Method:* Ultrasound can visualize the movement of vocal cords[13].
- *Conditions:* Useful in diagnosing conditions such as vocal cord paralysis [13].
- *Applications:* Particularly beneficial for patients with potential nerve damage due to surgical procedures or trauma.[13]

## Optic Nerve Sheath Diameter

The ocular anatomy on ultrasound is shown in **Figures 29A and B**.

### Measurement

*Method:* Measuring the diameter of the optic nerve sheath using ultrasound [16]

### Procedure

- *Positioning:* Patient lies supine with the head slightly elevated.
- *Transducer:* High-frequency linear probe (7.5–10 MHz)
- *Technique:* Gently place the probe on the closed eyelid using ample gel, identify the optic nerve sheath 3 mm behind the globe, and measure perpendicular to the optic nerve **(Fig. 30)**.[16]

### Interpretation

- *Normal range:* <5 mm in adults[16]
- *Elevated ICP:* Optic nerve sheath diameter (ONSD) >5.0 mm suggests increased ICP.[17]

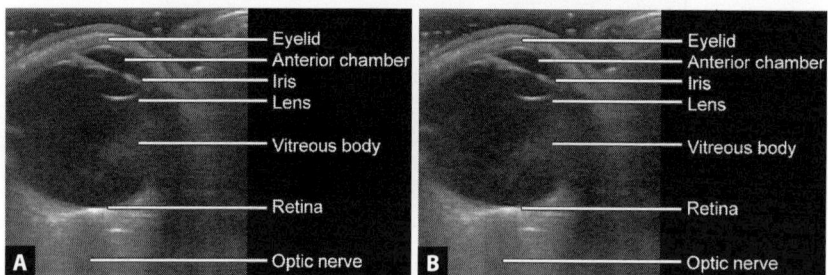

**Figs. 29A and B:** Ocular anatomy in ultrasound in and transverse view.

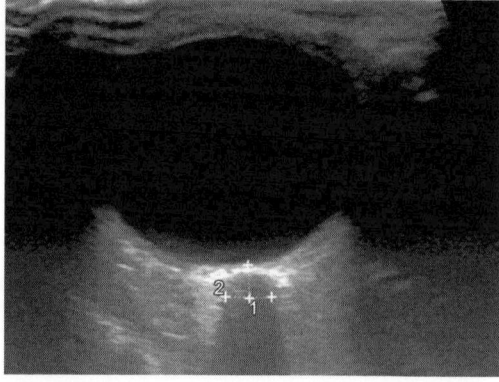

**Fig. 30:** Optic nerve sheath diameter measurement.

## Clinical Applications
- *Traumatic brain injury:* Rapid assessment of ICP[16]
- *Intracranial hemorrhage:* Monitoring ICP noninvasively[16]
- *Hydrocephalus:* Evaluating shunt function and monitoring ICP[16]

## Deep Vein Thrombosis and Ultrasound
Ultrasound is the primary diagnostic tool for detecting blood clots in deep veins, crucial for preventing complications like pulmonary embolism (PE).[18]

## Ultrasound Technique for Deep Vein Thrombosis
- *Venous ultrasound:* Imaging deep veins to identify thrombi
- *Key veins:* Femoral, popliteal, and calf veins **(Fig. 31)**

### Procedure
- *Patient positioning:* Supine with the leg slightly rotated outward[18]
- *Transducer selection:* Use a high-frequency linear probe (7.5-10 MHz) for superficial veins and a lower-frequency curvilinear probe (5-7.5 MHz) for deeper veins[18].
- *Compression technique:*
  - *Method:* Apply the probe transversely along the vein, gently compress every few centimeters
  - *Normal vein:* Compresses completely[18]
  - *Thrombus:* Prevents full compression[18]

### Interpretation
- *Compressibility:* A noncompressible vein suggests a thrombus[18]
- *Echogenicity:* Thrombus is seen as an echogenic area **(Fig. 32)**[18]

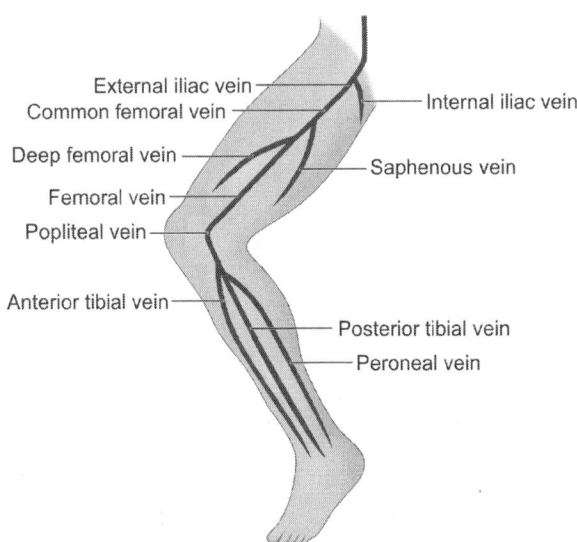

**Fig. 31:** Schematic diagram representing the venous system of the lower extremity.

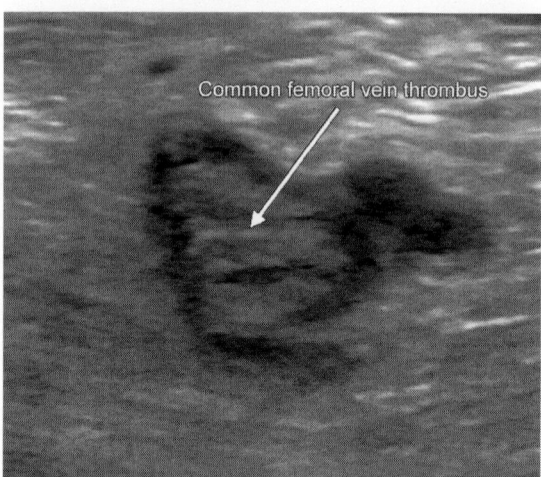

**Fig. 32:** Thrombus in the common femoral vein.

- *Flow characteristics:* Doppler ultrasound to assess blood flow; absence or reduced flow indicates thrombus[18]

## Clinical Applications

- *Symptomatic DVT:* Diagnosing leg pain, swelling, and erythema
- *Asymptomatic screening:* High-risk patients like those undergoing major surgery or with prolonged immobility
- *Follow-up:* Monitoring response to anticoagulation therapy and thrombus resolution

## Ultrasound in Abdominal Examination

### Procedure

- *Patient positioning:* Supine or left lateral decubitus for specific views.
- *Transducer selection:* Low-frequency curvilinear probe (2–5 MHz) for deep structures.
- *Scanning technique:*
    - *Right upper quadrant (RUQ):* Liver, gallbladder, right kidney, and Morison's pouch **(Fig. 33)**
    - *Left upper quadrant (LUQ):* Spleen, left kidney, and splenorenal recess **(Fig. 34)**
    - *Pelvis:* Bladder, pouch of Douglas, or rectovesical pouch **(Figs. 35 and 36)**
    - *Cardiac views:* Subxiphoid four-chamber view for pericardial effusion
    - *Lungs:* Pneumothorax and pleural effusion evaluation.

## Ultrasound in Lung Examination

A typical ultrasound image of the lung is seen with the hyperechoic pleural line reflecting the "back of a bat", and the hypoechoic rib shadows on either side reflect the "wings of the bat", hence the term Batwing sign for a normal lung **(Figs. 37A and B)**.

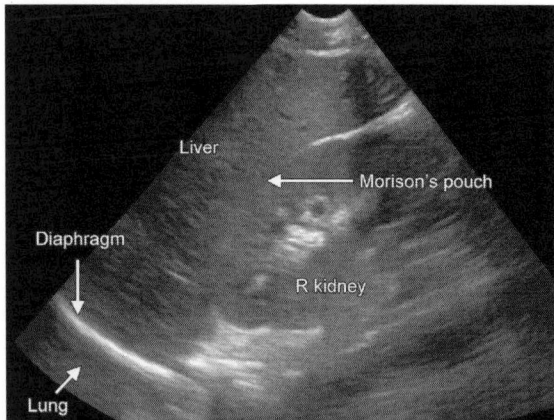

**Fig. 33:** Ultrasound scan of the right upper quadrant of the abdomen.

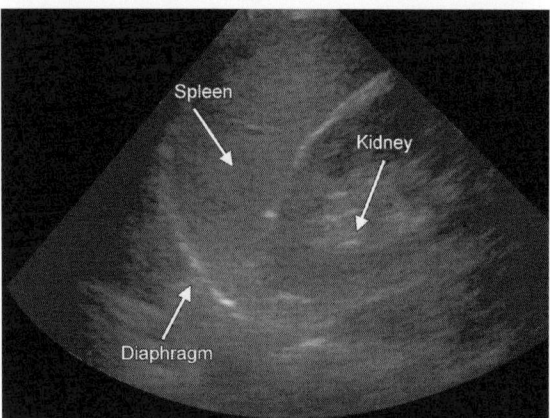

**Fig. 34:** Ultrasound scan of the left upper quadrant of the abdomen.

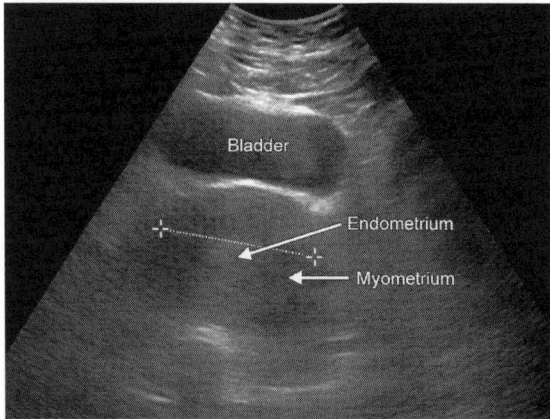

**Fig. 35:** Ultrasound scan of the female pelvis in the longitudinal view.

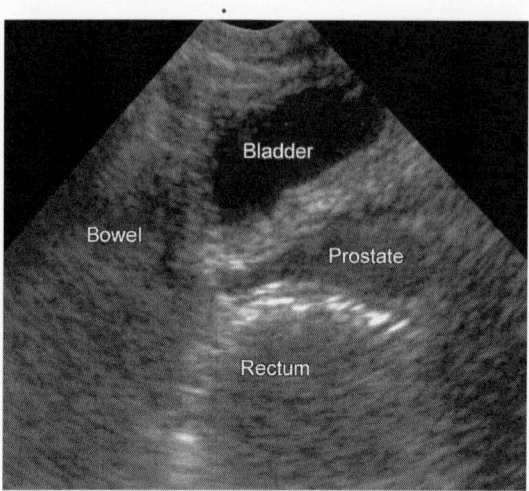

**Fig. 36:** Ultrasound scan of the male pelvis in the longitudinal view.

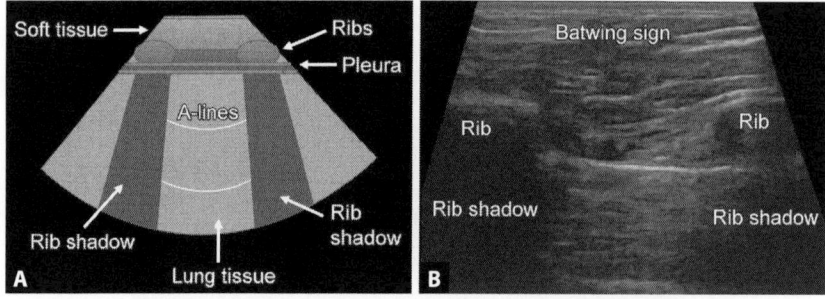

**Figs. 37A and B:** Normal ultrasound of the lung depicting the Batwing sign.

Pneumothorax is depicted by the absence of lung sliding and a barcode sign (**Figs. 38 and 39**). When lung sliding is abolished, a barcode or stratosphere sign is seen in patients with pneumothorax, and parallel hyperintense lines replace the normal aerated lung's sand-like appearance beneath the pleural line.

*Tension pneumothorax:* Recognized by the absence of lung sliding and the presence of lung point. Ultrasound aids in safe decompression during critical conditions.

## Limitations and Competencies in Protocol-driven Point-of-care Ultrasound

Point-of-care ultrasound is an increasingly utilized tool in medical practice due to its versatility, immediacy, and noninvasive nature. Despite its advantages, healthcare providers must recognize inherent limitations and required competencies to ensure accurate and effective use.

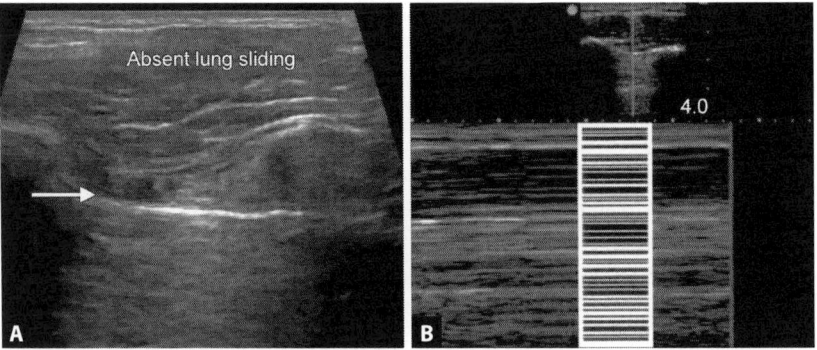

**Figs. 38A and B:** Lung ultrasound showing absence of lung sliding and barcode sign.

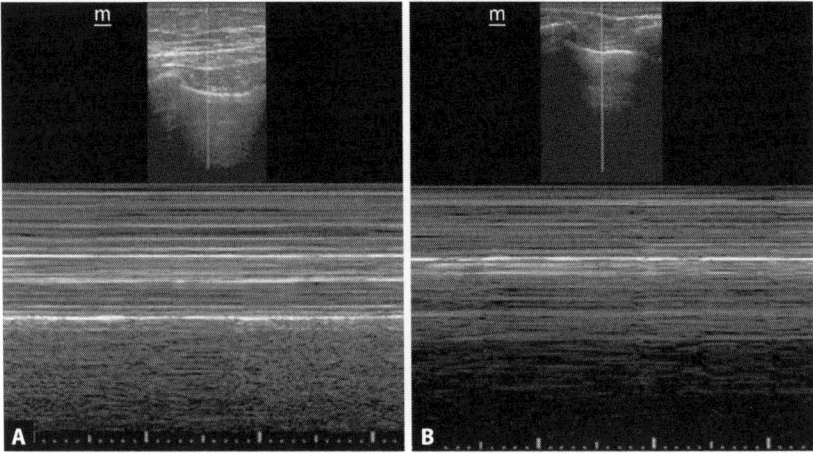

**Figs. 39A and B:** Anterior pulmonary window (M-mode).
(A) Seashore sign; (B) barcode (stratosphere) sign.

## Limitations

- *Operator dependence:* The accuracy of POCUS heavily relies on the operator's skill and experience. Inexperienced users may misinterpret findings, leading to incorrect diagnoses and inappropriate management.
- *Limited field of view:* Compared to traditional ultrasound machines, POCUS devices typically provide a limited field of view, which may result in incomplete assessments.
- *Technological constraints:* Portable ultrasound machines may have lower image resolution and fewer advanced features than larger, more sophisticated systems in radiology departments.
- *Patient-specific challenges:* Factors such as obesity, subcutaneous emphysema, and other patient-specific conditions can degrade image quality and limit the utility of POCUS.

- *Focused nature of examinations:* POCUS is designed for concentrated examinations rather than comprehensive evaluations, sometimes resulting in missed diagnoses outside the specific area of interest.

## Competencies

- *Training and certification:* Effective use of POCUS requires formal training and certification. Providers must undergo rigorous education to develop accurate image acquisition and interpretation skills.
- *Understanding indications and limitations:* Providers must be well-versed in the appropriate indications for POCUS and its limitations to avoid misuse and overreliance on the modality.
- *Skill in image acquisition:* Competent operators must acquire clear, diagnostic-quality images under various clinical conditions.
- *Interpretation proficiency:* Accurate interpretation of POCUS findings is crucial. Providers must be able to distinguish normal from pathological findings and recognize artifacts that could lead to diagnostic errors.
- *Clinical integration:* Competent use of POCUS involves integrating ultrasound findings with clinical examination and other diagnostic tools to form a comprehensive assessment and management plan.

## Protocol-driven POCUS

Protocol-driven POCUS involves standardized protocols for conducting and interpreting ultrasound examinations, ensuring consistency and reliability across providers and clinical settings.

## Advantages of Protocol-driven POCUS

- *Standardization:* Protocols standardize the approach to POCUS, reducing variability and increasing diagnostic accuracy and reproducibility.
- *Training and education:* Protocols provide a framework for training, ensuring that all practitioners achieve a minimum competency level.
- *Quality control:* Standardized protocols facilitate quality control and audit processes, helping to identify and rectify deviations from best practices.
- *Efficiency:* Protocol-driven POCUS can streamline workflows, allowing for rapid and focused assessments in critical situations.

## Examples of Protocol-driven POCUS

- *Focused Assessment with Sonography for Trauma:* A protocol used in trauma settings to quickly assess for free fluid in the abdomen and pericardium, indicating potential internal bleeding.
- *Lung ultrasound protocols:* Protocols such as the BLUE protocol (Bedside Lung Ultrasound in Emergency) guide evaluating patients with respiratory distress.
- *Cardiac ultrasound protocols:* Protocols such as the FATE (Focused Assessed Transthoracic Echocardiography) guide the assessment of cardiac function and pathology in emergency settings.

## ◼ CONCLUSION

The POCUS is an indispensable tool in clinical practice, providing immediate diagnostic information that enhances patient care. Mastery of ultrasound physics, knobology, and sonoanatomy is crucial for effective use. POCUS applications in vascular access and lung, cardiac, and renal assessments demonstrate its broad utility in various clinical scenarios.

## ◼ REFERENCES

1. ICM Teaching. (2011). Lung Ultrasound. Available from: https://www.icmteaching.com/ultrasound/lung%20ultrasound/ [Last accessed August, 2024]
2. Bouhemad B, Zhang M, Lu Q, Rouby JJ. Clinical review: Bedside lung ultrasound in critical care practice. Ann Intensive Care. 2014;4:1.
3. Reiterer F, Sivri T, Messmer AS, Meuli RA. Lung ultrasound: An essential tool for a critical care physician. Front Pediatr. 2020;8:458.
4. Medical Trade Hub. 3.0 MHz Cardiac Phased Array Probe. Available from: https://www.medicaltradehub.com/product/3-0-mhz-cardiac-phased-array-probe-for-code-33951-2/ [Last accessed August, 2024].
5. Majmundar M, Doshi R, Kumar A. Long-term outcomes with catheter ablation of atrial fibrillation: A review of current literature and emerging data. J Interv Card Electrophysiol. 2020;59(2):133-40.
6. Debasis M, Panda S. Role of lung ultrasound in diagnosis of COVID-19. J Clin Diagn Res. 2020;14(7):OE01-3.
7. Pogorelić Z, Domazet I, Jerončić A, Šušnjar T, Borić M, Batinica S. The application of lung ultrasound in COVID-19 patients. PLoS One. 2022;17(3):e0265101.
8. POCUS 101. Point-of-Care Ultrasound Training and Resources. Available from: https://www.pocus101.com/ [Last accessed August, 2024].
9. Santana PV, Cardenas LZ, Albuquerque ALP, Carvalho CRR, Caruso P. Diaphragmatic ultrasound: A review of its methodological aspects and clinical uses. J Bras Pneumol. 2020;46:e20200064.
10. Mohammad Abdelfattah W, Mohiedden O, Saad-eldeen Elgammal S, Mohammad Elsayed K, Said Mowafy SM, Mohammad Abdalla R. Distensibility index of inferior vena cava and pulse pressure variation as predictors of fluid responsiveness in mechanically ventilated shocked patients. J Emerg Med Trauma Acute Care. 2020:1-13.
11. Lichtenstein DA. Lung ultrasound in the critically ill. Ann Intensive Care. 2014;4:1.
12. Lichtenstein DA. BLUE-protocol and FALLS-protocol: Two applications of lung ultrasound in the critically ill. Chest. 2015;147:1659-70.
13. Gottlieb M, Holladay D, Burns KM, Nakitende D, Bailitz J. Ultrasound for airway management: An evidence-based review for the emergency clinician. Am J Emerg Med. 2020;38(5):1007-13.
14. Ramsingh D, Frank E, Haughton R, Schilling J, Gimenez KM, Banh E, et al. Auscultation versus point-of-care ultrasound to determine endotracheal versus bronchial intubation: A diagnostic accuracy study. Anesthesiology. 2016;124(5):1012-20.
15. Kim DH, Jun JS, Kim, R. Ultrasonographic measurement of the optic nerve sheath diameter and its association with eyeball transverse diameter in 585 healthy volunteers. Sci Rep.2017;7:15906.
16. Dubourg J, Javouhey E, Geeraerts T, Messerer M, Kassai B. Ultrasonography of optic nerve sheath diameter for detection of raised intracranial pressure: a systematic review and meta-analysis. Intensive Care Med. 2011;37(7):1059-68.
17. Komut E, Kozacı N, Sönmez BM, Yılmaz F, Komut S, Yıldırım ZN, et al. Bedside sonographic measurement of optic nerve sheath diameter as a predictor of intracranial pressure in ED. Am J Emerg Med. 2016;34(6):963-7.

18. Di Nisio M, van Es N, Büller HR. Deep vein thrombosis and pulmonary embolism. Lancet. 2016;17;388(10063):3060-73.
19. Kesieme E, Kesieme C, Jebbin N, Irekpita E, Dongo A. Deep vein thrombosis: a clinical review. J Blood Med. 2011;2:59-69.
20. Bernardi E, Camporese G. Diagnosis of deep-vein thrombosis. Thromb Res. 2018;163:201-6.
21. Kirkpatrick AW, Sirois M, Laupland KB, oldstein L, Brown DR, Simons RK, et al. Prospective evaluation of hand-held focused abdominal sonography for trauma (FAST) in blunt abdominal trauma. Can J Surg. 2005;48(6):453-60.
22. Blaivas M, Sierzenski PR. Extended focused assessment with sonography for trauma (EFAST): Utility in trauma care. J Trauma. 2002;53(2):380-4.
23. Nandipati KC, Allamaneni S, Kakarla R, et al. Extended focused assessment with sonography for trauma (EFAST) in the diagnosis of pneumothorax: experience at a community based level I trauma center. Injury. 2011;42(5):511-4.
24. Caldas J, Rynkowski CB, Robba C. POCUS, how can we include the brain? An overview. J Anesth Analg Crit Care. 2022;2:55.
25. Ávila-Reyes D, Acevedo-Cardona AO, Gómez-González JF, Echeverry-Piedrahita DR, Aguirre-Flórez M, Giraldo-Diaconeasa A. Ultrasound in cardiac arrest: Narrative review article. Ultrasound J. 2021;13:46.

# CHAPTER 18

# Current Concepts in the Management of Septic Shock

*Ramprasad Matsa*

## ABSTRACT

Sepsis is a clinical syndrome encompassing physiologic and biological abnormalities caused by a dysregulated host response to infection. Sepsis progression into septic shock is associated with significant increase in mortality, hence the importance of early identification and treatment. Surviving sepsis campaign (SSC), has been instrumental in developing and updating sepsis guidelines over the last two decades. The principles of management of patients in septic shock would include source control and treating underlying infection, haemodynamic stabilisation (resuscitation) and modulation of the host response. Although such principles exist, the rationalising such management principles to the individual patients and monitoring them is the key for the better outcomes. The recent advancements in resuscitation monitoring especially the use of ultrasound, and use of blood purification techniques are promising however to need further evaluation for routine application. in the This review elaborates the key principles and their supporting evidence to advocate the clinicians to optimise the management.

**Keywords:** Sepsis; Septic shock; Vasopressors; Inotropes; Early goal-directed therapy; Surviving sepsis campaign; Crystalloids; Colloids; Corticosteroids; Blood purification; Antibiotics; Corticosteroids

## KEY POINTS

- Septic shock is a subset of sepsis characterised by profound hypotension and lactate elevation, due to circulatory and cellular metabolic derangements.
- Main stay of septic shock management involves early source control and antimicrobial therapy, prompt resuscitation and control of dysregulated host immune response with immunomodulatory medications.
- Crystalloid fluid resuscitation and, if no improvement in shock state, vasoactive medications should be started early to maintain mean arterial pressure and hence perfusion.
- Noradrenaline remains the first-choice vasoactive agent in septic shock.
- Diligent antibiotic stewardship should be a standard process of care in patients with sepsis.
- Blood purification techniques should be carefully considered in selected group of septic shock patients.

## INTRODUCTION

Sepsis is defined as a life-threatening organ dysfunction due to a dysregulated host immune response to infection.[1] Septic shock is defined as a subset of sepsis in which underlying circulatory and cellular metabolism abnormalities are profound enough to increase mortality substantially. Currently, the hospital mortality rate secondary to septic shock is >40%.[2] Such patients have persistent hypotension despite adequate volume resuscitation, need vasopressor therapy, and increased lactate (>2 mmol/L or >18 mg/dL) levels.[1] The pathophysiological process and their therapeutic targets of sepsis and septic shock have been highly researched. The recent surviving sepsis campaign (SSC) provides evidence-based guidelines on identifying and treating these patients.[3] This review highlights the contemporaneous principles in managing patients with septic shock.

## PATHOPHYSIOLOGIC PRINCIPLES

Septic shock is a distributive type of shock, unlike other shock states. The process starts with an inflammatory stimulus (endotoxin) that triggers the production of inflammatory mediators [e.g., tumor necrosis factor (TNF) and interleukin 1]. The cytokines can lead to neutrophil—endothelial cell adhesion, activate the clotting mechanism, and generate microthrombi. They also release numerous other inflammatory mediators (leukotrienes, lipoxygenase, and IL-2). These mediators cause a rise in capillary permeability and result in a reduction in peripheral vascular resistance.[4] This results in a fall in venous return and a reduction in afterload. To compensate for the decrease in stroke volume, the heart rate rises, i.e., compensated septic shock. This hyperdynamic state is characteristic of septic shock. When the shock progresses, increased endogenous catecholamine production increases peripheral vascular resistance. The body adapts to this fall in cardiac output by shunting blood away from non-vital tissues [gastrointestinal (GI) tract, kidneys, muscle, and skin] to the vital tissues (brain and heart). Later, cardiac output may decrease, blood pressure falls, and typical features of hypoperfusion appear (progressive shock).[5] Decreased perfusion to the vital organs leads to their dysfunction (multiple organ dysfunction), and eventually, death ensues. It is imperative to initiate appropriate treatment measures with therapy based on the pathophysiology and continuum of septic shock.

Therefore, the principles in the management of patients with septic shock **(Flowchart 1)** should include:
1. Treatment and control of the infective process
2. Shock resuscitation and restoration of perfusion
3. Modulation of host response.

## TREATMENT AND CONTROL OF INFECTIVE PROCESS

The cornerstone in managing patients with septic shock is treating the underlying source of infection, as it is the primary cause of sepsis origin and immune dysregulation. The SSC guidelines recommend administering early antimicrobial therapy to patients with septic shock, ideally within 1 hour.[3] Recent studies have shown that delayed antibiotic delivery increases mortality in patients with septic shock as the progress from sepsis to septic shock is not hindered.[6,7] All attempts should be made to identify and eradicate the source, which may involve drainage or debridement of the infective foci, and to assess and/or remove indwelling devices and foreign bodies if necessary.

**Flowchart 1:** Principle of management of septic shock.

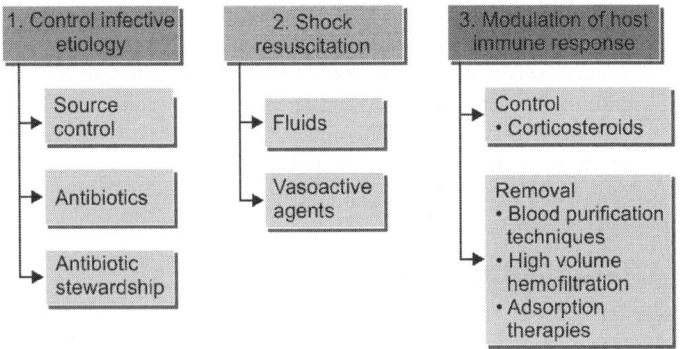

The choice of antimicrobial therapy is the key and impacts mortality.[8] Patient's background comorbidities, immunocompromise, presence of indwelling devices, history of ongoing/previous infections (especially with multidrug-resistant microorganisms), previous antibiotic administration, and the site of current infection should be accounted for while selecting the empirical antibiotics.[9] Special considerations should be given in patients with resistant microbes such as Methicillin-resistant *Staphylococcus aureus* (MRSA), multi-drug resistant (MDR), gram-negative rods (GNR), etc. The choice of antibiotics must consider local antibiogram and common community infections. Patients with neutropenia and organ transplant recipients are at an increased risk of fungal infections. They should be regarded as antifungal agents as the mortality in septic shock in such patients is extremely high.

## ■ SHOCK RESUSCITATION

### Principles

Initial resuscitation is primarily aimed at restoring hypovolemia in patients with septic shock, which can be relative or absolute. Absolute hypovolemia in such patients can result from external fluid losses (diarrhea, perspiration, etc.) due to their disease state. However, dysregulated inflammatory response and its effects on glycocalyx and endothelium alter microcirculation, resulting in relative hypovolemia due to processes such as capillary leak and vasodilatation.[10] These mechanisms lead to reduced stress volume, a reduction in the venous return, decreased preload, and reduced cardiac output.[11]

If the circulatory blood volume is adequately augmented and the pressure gradient for venous return exceeds the central venous pressure (CVP), fluid resuscitation benefits.[11] The resultant improvement in cardiac output restores the mean arterial pressure (MAP) and improves microcirculatory flow and perfusion pressure. This reduces the risk of tissue hypoperfusion and ischemic damage.[12] Fluid resuscitation also leads to renal function restoration and acid-base balance stabilization, resulting in cellular homeostasis and improving microvascular integrity and endothelial function.[5] The current SSC guidelines "strongly" recommend that at least 30 mL/kg of IV crystalloids be administered within the first 3 hours, despite "low-quality evidence" of a benefit.[3]

Although early intravenous fluid resuscitation is recommended in septic shock, patients who receive excess fluid have a poor outcome, including mortality. Excess fluid resuscitation may harm by causing extravasation of fluid, thereby decreasing venous return, impairing tissue perfusion, and no significant increase in end-diastolic volume.[12] Excess fluid resuscitation can also lead to endothelial shear stress, increased nitric oxide release and vasodilation, and decreased systemic vascular resistance (SVR).[11] Furthermore, sepsis alters vascular permeability, and as a result, only 5% of the fluid volume administered remains intravascular after 90 minutes in critically ill patients.[12] Therefore, optimal fluid resuscitation is about delivering the right amount of fluid. There are various parameters to guide fluid resuscitation, including point-of-care ultrasound (POCUS).

## Assessment of Fluid Responsiveness

Predicting fluid responsiveness in critically ill patients is essential to optimizing fluid therapy and avoiding the adverse effects of under or over-resuscitation. The choice of measuring fluid responsiveness depends upon the individual patient's clinical context, operator skills, and the availability of resources. Although static preload indices, such as CVP and pulmonary capillary wedge pressure (PCWP), have been widely used in clinical practice, they are poor predictors of fluid responsiveness.[13,14]

Amongst many, the dynamic indices that are commonly used in the contemporary practice are:

### Passive Leg Raising

Passive raising of the legs (PLR) at 45° should increase the cardiac output by 10 %, and the maximal effect occurs at 30–90 seconds and then return to baseline. The change in the cardiac output can measured as pulse pressure variation (PPV), or echocardiographic demonstration of velocity time integral (VTI), carotid Doppler flow, etc. However, the limitations of its use are its unreliability in intra-abdominal hypertension and its practicality when used in certain disease conditions such as raised intracranial pressure or pulmonary edema.

### End-expiratory Occlusion Test

The principle behind end-expiratory occlusion test (EEOT) is that occluding the circuit at the end of expiration prevents the cyclic effect of inspiration from reducing left cardiac preload and acts like a fluid challenge. It is performed with occluding at expiration (expiratory hold) for a 15-second period, which can increase the pulse pressure or cardiac index with reasonable accuracy. However, the patients must tolerate 15-second ventilatory interruption, which may be difficult in severe hypoxemic states. Moreover, the test relies less on low-compliance lung states such as acute respiratory distress syndrome (ARDS). The other limitation is that this test requires a real-time carbon monoxide (CO) monitor, as the effect lasts only a few seconds and should not be done in prone patients.

### Point of Care Ultrasound

Echocardiograms in assessing fluid responsiveness have gained momentum in the last decade. The most common echocardiographic assessments include the left ventricular outflow tract velocity time index (VTI), which allows the direct measurement of stroke volume and end-diastolic volume approximate preload. Inferior vena cava ultrasound is used to assess size and collapsibility index, which is increasingly used to assess fluid responsiveness. The current recommendation is inferior vena cava (IVC) diameter >2.1 cm or a collapsibility index of <50% with a sniff suggests high filling pressures.

Point-of-care lung ultrasound can quickly identify fluid overload by assessing a symmetrical B-line pattern. Recently, the venous excess ultrasound (VExUS) has been developed. This protocolized USG involves POCUS based measurements of IVC along with Doppler scans of portal, hepatic, and intrarenal veins. The VExUS grading score correlates with minimal, moderate, severe, or no venous congestion.

Although the currently available indices give the treating clinician an arbitrary understanding of the fluid status, their wider use is limited. Operator skills, resource availability, and most importantly, the need for more well-designed, robust studies are the reasons for the limitation of more comprehensive recommendations.

## Fluid Selection

The ideal fluid for resuscitation in shock should be similar to plasma, not alter the pH state and improve perfusion. The two major categories of fluids used for resuscitation are colloids and crystalloids.

Crystalloids are commonly used as first-line resuscitation fluids. The crystalloids exist as balanced and unbalanced solutions. Balanced solutions have an ion difference close to 24 mEq/L, and their chloride content is similar to that of plasma (98–112 mmol/L). To maintain electroneutrality (a balance between positive and negative anions), balanced solutions contain buffers such as bicarbonate, lactate, acetate, or gluconate.[15] On the contrary, 0.9% normal saline (NS) is an unbalanced crystalloid, though it is isotonic, as it does not contain an organic anion as an acid buffer. Its chloride concentration is higher than that of the plasma and thus can cause hyperchloremic metabolic acidosis and potentially lead to acute kidney injury and altered inflammatory response.[16] The high chloride concentration causes vascular smooth muscle contraction and exaggerates norepinephrine and angiotensin II-induced vasoconstriction, resulting in acute kidney injury (AKI) secondary to reduced perfusion.[17]

Commercially available balanced solutions are lactated Ringer's, Hartmann's solution, Plasma-Lyte, and Normosol. The 2021 SSC guidelines suggest using balanced crystalloids instead of normal saline for resuscitation, but the evidence is weak. Two extensive, randomized control studies published after the SSC guidelines (BaSICS and PLUS) showed similar outcomes between balanced solutions and saline in critically ill patients. Hence, there is little evidence to strongly recommend balanced crystalloids over normal saline across a heterogeneous ICU population.[17,18]

Albumin is a non-synthetic colloid. The theoretical advantage of albumin over crystalloids is its effect on maintaining oncotic pressure, which has the added benefit of better volume expansion. The 2021 SSC guidelines also suggest using albumin in patients who received large volumes of crystalloids, but the evidence needs to be stronger. So far, studies have not shown any improvement in mortality; however, they did not show any harm either.[19,20] Hence, the current use of albumin is restricted to the recommendation as suggested in SSC guidelines and has a role in resuscitation in patients with decompensated liver disease. Currently, no other colloid but albumin is recommended in shock resuscitation due to its harmful effects.

## Optimal Blood Pressure Target

Surviving Sepsis Campaign guideline recommends an ideal mean arterial pressure (MAP) target to aim during resuscitation of ≥65 mm Hg; when this cannot be achieved by initial fluid resuscitation, a vasoactive agent should be started. However, a recent randomized clinical trial (RCT) demonstrated that a 60–65 mm Hg MAP in patients over 65 years with septic shock made no difference in 90-day mortality.[21] Similarly, patients with hypertension may require a higher target MAP. The understanding of autoregulation of blood flow in the vascular beds of major organs leads to the basis of target MAP. Moreover, tissue perfusion reduces linearly as blood pressure drops below a crucial level. Therefore, the treating clinician should consider factors other than target MAP during shock resuscitation, such as urine output, mental state, and cutaneous perfusion (capillary refill time).

The decision to start vasopressors early should be considered in cases of profound hypotension. The importance of diastolic blood pressure (DBP) has been reviewed in some studies, to guide the decision to start vasopressors. DBP is determined by vascular tone and the decay time of aortic blood volume. In sepsis, a low DBP often reflects severe vasodilation and is associated with increased mortality.[22] Therefore, it is appropriate to initiate vasopressors when DAP is very low, e.g., <45 mm Hg.

## Vasoactive Agents

The pathophysiology behind septic shock involves loss of vasomotor tone with consequent systemic vasodilation, hypotension, and tissue hypoperfusion.[23] This effect can persist even after adequate fluid resuscitation and is called persistent hypotension. Such patients can also have myocardial depression secondary to sepsis. Vasopressors and inotropes increase the cardiac output and arterial pressure to restore tissue oxygen delivery. The choice of vasoactive agents would be guided by the parameters, including cardiac contractility, etc., although the SSC guidelines recommend noradrenaline as the first-line agent.

### Noradrenaline

Noradrenaline (NA) is an α-1/β-1 adrenergic agonist. It improves myocardial contractility and cardiac output without increasing the heart rate. NA also increases the filling pressure through the venoconstrictive effect and redistribution of blood flow. Early administration of NA (0.1–1.2 µg/kg/minute) decreases intensive care unit (ICU) stay length and improves outcomes in patients with septic shock.[24,25] Moreover, early NA administration successfully resuscitates the microcirculation by improving tissue perfusion and oxygenation.[26] At early stages of shock, prompt NA infusion increases the arterial diastolic pressure and, thereby, the coronary perfusion due to its action through the β-adrenergic receptors of cardiac myocytes.[26]

### Vasopressin

Vasopressin (VA) is a long-acting endogenous hormone. In addition to its vasopressor ($V_1$ receptors) properties, vasopressin is a hormone that influences kidney function ($V_2$ receptors) and water metabolism. The underlying concept is that exogenous vasopressin administration in patients with sepsis can substitute for inadequate vasopressin levels in patients with septic shock.[27] According to the

SSC's recommendations, it can be administered at a dose of 0.25–0.5 μg/kg/minute to supplement NA as a *second-line* agent to achieve the target MAP and reduce the side effects of adrenergic overload.[3] Recent evidence suggests that early administration of vasopressors in patients with septic shock may improve kidney function, increase urine output, decrease fluid requirements, and decrease edema formation.[27-30]

## Adrenaline

Adrenaline is a non-selective adrenergic agonist with potent β-1 and moderate α-1 and β-2 receptor activity. Through β1 receptor stimulation, adrenaline increases the myocardial contractility and heart rate. Stimulation α1 receptors increase systemic vascular resistance through peripheral vasoconstriction. Adrenaline should be considered as a *third-line* treatment for septic shock. Its use is currently limited to inadequate MAP levels despite NE and VA administration.[3] Due to its significant β-adrenergic effect, adrenaline is indicated in cases of cardiac dysfunction. However, its administration may lead to more adrenergic side effects, such as tachycardia, tachyarrhythmia, and increased blood lactate concentrations.

## Newer Vasoactive Agents

### Angiotensin II

Angiotensin II causes vasoconstriction by stimulating the renin-angiotensin system and is currently Food and Drug Administration (FDA)-approved. In the recent trial (ATHOS -3), 70% of the patients in the intervention group (angiotensin II) achieved the desired primary endpoint (MAP increase of at least 10 mm Hg or 75 mm Hg) compared to that of the patients in the control group (placebo). However, the study showed no difference in mortality.[31] Although angiotensin II is gaining popularity, especially after the FDA approval, more evidence is needed to deliberate this in usual practice.

### Selepressin

Selepressin is a selective vasopressin $V_{1a}$ receptor agonist that reduces vasodilatation and vascular leakage secondary to sepsis. A large multicenter trial (SEPSIS-ACT) compared selepressin versus placebo when added to patients in septic shock who were on noradrenaline. The study failed to show any difference between ventilator and vasopressor-free days with its use.[32] Selepressin currently does not have FDA approval. The 2021 SSC guidelines recommended against using selepressin as a first-line therapy, but the evidence is weak.

### Methylene Blue

Methylene blue (MB) is a thiazine dye used to treat methemoglobinemia. MB exerts an indirect vasoconstrictor effect through several mechanisms. Methylene blue inhibits nitrous oxide (NO)-induced guanylate cyclase activation, thereby preventing smooth muscle relaxation. MB also selectively inhibits iNOs and can scavenge NO.[33] To date, the evidence level for using MB in septic shock outside of a research protocol needs to be higher. Methylene blue can cause falsely low oxygen saturation as it can absorb emitted light. Other adverse effects include methemoglobinemia and pulmonary vasoconstriction.

## MODULATION OF HOST RESPONSE

### Steroids

Corticosteroids regulate the immune response and reduce the generation of inflammatory agents. This is particularly significant in the context of septic shock, as hypotension occurs because of vasoplegia due to excessive release of pro-inflammatory cytokines. Corticosteroids, therefore, are currently used as an adjunctive therapy in septic shock. Moreover, in septic shock, the anti-inflammatory properties of corticosteroids improve the blood vessels' responsiveness to vasoconstrictors.[34]

A systematic review and meta-analysis, including 37 RCTs, suggested a reduced 28-day mortality with corticosteroid use compared with a placebo in adults with sepsis.[35] A Cochrane meta-analysis by Annane et al., including 61 RCTs ($n = 12,192$), also suggested that corticosteroids probably reduced 28-day and hospital mortality.[36] However, another systematic review and meta-analysis, including 22 RCTs ($n = 7,297$), found no difference in mortality between corticosteroids and placebo. Low-dose corticosteroid use was, however, associated with reduced shock duration, mechanical ventilation, and ICU length of stay in septic shock patients.[37] Based on the results, the current SSC guidelines included a weak recommendation on corticosteroid administration at a dose of 200 mg of hydrocortisone (given as 50 mg intravenously every 6 hours) for patients in septic shock requiring relatively high doses of noradrenaline to maintain arterial pressure, approaching or exceeding 0.25 µg/kg/minute.[3]

### Extracorporeal Blood Purification

#### General Principles

Extracorporeal blood purification techniques have been proposed as adjunctive therapy in sepsis. The pathophysiologic process in the transition from an infection, deteriorating to septic shock and multiple organ dysfunction, is primarily due to the endotoxin from the antigen (infective agent) and their resultant modulation and release of inflammatory mediators. This extracorporeal blood purification technique is based on the principle that removing such bacterial toxins or inflammatory mediators (individually or both) could attenuate sepsis-related organ dysfunction and vasomotor failure, thereby reducing morbidity and mortality.[38] Moreover, a reduction in the concentration of cytokines in tissues would further reduce the production of local cytokines, thus reducing the overall cytokine load. Extracorporeal blood purification also increases the lymphatic flow rate, which allows cytokines in tissues to be removed (mediator delivery hypothesis).[38] With the remit of this review, the focus is made on high-volume hemofiltration (HVHF) and hemadsorption techniques.

#### High-volume Hemofiltration

Continuous hemodialysis or hemodiafiltration with high filtration volume is commonly used for extracorporeal removal of small molecules. In hemofiltration, dissolved substances are transported by convection with a solvent across a semipermeable membrane (ultrafiltration) through a positive transmembrane gradient. The solvent's clearance in this process depends on the ultrafiltration rate, sieving properties of the membrane for the solute, and the solute's molecular size.

High-volume hemofiltration (35 mL/kg/hour) and very-high-volume hemofiltration (45 mL/kg/hour) are used for immunomodulation in sepsis to eliminate inflammatory mediators through convection. Although most inflammatory molecules are medium-molecular substances and theoretically, can be removed by this technique, their endogenous release rate in sepsis is significantly higher than that of uremic toxins. The studies have not demonstrated a significant impact of high-volume hemofiltration on patient outcomes in septic shock.[39,40]

## Hemadsorption

Hemadsorption is a technique that involves the placement of a sorbent cartridge in direct contact with blood *via* an extracorporeal circuit. The characteristics of the sorbents can lead to the capture and removal of the endotoxins. The different sorbents could also target high-molecular-weight molecules, usually not captured by conventional hemofilters (Polymyxin B-immobilized fiber columns) or circulating cytokines (CytoSorb®) or both (oXiris®).

## Removal of Endotoxins

Lipopolysaccharide (LPS) is an endotoxin in cases of Gram-negative sepsis. LPS triggers the activation of the inflammatory cascade. Polymyxin B (PMX), a cyclic lipophilic peptide antibiotic, neutralizes LPS due to its high affinity for the lipid A moiety of endotoxin. Due to this characteristic, its use has been advocated in treating only septic shock caused by Gram-negative bacteria. Two RCTs (ABDO-MIX and EUPHRATES) evaluated PMX hemadsorption in patients with abdominal sepsis and delivered inconclusive results.[41,42] However, The EUPHRATES trial subgroup analysis showed a reduction in mortality in a subset of patients with endotoxin activity assay (EAA) >0.6–0.89.[42] Therefore, using PMX remains a highly considered option and should be investigated further.[43]

## Removal of Cytokines

CytoSorb® device utilizes a nonselective hemadsorption process. It is integrated into a conventional extracorporeal system, such as continuous renal replacement therapy (CRRT), and the patient's blood is passed over the adsorptive surface of the cartridge. CytoSorb® represents an evolution of coupled plasma filtration and adsorption. This device facilitates the selective adsorption of various substances and molecules within the range of ~5–60 kDa, depending on their plasma concentration. Substances such as free hemoglobin, myoglobin, bilirubin, bile acids, bacterial toxins (excluding endotoxin), activated complement components, some drugs, cytokines, and inflammatory mediators can also be absorbed. However, the studies have had inconclusive and/or variable results. Hence, their use of this mode of therapy as an initial line of management in septic shock is not recommended but can be considered as an adjunctive therapy.[44]

## Combination Methods

oXiris® technique involves the simultaneous removal of inflammatory mediators, endotoxin, fluid, and uremic toxins on the passage of blood through the inherent hydrogel structure of the AN69 membrane. A recent meta-analysis of compiled clinical data from 10 cohort studies and four RCTs encompassing 695 patients with sepsis undergoing CRRT suggested potential benefits by reduction in mortality, catecholamine requirement, and length of ICU stay with its use.[45] However, the studies' quality was deficient to draw definitive conclusions about making its use routine in patients with septic shock. Still, it can be considered as an adjunctive therapy.

The effectiveness of such blood purification techniques should be weighed against their safety. Blood purification techniques may inadvertently remove beneficial substances, such as essential proteins, immune cells, etc. They also affect drug levels, especially antibiotics and can potentially lead to negative consequences. The other adverse effects involve bleeding due to anticoagulation and hemodynamic instability. These treatments are less accessible, resource-intensive, and require specialized equipment and personnel. To confirm the efficacy and safety of these techniques, well-designed RCTs are needed.

## ■ CONCLUSION

The review highlights the process of contemporary care for patients with septic shock. Coordination of care is essential in such patients as the delivery of shock resuscitation is time-critical. There is a clear message that excess fluid is dangerous to the patients, and early introduction of vasoactive drugs is pertinent in such patients. The treating clinicians should endorse appropriate targets and the patient's response to such targets. Modulation of immune response is gaining significant importance. Although the science of extracorporeal blood purification is acceptable and has shown some promising results in relatively controlled, carefully selected conditions of early-phase clinical trials, none has been shown to have a convincing beneficial effect on survival in large-scale RCT. Therefore, their use should be considered in carefully selected patients as an adjunct.

Sepsis and septic shock are a complex phenomenon that results not just because of an infection but also abnormal regulation of immunological pathways, which then is phenotypically represented as multi-organ failure and shock state. Such complex regulatory pathways and cell signaling are heterogeneous in different patient groups. Therefore, their response to formalized management protocols must be more consistent. This is reflected very well in most studies that have generated variable results that investigated the efficacy and safety of a specific treatment and their response to this broad cohort. Therefore, the management of patients with septic shock must be individualized and tailored to the patient's responses. Precision medicine principles involve phenotyping, characterizing metabolomics, and delivering a personalized management process. Therefore, the future is about developing pathobiological models with defined therapeutic targets.

## ■ REFERENCES

1. Singer M, Deutschman CS, Seymour CW, Singer M, Deutschman CS, Seymour CW, Shankar-Hari M, Annane D, Bauer M, et al. The third international consensus definitions for sepsis and septic shock (sepsis- 3). JAMA. 2016;315(8):801-10.
2. Fleischmann C, Scherag A, Adhikari NK, Hartog CS, Tsaganos T, Schlattmann P, et al. Assessment of global incidence and mortality of hospital-treated sepsis. Current estimates and limitations. Am J Respir Crit Care Med. 2016;193(3):259-72.

3. Evans L, Rhodes A, Alhazzani W, Antonelli M, Coopersmith CM, French C, et al. Surviving sepsis campaign: International guidelines for management of sepsis and septic shock 2021. Intensive Care Med. 2021;47(11):1181-247
4. Venet F, Monneret G. Advances in the understanding and treatment of sepsis-induced immunosuppression. Nat Rev Nephrol. 2018;14:121-37.
5. Lundy DJ, Trzeciak S. Microcirculatory dysfunction in sepsis. Crit Care Clin. 2009;25:721-31.
6. Im Y, Kang D, Ko RE, Lee YJ, Lim SY, Park S, et al. Time-to-antibiotics and clinical outcomes in sepsis and septic shock patients: a prospective nationwide multicenter cohort study. Crit Care. 2022;26(1):19.
7. Bisarya R, Song X, Salle J, Liu M, Patel A, Simpson SQ. Antibiotic timing and progression to septic shock among patients in the ED with suspected infection. Chest. 2022;161(1):112-20.
8. Kumar A, Ellis P, Arabi Y, Roberts D, Light B, Parrillo JE, et al. Initiation of inappropriate antimicrobial therapy results in a fivefold reduction of survival in human septic shock. Chest. 2009;136(5):1237-48.
9. Taplitz RA, Kennedy EB, Bow EJ, Crews J, Gleason C, Hawley DK, et al. Outpatient management of fever and neutropenia in adults treated for malignancy: American Society of Clinical Oncology and Infectious Diseases Society of America Clinical Practice Guideline Update. J Clin Oncol. 2018;36(14):1443-53.
10. De Backer D, Cecconi M, Lipman J, Machado F, Myatra SN, Ostermann M, et al. Challenges in the management of septic shock: A narrative review. Intensive Care Med. 2019;45(4):420-33.
11. Brown RM, Semler MW. Fluid management in sepsis. J Intensiv Care Med. 2019;34:364-73.
12. Malbrain MLNG, Van Regenmortel N, Saugel B, De Tavernier B, Van Gaal PJ, Joannes-Boyau O, et al. Principles of fluid management and stewardship in septic shock: It is time to consider the four D's and the four phases of fluid therapy. Ann Intensiv Care. 2018;8(1):66.
13. ProCESS Investigators; Yealy DM, Kellum JA, Huang DT, Barnato AE, Weissfeld LA, et al. A randomized trial of protocol-based care for early septic shock. N Engl J Med. 2014;370(18):1683-93.
14. ARISE Investigators; ANZICS Clinical Trials Group; Peake SL, Delaney A, Bailey M, Bellomo R, et al. Goal-directed resuscitation for patients with early septic shock. N Engl J Med. 2014;371(16):1496-1506.
15. Myburgh JA, Mythen MG. Resuscitation fluids. N Engl J Med. 2013;369:1243-51.
16. Jaynes MP, Murphy CV, Ali N, Krautwater A, Lehman A, Doepker BA. Association between chloride content of intravenous fluids and acute kidney injury in critically ill medical patients with sepsis. J Crit Care. 2018;44:363-7.
17. Finfer S, Micallef S, Hammond N, Navarra L, Bellomo R, Billot L, et al. Balanced multielectrolyte solution versus saline in critically ill adults. N Engl J Med. 2022;386(9):815-26.
18. Zampieri FG, Machado FR, Biondi RS, Freitas FGR, Veiga VC, Figueiredo RC, et al. Effect of intravenous fluid treatment with a balanced solution vs. 0.9% saline solution on mortality in critically ill patients: The BaSICS randomized clinical trial. JAMA. 2021;326(9):818-29.
19. Dubois MJ, Orellana-Jimenez C, Melot C, De Backer D, Berre J, Leeman M, et al. Albumin administration improves organ function in critically ill hypoalbuminemic patients: a prospective, randomized, controlled, pilot study. Crit Care Med. 2006;34(10):2536-40.
20. Caironi P, Tognoni G, Masson S, Fumagalli R, Pesenti A, Romero M, et al. Albumin replacement in patients with severe sepsis or septic shock. N Engl J Med. 2014;370(15):1412-21.

21. Lamontagne F, Richards-Belle A, Thomas K, Harrison DA, Sadique MZ, Grieve RD, et al. Effect of reduced exposure to vasopressors on 90-day mortality in older critically ill patients with vasodilatory hypotension: a randomized clinical trial. JAMA. 2020;323(10):938-49.
22. Ospina-Tascón GA, Teboul JL, Hernandez G, Alvarez I, Sánchez-Ortiz AI, Calderón-Tapia LE, et al. Diastolic shock index and clinical outcomes in patients with septic shock. Ann Intensive Care. 2020;10(1):41.
23. Vincent JL, DeBacker D. Circulatory shock. N Engl J Med. 2013;369:1726-34.
24. Hernández G, Teboul JL, Bakker J. Norepinephrine in septic shock. Intensive Care Med. 2019;45:687-89.
25. Boyd JH, Forbes J, Nakada TA, Walley KR, Russell JA. Fluid resuscitation in septic shock: a positive fluid balance and elevated central venous pressure are associated with increased mortality. Crit Care Med. 2011;39(2):259-65.
26. Hamzaoui O, Jozwiak M, Geffriaud T, Sztrymf B, Prat D, Jacobs F, et al. Norepinephrine exerts an inotropic effect during the early phase of human septic shock. Br J Anaesth. 2018;120(3):517-24.
27. Huang H, Wu C, Shen Q, Xu H, Fang Y, Mao W. The effect of early vasopressin use on patients with septic shock: A systematic review and meta-analysis. Am J Emerg Med. 2021;48:203-8.
28. Russell JA, Walley KR, Singer J, Gordon AC, Hébert PC, Cooper DJ, et al. Vasopressin versus norepinephrine infusion in patients with septic shock. N Engl J Med. 2008;358(9):877-87.
29. Cioccari L, Jakob SM, Takala J. Should vasopressors be started early in septic shock? Semin Respir Crit Care Med. 2021;42:683-8.
30. Ospina-Tascón GA, Hernandez G, Alvarez I, Calderón-Tapia LE, Manzano-Nunez R, Sánchez-Ortiz AI, et al. Effects of very early start of norepinephrine in patients with septic shock: A propensity score-based analysis. Crit Care. 2020;24(1):52.
31. Wieruszewski PM, Bellomo R, Busse LW, Ham KR, Zarbock A, Khanna AK, et al. Initiating angiotensin II at lower vasopressor doses in vasodilatory shock: An exploratory post-hoc analysis of the ATHOS-3 clinical trial. Crit Care. 2023;27(1):175.
32. Laterre PF, Berry SM, Blemings A, Carlsen JE, François B, Graves T, et al. Effect of selepressin vs. placebo on ventilator- and vasopressor-free days in patients with septic shock: The SEPSIS-ACT randomized clinical trial. JAMA. 2019;322(15):1476.
33. Tchen S, Sullivan JB. Clinical utility of midodrine and methylene blue as catecholamine sparing agents in intensive care unit patients with shock. J Crit Care. 2020;57:148-56.
34. Heming N, Sivanandamoorthy S, Meng P, Bounab R, Annane D. Immune effects of corticosteroids in sepsis. Front Immunol. 2018;9:1736.
35. Fang F, Zhang Y, Tang J, Lunsford LD, Li T, Tang R, et al. Association of corticosteroid treatment with outcomes in adult patients with sepsis: a systematic review and meta-analysis. JAMA Intern Med. 2019;179(2):213-23.
36. Annane D, Bellissant E, Bollaert PE, Briegel J, Keh D, Kupfer Y, et al. Corticosteroids for treating sepsis in children and adults. Cochrane Database Syst Rev. 2019;12(12):CD002243.
37. Rygård SL, Butler E, Granholm A, Møller MH, Cohen J, Finfer S, et al. A. Low-dose corticosteroids for adult patients with septic shock: A systematic review with meta-analysis and trial sequential analysis. Intensive Care Med. 2018;44(7):1003-16.
38. Monard C, Rimmelé T, Ronco C. Extracorporeal blood purification therapies for sepsis. Blood Purif. 2019;7(Suppl. 3):1-14.
39. Joannes-Boyau O, Honore PM, Perez P, Bagshaw SM, Grand H, Canivet JL, et al. High-volume versus standard-volume haemofiltration for septic shock patients with acute kidney injury (IVOIRE study): a multicentre randomized controlled trial. Intensive Care Med. 2013;39(9):1535-46.

40. VA/NIH Acute Renal Failure Trial Network; Palevsky PM, Zhang JH, O'Connor TZ, Chertow GM, Crowley ST, et al. Intensity of renal support in critically ill patients with acute kidney injury. N Engl J Med. 2008;359(1):7-20.
41. Payen D, Dupuis C, Deckert V, Pais de Barros JP, Rérole AL, Lukaszewicz AC, et al. Endotoxin mass concentration in plasma is associated with mortality in a multicentric cohort of peritonitis-induced shock. Front Med. 2021;8:749405.
42. Dellinger RP, Bagshaw SM, Antonelli M, Foster DM, Klein DJ, Marshall JC, et al. Effect of targeted polymyxin B hemoperfusion on 28-day mortality in patients with septic shock and elevated endotoxin level: The EUPHRATES randomized clinical trial. JAMA. 2018;320(14):1455-63.
43. Shoji H, Opal SM. Therapeutic rationale for endotoxin removal with polymyxin B immobilized fiber column (PMX) for septic shock. Int J Mol Sci. 2021;22:2228.
44. Becker S, Lang H, Vollmer Barbosa C, Tian Z, Melk A, Schmidt BMW. Efficacy of CytoSorb®: a systematic review and meta-analysis. Crit Care. 2023;27(1):215.
45. Wang G, He Y, Guo Q, Zhao Y, He J, Chen Y, et al. Continuous renal replacement therapy with the adsorptive oXiris filter may be associated with the lower 28-day mortality in sepsis: A systematic review and meta-analysis. Crit Care. 2023;27(1):275.

# CHAPTER 19

# Perioperative ECMO Support: A Primer for Anesthetists

*Ujwal Dhundi, Praveen Kumar G, Vivek Kakar*

## ABSTRACT

Following decades of technological innovation and clinical improvements in critical care practice, extracorporeal membrane oxygenation (ECMO) is not only saving the lives of patients with refractory respiratory and/or cardiac failure but also allowing our surgical (and interventional) colleagues to spread their wings and take on cases that were previously deemed either technically impractical or clinically very high risk.

The critical care physicians in tertiary ECMO centers have already taken the lead in developing their ECMO programs; its increasing use de novo in the operating rooms (ORs) necessitates that the anesthesiologists involved in these cases also become familiar with ECMO. ECMO is a complex therapy with steep learning curves and multiple potential complications. Therefore, hospitals should implement formal training programs for ECMO specialists and regular mechanisms of maintaining skills in each area where they will be used.

**Keywords:** Extracorporeal membrane oxygenation; Perioperative ECMO; ECMO for anesthetists

## KEY POINTS

- Extracorporeal membrane oxygenation (ECMO) is being used for an increasing number of indications in operating rooms (Ors), for complex procedures, and procedures on high-risk patients.
- Patients already on ECMO in critical care may also need elective or emergent procedures in OR/catheterization laboratory (Cath Lab).
- Anesthesiologists must become familiar with ECMO, seek formal training, and lead the perioperative planning and management of patients undergoing these procedures.
- ECMO is a complex and resource-intensive therapy, and close multidisciplinary coordination is essential at every stage to limit complications and achieve the best outcomes.

## ■ INTRODUCTION

Extracorporeal membrane oxygenation has existed for over 50 years, but its use in the adult population has risen sharply over the past two decades. In addition to the traditional indications such as acute and acute-on-chronic cardiac and or respiratory failure, there is an ever-growing list of other scenarios where its use has been reported, including complex or high-risk procedures in the OR and Cath Lab. Several centers initiate ECMO in the OR, and patients already established on ECMO may also need to visit the OR for planned or emergent procedures. Therefore, the modern anesthetist must be well-versed with the fundamental principles of ECMO, familiar with the equipment, and trained in timely and effective troubleshooting. In addition, they must also be familiar with the nuances of perioperative management of ECMO patients.

# EXTRACORPOREAL MEMBRANE OXYGENATION FUNDAMENTALS

## What is ECMO?

Extracorporeal Membrane Oxygenation, or extracorporeal life support (ECLS), is a life-saving therapy that can support patients with advanced respiratory failure or cardiogenic shock, refractory to conventional medical management. It is similar to the traditional cardiopulmonary bypass machine used by cardiothoracic surgeons in the OR for decades. Still, technological advancements have allowed it to be packaged into a miniaturized and yet sophisticated form **(Figs. 1A and B)**, and the advancements in various fields of medicine have allowed it to be safely used at the bedside for longer durations.[1]

## Brief History

Development of ECMO began once significant technical and clinical advancements were made in the field of cardiopulmonary bypass.[2] ECMO use in adults was first reported in a polytrauma patient in 1971,[3] and even after a United States National Institute of Health (NIH) funded randomized controlled trial that followed failed to show any benefit[4] enthusiasm for demonstrating the perceived benefits of this therapy continued with further studies.[5] The clinical practices and technology available then differed significantly from today, e.g., mechanical ventilation, anticoagulation, etc. Over the past five decades, the technology and the materials used for ECMO have continually evolved. The cannulae are coated with biologically inert substances that resist activation of the coagulation and inflammation pathway; centrifugal pumps

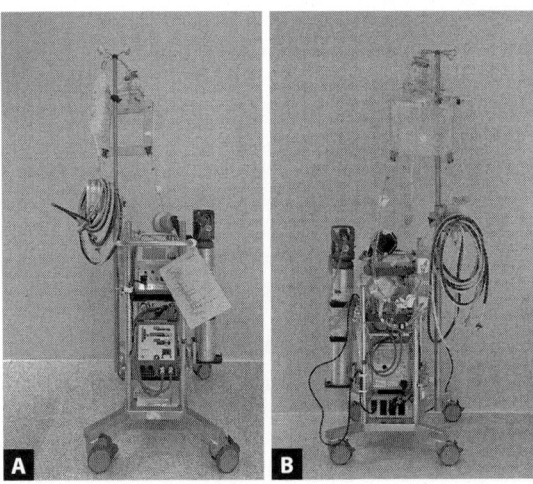

**Figs. 1A and B:** Modern extracorporeal membrane oxygenation (ECMO) machine.

that are magnetically levitated and less traumatic to blood cells; and integrated multi-parameter monitoring despite a more compact physical form factor have made ECMO much safer.[6] Clinical care of ECMO patients has also improved over the same period with safer ventilatory management,[7,8] safer anticoagulation protocols with the availability of point-of-care testing,[9] and an overall improvement in critical care standards.[10] Ultrasound-guided percutaneous cannulation, better anticoagulation protocols, more accessible ECMO training, the ability to safely rehabilitate patients, and the possibility of bridging select patient groups to destination devices or therapies have also contributed to better outcomes.

The CESAR (Conventional ventilation or ECMO for Severe Adult Respiratory failure) trial that pitched venovenous ECMO (VV ECMO) against the prevalent standard of care for patients with acute respiratory distress syndrome (ARDS) recruited 90 patients in each arm across the participating centers in the United Kingdom (UK) and demonstrated a 16% absolute risk reduction in mortality for patients referred to an ECMO center.[11] Its findings were immediately validated by observational data published during the flu pandemic.[12] Even though the EOLIA trial published in 2019[13] could not reproduce the results of the CESAR trial, this has not dulled the enthusiasm for VV ECMO, as evidenced by the number of ECMO centers and annual ECMO runs that have grown significantly since 2009.[14] While the excitement for VV ECMO has also increased the use of venoarterial ECMO (VA ECMO) for patients with cardiogenic shock, several recent trials have failed to show significant benefits over standard medical therapy.[15,16] VA ECMO has also been used to resuscitate patients with cardiac arrest refractory to conventional cardiopulmonary resuscitation, also referred to as extracorporeal cardiopulmonary resuscitation (ECPR). A small trial from Minnesota showed significantly improved outcomes in patients with refractory ventricular fibrillation (VF).[17] However, several other trials since then have yet to show any benefit.[18,19] Regardless, the updated American Heart Association (AHA) guidelines suggest considering ECPR in centers with access to VA ECMO and the capability to initiate it rapidly in patients with refractory cardiac arrest.[20]

## ECMO Modalities

Broadly, there are two main types of ECMO: VV ECMO and VA ECMO. As the name suggests, VV ECMO draws blood out of the patients' venous system, usually the vena cava, and returns it to the venous system. It is used in patients with respiratory failure resulting in refractory hypoxia and or hypercapnic acidosis despite maximum medical therapy. VA ECMO also draws blood out of patients' venous system but returns it to the patients' arterial system, usually the aorta. VA ECMO supports patients with cardiogenic shock refractory to maximum medical therapy, although it can also support patients with combined cardiorespiratory failure. The indications for using VV ECMO and VA ECMO are shown in **Box 1 and Table 1**, respectively.

## ECMO Cannulation and Configurations

Each ECMO type can achieve its goal using various cannulation strategies to access the venous and/or arterial system, also known as ECMO configurations. ECMO cannulae come in multiple sizes from different manufacturers, with various coatings to make them biologically inert, relatively, and most cannulae are wire-reinforced. The cannula used to draw the blood out of a patient is called an "access", "drainage", or "venous" cannula. These are usually long and wide (we use 38 cm and 55 cm lengths, up to 29 Fr in diameter), with several side holes along the length near the tip for adequate drainage. The cannula that is used to return blood to the patient is called a "return" or "arterial" cannula, and these are much shorter and thinner (we use 15 cm and 23 cm lengths, up to 21 Fr), with only a few holes at the tip of the cannula. Venovenous ECMO can be accomplished using the following configurations:

- *Femoral-jugular VV ECMO:* The access cannula is placed in the inferior vena cava via one of the femoral veins, with the tip close to the right atrium. The return cannula is placed in the superior vena cava, accessed via one of the jugular veins.
- *Femorofemoral VV ECMO:* The access and return cannula are placed in the inferior vena cava, with the access cannula tip lower than the return cannula's tip.

**BOX 1:** Indications for use of venovenous extracorporeal membrane oxygenation (VV ECMO) in the operating room (OR).

*Extremely difficult or impossible management of airway and ventilation:*
- Tracheoesophageal fistula[21]
- Resection of airway masses
- Tracheobronchial resections
- Severe airway trauma or airway disruption
- Risk of airway obstruction[22–25]
- Large bronchopleural fistula[26]
- Complete or near complete airway occlusion with foreign body aspiration[27]
- Airway compression due to intrinsic/extrinsic compressive lesions like mediastinal masses[28]
- Severe tracheomalacia[29]

*Management of the patient with underlying parenchymal lung disease:*
- Complex lung resection[30]
- Peri-lung transplant surgery[31]

**TABLE 1:** Indications for use of venoarterial extracorporeal membrane oxygenation (VA ECMO) in the operating room (OR).

| Specialty | Procedure | Specific consideration |
|---|---|---|
| Airway and thoracic surgery | • Major carinal resection<br>• Complex lung resection<br>• Risk of airway obstruction<br>• Major tracheobronchial tree disruption in trauma[24,32] | For hemodynamic and gas exchange support during the major vessel resection or compression and risk of airway obstruction |
| Abdominal surgery | Resection of pheochromocytoma with refractory cardiogenic shock or malignant arrhythmia[33] | |
| Obstetrics | • Peripartum cardiomyopathy<br>• Acquired cardiomyopathy<br>• Amniotic fluid embolism<br>• Pregnancy with pulmonary hypertension[34–36] | Insert sheaths in groins preemptively |

*Contd...*

*Contd...*

| Specialty | Procedure | Specific consideration |
|---|---|---|
| Interventional cardiology | • TAVR<br>• MitraClip<br>• Ventricular tachycardia ablation[37–40] | Initiate ECMO preprocedure or insert the sheaths in the groin for rapid initiation if needed intraprocedure |
| Miscellaneous | • Massive pulmonary embolism<br>• ECPR<br>• Organ donation[41–44] | • Intraoperative resuscitation<br>• Salvage ECMO for unstable brain dead donors, and ECMO-assisted DCD donation |
| Anesthetic emergencies | Malignant hyperthermia[45]<br>Local anesthetic systemic toxicity[46]<br>Takotsubo cardiomyopathy[47]<br>Anaphylaxis[48]<br>Fat embolism[49] | |

(DCD: donor after circulatory death; ECPR: extracorporeal cardiopulmonary resuscitation; TAVR: transcatheter aortic valve replacement)

In both above configurations, the tips of the access and return cannula must be at least 10–15 cm apart to avoid draining the well-oxygenated blood returning to the patient's circulation back into the machine. This creates an inefficient gas exchange mechanism called recirculation, which is clinically observed by seeing both the access and return blood of similar, bright red (well-oxygenated) color. This issue is only relevant to patients on VV ECMO.

- *Jugular-bicaval VV ECMO:* Some companies have devised specially designed cannulae with access and return lumens built into a single cannula. The cannula is placed via the jugular vein (most often right), and the tip is positioned under fluoroscopy and transesophageal echocardiography (TEE) into the inferior vena cava. The return opening must be placed in the right atrium facing the tricuspid valve. The proposed benefit of this strategy is to allow better mobilization by using a single cannulation site, avoiding the lower limbs, especially in patients where rehabilitation may be the key to their overall outcomes, e.g., patients awaiting a lung transplant. Several centers routinely and safely ambulate their patients with femoral cannulations.[50]

Venoarterial ECMO can be accomplished using the following configurations:

- *Peripheral VA ECMO:* The access cannula is placed in the inferior vena cava via one of the femoral veins, and the tip is usually positioned near the right atrium. However, there is some evidence in support of advancing the tip into the superior vena cava.[51] The return cannula is placed in the descending aorta and accessed via one of the common femoral arteries. This predisposes the limb with the arterial cannulation to limb ischemia by restricting the forward flow of blood. The insertion of another smaller cannula must mitigate this problem, called the "distal perfusion cannula" (DPC) into the superficial femoral artery or the popliteal artery, toward the foot ("anterograde") or in one of the foot arteries,

dorsalis pedis or posterior tibial, toward the heart. This cannula is fed from the oxygenated blood being returned to the patient. The flow of blood retrogradely in the aorta against the failing heart increases the left ventricular afterload. It predisposes these patients to left ventricular distension and pulmonary edema, which has been repeatedly shown to result in poor outcomes.[52] This problem can be mitigated by preemptively using a left ventricle (LV) off-loading strategy.
- However, the jury is still out on the best option [we used an intra-aortic balloon pump (IABP) for all our patients].[53] Although VA ECMO can support gas exchange, in some patients with combined cardiopulmonary failure, where the heart has started to recover but the lungs are still poorly functioning; there is the risk of poorly oxygenated blood being pumped by the recovering or recovered heart into the coronaries, upper limbs, and the brain. In contrast, the well-oxygenated blood is being supplied to the rest of the body by VA ECMO. This is also known as the Harlequin syndrome, the North–South syndrome, or differential hypoxia. Patients with peripheral VA ECMO must always have a right radial arterial line (the brachiocephalic trunk is the first vessel coming off the aorta) and cerebral oximetry in place to facilitate timely detection of this physiology. The use of the axillary artery has been reported to avoid the complications reported with femoral cannulations.[54]
- *Central VA ECMO:* Patients who develop refractory cardiogenic shock with their chest open, most often the postcardiotomy patients, failing to come off the cardiopulmonary bypass, are often continued on the operative cannulation strategy involving the biatrial access and ascending aorta return cannula, with the cannula then connected to an ECMO machine as opposed to the cardiopulmonary bypass machine. In these cases, the chest is usually left open in anticipation of myocardial recovery, allowing ECMO to be removed and the chest to be closed in a few days. However, the use of central VA ECMO for more extended periods has also been reported, with the chest closed and cannulae tunneled out either superiorly or inferiorly.[55] Increasingly, many centers are moving toward peripheral VA ECMO cannulation, even for postcardiotomy cardiogenic shock.[56]

There is good evidence of better outcomes with percutaneous cannulation compared to surgical cutdown.[57] However, in cases with severe peripheral vascular disease or small-caliber vessels, it may be advisable to get a vascular surgeon involved and consider a surgical cutdown with the placement of a cannula using a synthetic graft.[58] Whether the cannulation is achieved percutaneously, using an ultrasound-guided, Seldinger-based technique, or a surgical cutdown, it does not affect the classification of ECMO type or configuration. There has been an attempt to standardize the terminology used for types and configurations of ECMO, incorporating a choice of cannula size and site. Still, it has not become standard practice yet. A detailed discussion on this subject is beyond the scope of this chapter; the reference has been included for further reading.[59]

## ECMO Circuit and Basic Physiology

All ECMO circuits have similar components and basic designs. Blood is drawn out of a patient's venous system via an access cannula, with the help of a pump, circulated the circuit through an oxygenator (or the "membrane lung") before returning to the patient's venous or arterial system. A schematic diagram of a basic ECMO circuit is shown in **Figure 2**. The pump used in most machines is centrifugal, often magnetically

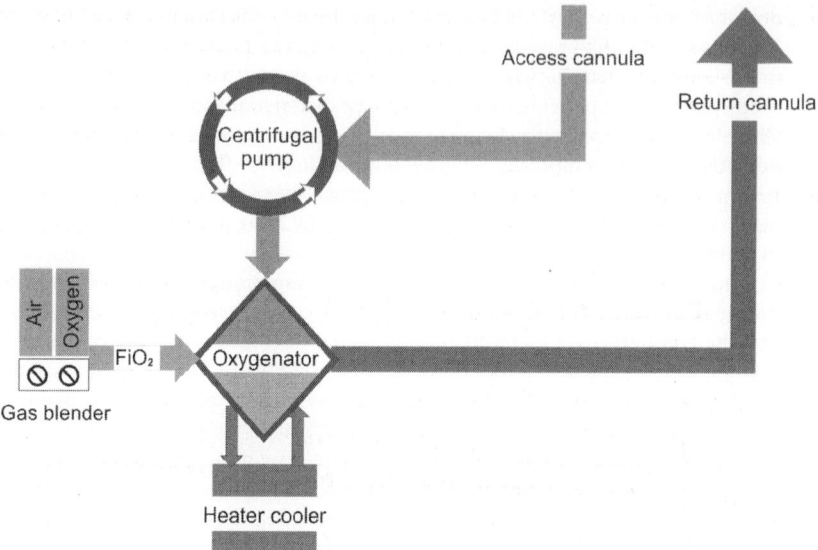

**Fig. 2:** Schematic diagram of a basic extracorporeal membrane oxygenation (ECMO) circuit. ($FiO_2$: fraction of inspired oxygen)

levitated, and hence much less traumatic to the blood cells than a roller pump used in cardiopulmonary bypass machines and some of the older ECMO machines. The oxygenator is the critical component and the basis of ECMO therapy. It is made up of tightly packed hollow fibers, most often made of polymethylpentene (PMP) that is gas permeable and participates in gas exchange and temperature regulation of the blood flowing through it, determined by the oxygen content of the gas (sweep gas) it receives from the device called the blender, and the temperature of the water that it receives from a device called the heater-cooler.

- Oxygenation depends on the blood flow rate through the oxygenator, the blood's hemoglobin content, and the sweep gas's oxygen fraction. Decarboxylation depends on the partial pressure of the carbon dioxide in the blood coming into the oxygenator and the sweep gas flow rate.[60]
- The centrifugal pump in the ECMO circuit provides hemodynamic support to the patient when the blood is returned to the aorta. The difference is that it is nonpulsatile; in the case of peripheral VA ECMO, it is retrograde, i.e., toward the heart.[61]

The oxygenator is also called the membrane lung, but compared to the native lung, which has a surface area of up to 140 $m^2$, the membrane lung's surface area is only up to 2 $m^2$.

## Indications and Patient Selection

Extracorporeal membrane oxygenation is not a cure, but it helps keep patients alive, who are otherwise almost certainly looking at death, which allows time for spontaneous recovery or for procedures that may aid recovery. The indications for ECMO have continued to expand in recent years, but it is advisable to think of ECMO indication in any case using the following framework:

- *Bridge to recovery:* ECMO in patients where there is a reasonable expectation of full or sufficient recovery that will allow separation from ECMO, e.g., bacterial or viral pneumonia leading to ARDS, viral myocarditis, or toxic exposure leading to cardiogenic shock, ECMO for patients who develop refractory cardiac arrest due to STEMI (ST-elevation myocardial infarction) but after complete revascularization (also known as ECPR), etc.
- *Bridge to definitive treatment:* ECMO may also be used in patients who can recover fully or enough to be separated from ECMO, but that may require one of the following:
  - Therapeutic procedures, e.g., valve replacement (open or percutaneous), coronary revascularization, or treatment of complications of myocardial infarction.
  - Lung and or heart transplant in patients with advanced lung and or heart disease that have already undergone necessary multidisciplinary discussion and workup and are ideally already active on the transplant list.
  - Ventricular assist device(s), either as a destination therapy or as a bridge to heart transplant.
- *Bridge to decision:* Often, the clinical situation is not as black and white as the above two scenarios, and trained clinical judgment of the multidisciplinary team may decide to proceed with ECMO even though it is not clear if recovery is possible and although no transplant workup has been done, no obvious contraindication is apparent at the time.
- *Periprocedural ECMO:* Given the increasing ease and comfort of various teams in tertiary hospitals with ECMO therapy, it is also starting to be used to facilitate an expanding set of procedures that may have previously been turned down due to prohibitive risk, e.g., transcatheter aortic valve replacement (TAVR), complex percutaneous coronary intervention (PCI), ventricular tachycardia (VT) ablation, etc. It is also used to make it easier to perform some surgical procedures, e.g., major airway tumors or trauma.

## Contraindications

Patients who refuse to accept ECMO therapy and are unlikely to benefit based on the above framework should not be offered ECMO. Published reports are increasingly challenging several of the criteria previously considered absolute contraindications based on age, weight, access restrictions, suitability for anticoagulation, or willingness to accept a blood transfusion, so it largely depends on individual centers' experience and policy.

## Anticoagulation

Anticoagulation is essential to prevent thromboembolic complications of ECMO therapy and is the current standard of care.[62] Patients on VA ECMO are at a greater risk of arterial thromboembolism, while VV ECMO patients have a greater incidence of venous thromboembolis.[63] Patients typically receive a 50-100 U/kg bolus dose of unfractionated heparin (UFH) at the time of cannulation, followed by an infusion targeting activated clotting time (ACT), active partial thromboplastin time (aPTT), or anti-factor Xa. Targets are higher for patients on VA ECMO (aPTT 60-80 s) than VV ECMO (40-60 s). There are several reports of patients on ECMO, specifically

VV ECMO, where anticoagulation has had to be held for extended periods for a variety of reasons (major bleeding, neurotrauma), and patients have suffered no harm.[64] For patients with heparin-induced thrombocytopenia, argatroban or bivalirudin may be used.[65]

## Weaning from ECMO

Patients are weaned off ECMO support when the underlying condition is reversed, and other organ systems also function well. This involves progressive weaning of the sweep gas flow rate and oxygen content in patients on VV ECMO[66] and weaning the blood flow rate in patients on VA ECMO.[67]

## ■ PERIOPERATIVE MANAGEMENT OF ECMO PATIENTS

As discussed, an anesthetist may interface with ECMO in procedural areas in several ways:
- ECMO initiation
- Procedures on ECMO patients
- ECMO decannulation

## ECMO Initiation

Even if the patient is being cannulated for a few hours to facilitate a procedure, the same level of attention to detail, bearing in mind the following:
- Even though ECMO cannulation is an extension of the traditional Seldinger technique-based vascular access, and the expertise has been reported across several specialties, including cardiothoracic and vascular surgery, anesthesia and critical care, interventional cardiology, interventional radiology, and emergency physicians, the hospitals must specify the training and onboarding route to ECMO cannulation competency in their policy.
- The ECMO configuration will largely depend on the proposed procedure. For example, a femorofemoral VV ECMO will be more suitable for major thoracic and upper airway surgeries.
- Cannulation must be ultrasound, echocardiography, or fluoroscopy-guided; hence, these competencies must be part of the training program.
- Percutaneous cannulation should be the default approach unless otherwise indicated, e.g., severe peripheral vascular disease.
- Cannula sizes must be able to support the anticipated need based on patient size, underlying heart and or lung function, and likely complications of the planned procedure. Current recommendations for desired ECMO flow for patients receiving VV ECMO and VA ECMO are based on the fact that their underlying heart and or lungs are completely failing, and ECMO must sufficiently replace those functions, as opposed to ECMO initiation for high-risk procedures in otherwise stable patients. Most manufacturers provide a datasheet with information on flows and pressure drops across their selection of ECMO cannula, which follows the Hagen–Poiseuille Law.
- The cannulae must be adequately secured with appropriately resilient suture material at the insertion site and several anchor points along their length and covered with transparent dressings.

- The possibility of limb ischemia must be anticipated and addressed at the outset in patients receiving peripheral VA ECMO. Patients may tolerate short procedures requiring only a small-caliber arterial cannula (15 Fr). If a bigger arterial cannula is required or if the patient has severe peripheral vascular disease, the insertion of a DPC may be necessary to prevent limb ischemia. Regardless of the selected approach, throughout the procedure, color, warmth, Doppler signals, and near-infrared spectroscopy (NIRS) should be closely monitored for the adequacy of limb perfusion.
- Occasionally, patients undergoing coronary or structural interventions in the Cath Lab or undergoing major surgeries in the OR will suddenly decompensate, e.g., coronary dissection, refractory VT/VF, pulmonary embolism, etc. Hospitals should have a policy on escalation of such cases appropriately to their "Shock Teams" and set criteria for determining candidacy for mechanical circulatory support (MCS).
- ECMO in patients with refractory cardiac arrest poses several unique challenges, a discussion that is outside the scope of this chapter.

## Procedures on ECMO Patients

### Preoperative Assessment and Planning

Standard preoperative assessment and planning applies as much to these patients, with perhaps more attention to detail. The perioperative plan must be collaboratively developed and shared with the entire team, which includes the proceduralist, anesthetist, critical care physician, perfusionist, and OR nurses. The team and plan will depend on whether the patient is receiving ECMO in the OR, e.g., high-risk TAVR, or is already on ECMO in intensive care unit (ICU) and needs to undergo a procedure in the OR, e.g., laparotomy for bowel ischemia.

The following should be established:
- Roles and responsibilities
- The ECMO plan includes the cannulation, configuration, estimated flow requirements, anticoagulation, relevant intraoperative considerations, and a postoperative plan for ECMO decannulation. It should be clear if ECMO will be needed from the outset or if it will be used only in the event of complications.
- Management of non-ECMO support in the perioperative period
- Goals of care and limits of escalation, which may include a review of the patient's comorbidities, baseline functional status, the severity of the current condition for which several outcome prediction scores may be used, and the patient's current or previously expressed wishes. It should also discuss the action plan if the patient deteriorates before the proposed procedure. Would they be an ECMO candidate as a bridge to the procedure?

### Intraoperative Care

- *Patient transfer:* Elective patients will present themselves to the OR. Still, the ECMO patients in the ICU must be transferred to the OR with appropriate staff and support according to the hospital policy, which should also include pre- and post-transfer safety checklists.
- *Anesthesia and analgesia:* Patients with VV ECMO may have very low minute ventilation, either due to underlying lung disease, e.g., severe ARDS, or due to

lack of ventilation for extended periods during major thoracic procedures, and patients on VA ECMO will have a significant proportion of blood flow bypass the lung. The efficacy of inhalational anesthesia and its titration may be challenging; hence, total intravenous anesthesia is prudent for patients undergoing ECMO procedures. ECMO adds 800–1,500 mL to the volume of distribution. The highly lipid-soluble and protein-bound drugs also have more significant sequestration in the ECMO circuit and often require higher doses, e.g., propofol, fentanyl, midazolam, dexmedetomidine, etc.[68-72] Neuromuscular blockers may have reduced clearance due to organ dysfunction, common in patients with ECMO.

- *Antibiotics:* Cephalosporins are the commonly used antibiotics for surgical prophylaxis, and their clearance is minimally affected by ECMO. They can be used in the usual doses for critically ill patients. Vancomycin has similar pharmacokinetics, but its clearance may be decreased in these patients, and the dosing interval should be adjusted. It is more prudent to have therapeutic drug monitoring in this situation.[73-76]
- *ECMO management:* The ECMO-specific management for both VA and VV ECMO patients is summarized in **Table 2**. Changes to ECMO blood flows significantly impact hemodynamics and biventricular function, so any adjustment to pharmacological support should coordinate with the changes to the ECMO settings. Likewise, changes to ECMO sweep gas flow rate, and fraction of inspired oxygen ($FiO_2$) can rapidly impact gas exchange, so such changes must be coordinated with any changes to the mechanical ventilation settings.

**TABLE 2:** Balancing extracorporeal membrane oxygenation (ECMO) versus non-ECMO support in operating room (OR).

|  | VA ECMO | VV ECMO |
|---|---|---|
| Hemodynamics | • ECMO blood flow (EBF) directly influences the hemodynamic parameters (MAP, CVP, PAP)<br>• EBF requirements will be higher in patients with cardiogenic shock and or higher body mass compared to those undergoing elective procedures in OR<br>• Flows should be titrated to MAP and perfusion endpoints, e.g., lactate, $MvO_2$, etc., and appropriate targets must be reviewed by the team on a case-by-case basis | • ECMO Blood Flow (EBF) has no impact on the hemodynamics of a patient on VV ECMO<br>• Patients with end-stage lung disease or severe ARDS may have varying degrees of pulmonary hypertension, which may be sensitive to hypoxia, hypercapnia, and or acidosis. Worsening pH will impact the biventricular function and systemic hemodynamics<br>• VV ECMO flows should target to 60% of the patient's cardiac output to maintain adequate oxygenation<br>• For patients who require extracorporeal $CO_2$ removal, lower ECMO flows can be tolerated |

*Contd...*

*Contd...*

|  | **VA ECMO** | **VV ECMO** |
|---|---|---|
| Gas exchange | • ECMO sweep gas adjustments can help with gas exchange<br>• Sweep gas $FiO_2$ will influence the oxygenation, while the sweep gas flow rate will influence the carbon dioxide clearance<br>• Patients with recovering or only moderately impaired LV but a diseased lung will be at risk of Harlequin syndrome, which should be monitored using ABGs from the right radial arterial line and cerebral NIRS monitoring, and the ventilator may also need to be optimized as needed | • Every ECMO setting influences the gas exchange<br>• Sweep gas $FiO_2$ and EBF will influence the oxygenation, while the sweep gas flow rate will influence the carbon dioxide clearance<br>• EBF that is at least two-thirds of the patient's native cardiac output will ensure oxygen saturation in 90 s (%)<br>• Patients with normal lungs undergoing elective procedures will contribute significantly to gas exchange, so any changes with ECMO settings may amplify the impact on gas exchange, therefore the anesthetist and perfusionist must jointly review ABGs and agree on any changes to the ventilator and or ECMO |
|  | All patients should receive protective lung ventilation with plateau pressure ≤25 $cmH_2O$, driving pressure ≤15 $cmH_2O$, tidal volumes ≤6 mL/kg predicted IBW, and individually titrated PEEP ||

(ABG: arterial blood gases; ARDS: acute respiratory distress syndrome; CVP: central venous pressure; $FiO_2$: fraction of inspired oxygen; IBW: ideal body weight; LV: left ventricle; MAP: mean arterial blood pressure; $MvO_2$: mixed venous oxygen saturation; NIRS: near-infrared spectroscopy; PAP: pulmonary artery pressure; PEEP: positive end-expiratory pressure; VA ECMO: venoarterial ECMO; VV ECMO: venovenous ECMO)

The teams managing the patient and ECMO must maintain good, closed-loop communication throughout the procedure.

- *Anticoagulation:* As discussed, anticoagulation may be safely withheld in many ECMO patients for extended periods, provided a reasonable ECMO flow rate is maintained, especially in VA ECMO [greater than 3–3.5 LPM (liter per minute)]. Discussion of the need for withholding anticoagulation should be a part of the preoperative planning, and the potential thromboembolic risk versus risk of bleeding during the surgery should be considered. In patients with heparin-induced thrombocytopenia, the thromboembolic risk is much higher in the absence of anticoagulation. Still, the bleeding risk is also much higher if the decision is made to continue anticoagulation with direct thrombin inhibitors during the surgery. Likewise, patients with existing thrombi, e.g., in the inferior vena cava or the ventricles, may require careful discussion of the risks involved. Therefore, decisions on anticoagulation must be made on a case-by-case basis. Where the decision has been made to withhold anticoagulation, heparin may be stopped 6 hours before the scheduled procedure. It is usually sufficient to prevent direct thrombin inhibitors for 6 hours before the surgery but may require longer if there is significant hepatic and or renal dysfunction. Anticoagulation is best monitored intraoperatively using ACT, complemented by frequent viscoelastic assessment [thromboelastography (TEG), rotational thromboelastometry (ROTEM)].

- *ECMO-specific monitoring:* Standard monitoring per the latest guidelines must be used in all ECMO patients, which should be sufficient for all patients on VV ECMO. For patients on VA ECMO, you also need to consider the following.
  - *Right radial arterial line:* The earliest evidence of Harlequin syndrome will be evident from a significant drop in partial pressure of oxygen ($pO_2$) in the right subclavian (therefore, the right radial). This is more likely in patients with reasonably functioning LVs undergoing major thoracic procedures on VA ECMO.
  - *NIRS:* A pair should always be applied to the forehead and calves. The forehead reading helps detect Harlequin SYNDROME or another sudden global cerebral event in time. The readings from the pads applied to calves can be used to monitor leg perfusion in patients with VA ECMO, both on the side of arterial cannulation and the contralateral side where an IABP or Impella may have been inserted.
  - Based on mechanical ventilator settings, the end-tidal $CO_2$ monitor may read lower than expected, as pulmonary blood flow is reduced and most gas exchange occurs at the oxygenator.
  - *Cardiac output monitoring:* A Swan–Ganz catheter is routinely used in patients on VA ECMO to monitor hemodynamics and biventricular function, titration of therapy continuously, and during ECMO weaning. Pulmonary artery catheter (PAC) insertion in VA ECMO patients may be challenging as much of the blood is diverted toward ECMO. Thermodilution measurements are not validated in ECMO, primarily if the thermal filament lies across the tricuspid valve as the injectate is unreliably distributed between the pulmonary artery and the ECMO cannula.[77]
  - Fick's estimate of cardiac output is also inaccurate, as gas exchange occurs both at the oxygenator and the lungs. Thermodilution and Fick's method can render an error of as high as 3 LPM if the ECMO flows are high.[78]
  - Mixed venous oxygen saturation from PACs may be a valuable target for monitoring.

## ECMO Troubleshooting

To ensure a consistent and systematic approach to all troubleshooting scenarios. Even though perfusionists will be at hand to help navigate any ECMO emergencies, all ECMO specialists should have access to troubleshooting protocols and undergo periodic refresher training for individual technical skills in a simulated team environment (role allocation, team dynamics, communications). **Table 3** gives a summary of standard alarms and recommended actions.

## ECMO Decannulation

The strategy for decannulation will depend on the ECMO modality and indication. For patients receiving ECMO in the OR for high-risk surgeries, the decision on the timing of decannulation should be a part of the preoperative plan. This may include decannulation by the surgeon or proceduralist at the end of the procedure or transfer to the ICU on ECMO for observation. Patients may sometimes be extubated before

**TABLE 3:** Basic extracorporeal oxygenation (ECMO) troubleshooting.

| Alarm/scenario | Possible causes | Management |
|---|---|---|
| Low venous pressure, or access line chattering/chugging | • Hypovolemia<br>• Access cannula malposition<br>• Access cannula kink<br>• High intrathoracic pressure, e.g., tension pneumothorax, repeated coughing and straining, etc.<br>• Cardiac tamponade<br>• Flows too high relative to cannula size | • Reduce EBF until line chugging or chattering stops<br>• Confirm and address the etiology, e.g., reposition the cannula, fluid bolus, insert bigger cannula, etc. |
| High pre-membrane pressure | Clots in the oxygenator or at the oxygenator inlet | • Inspect the oxygenator for clots<br>• Check for signs of intravascular hemolysis (platelets, PF-Hb)<br>• Check oxygenator function (pre-/post-oxygenator ABGs)<br>• Cut in a new oxygenator |
| High post-membrane Pressure | • Return line kink<br>• High systemic arterial pressures (in VA ECMO) | • Remove any kink in the return line<br>• Reduce ECMO flows or control elevated systemic arterial pressure (VA ECMO) |
| Gas failure | • Oxygen tank empty<br>• Gas tubing disconnected | • Replace the oxygen tank or connect to the wall supply<br>• Reconnect the gas tubing |
| Pump failure | • Mechanical failure<br>• Power failure | • Check power supply connection<br>• Use the hand-crank to maintain the EBF<br>• Cut in a new pump or switch to the backup ECMO machine |
| Air bubble detected | Air entrainment in the circuit, e.g., open line ports (CVC, PAC, CRRT, etc.), cracked circuit tubing, damaged ECMO membrane, etc. | • Visually inspect the entire circuit for evidence of air<br>• Use the machine-specific steps for de-airing the circuit<br>• If a large volume of air is entrained, cut in a new oxygenator or switch to the backup machine |

(CVC: central venous catheter; CRRT: continuous renal replacement therapy; PAC: pulmonary artery catheter; PF-Hb: plasma-free hemoglobin)

ECMO is gradually weaned off, e.g., major airway repair. Patients on VV ECMO can be safely decannulated by critical care physicians at the bedside with purse-string sutures for hemostasis followed by close observation for 24 hours. Although patients with peripheral VA ECMO are conventionally decannulated in the OR and undergo an open repair of the cannulated artery, anecdotal use of newer percutaneous closure devices suggests that they are probably superior to manual pressure,[79] even surgical decannulation. Still, enough data is not available to make a firm recommendation.

Since the decannulation of VA ECMO occurs in the OR and involves a transition of care from ICU to anesthesia, the OR teams must be familiar with the process of weaning and potential challenges. A patient's weaning readiness must be determined collectively by the ICU and other members of the shock team (heart failure, interventional cardiology, cardiac surgery). Patients are weaned by progressively reducing ECMO blood flow rate while closely monitoring the invasive systemic and pulmonary hemodynamics [central venous pressure (CVP), pulmonary artery pressure (PAP), cardiac output], perfusion indices (mixed venous saturation, lactate), and echocardiographic indices [right ventricle (RV) and LV ejection fraction (EF), left ventricular outflow tract (LVOT), velocity time integral (VTI)], and adjusting the pharmacological support to optimize these parameters. The challenges often arise from the fact that the ECMO blood flow rate cannot be lowered below or maintained below a certain level for long periods without increasing thromboembolic risk, and any delays between deemed decannulation readiness and subsequent transfer to OR for decannulation increase the likelihood of failure. Patients with VA ECMO are older and more fragile than VV ECMO patients; they will often have multi-organ failure in various stages of recovery, and several patients will need to come off on at least moderate support with multiple agents so expectations must be aligned between the critical care and OR team.

## ■ CONCLUSION

The rapidly evolving technology, standardized, evidence-based guidelines, and growing clinical expertise with ECMO and its various indications within critical care are also encouraging its use perioperatively to facilitate an increasing number of procedures that would have been declined previously on the grounds of the complexity of the procedure or the fragility of the patient. Even if patients receive ECMO only for a few hours in a procedural area, several challenges and complications may still occur, requiring attention to detail throughout. All OR staff who attend to ECMO patients must have a similar level of training and experience with all aspects of ECMO care, supported by simulation and practical refresher sessions completed at least twice a year. At the dawn of an era where ECMO is continually redefining what is feasible surgically, and it is likely to become an integral part of the OR skillset, anesthetists should prepare themselves adequately to embrace that future.

## ■ REFERENCES

1. Kakar V, North A, Bajwa G, Raposo N, Kumar PG. Long Runs and Higher Incidence of Bleeding Complications in COVID-19 Patients Requiring Venovenous Extracorporeal Membrane Oxygenation: A Case Series from the United Arab Emirates. Indian J Crit Care Med Peer-Rev Off Publ Indian Soc Crit Care Med. 2021;25(12):1452-8.
2. Hessel EA 2nd. A Brief History of Cardiopulmonary Bypass. Semin Cardiothorac Vasc Anesth. 2014;18(2):87-100.

3. Hill JD, O'Brien TG, Murray JJ, Dontigny L, Bramson ML, Osborn JJ, et al. Prolonged extracorporeal oxygenation for acute post-traumatic respiratory failure (shock-lung syndrome). Use of the Bramson membrane lung. N Engl J Med. 1972;286(12):629-34.
4. Zapol WM, Snider MT, Hill JD, Fallat RJ, Bartlett RH, Edmunds LH, et al. Extracorporeal membrane oxygenation in severe acute respiratory failure. A randomized prospective study. JAMA. 1979;242(20):2193-6.
5. Morris AH, Wallace CJ, Menlove RL, Clemmer TP, Orme JF, Weaver LK, et al. Randomized clinical trial of pressure-controlled inverse ratio ventilation and extracorporeal $CO_2$ removal for adult respiratory distress syndrome. Am J Respir Crit Care Med. 1994;149(2 Pt 1):295-305.
6. Betit P. Technical Advances in the Field of ECMO. Respir Care. 2018;63(9):1162-73.
7. Brower RG, Lanken PN, MacIntyre N, Matthay MA, Morris A, Ancukiewicz M, et al. National Heart, Lung, and Blood Institute ARDS Clinical Trials Network. Higher versus lower positive end-expiratory pressures in patients with the acute respiratory distress syndrome. N Engl J Med. 2004 Jul;351(4):327-36.
8. Amato MBP, Meade MO, Slutsky AS, Brochard L, Costa ELV, Schoenfeld DA, et al. Driving Pressure and Survival in the Acute Respiratory Distress Syndrome. N Engl J Med. 2015;372(8):747-55.
9. Rajsic S, Breitkopf R, Jadzic D, Popovic Krneta M, Tauber H, Treml B. Anticoagulation Strategies during Extracorporeal Membrane Oxygenation: A Narrative Review. J Clin Med. 2022;11(17):5147.
10. Vincent JL. Critical care--where have we been and where are we going? Crit Care. 2013;17Suppl 1(Suppl 1):S2.
11. Peek GJ, Mugford M, Tiruvoipati R, Wilson A, Allen E, Thalanany MM, et al. Efficacy and economic assessment of conventional ventilatory support versus extracorporeal membrane oxygenation for severe adult respiratory failure (CESAR): a multicentre randomised controlled trial. The Lancet. 2009;374(9698):1351-63.
12. Australia and New Zealand Extracorporeal Membrane Oxygenation (ANZ ECMO) Influenza Investigators; Davies A, Jones D, Bailey M, Beca J, Bellomo R, Blackwell N, et al. Extracorporeal Membrane Oxygenation for 2009 Influenza A(H1N1) Acute Respiratory Distress Syndrome. JAMA. 2009;302(17):1888-95.
13. Combes A, Hajage D, Capellier G, Demoule A, Lavoué S, Guervilly C, et al.; EOLIA Trial Group, REVA, and ECMONet. Extracorporeal Membrane Oxygenation for Severe Acute Respiratory Distress Syndrome. N Engl J Med. 2018;378(21):1965-75.
14. Extracorporeal Life Support Organization. ELSO Annual Report 2023. Available from https://www.elso.org/aboutus/annualreport/annualreport2023.aspx [Last accessed July, 2024].
15. Ostadal P, Rokyta R, Karasek J, Kruger A, Vondrakova D, Janotka M, et al. ECMO-CS Investigators. Extracorporeal Membrane Oxygenation in the Therapy of Cardiogenic Shock: Results of the ECMO-CS Randomized Clinical Trial. Circulation. 2023;147(6):454-64.
16. Banning AS, Sabaté M, Orban M, Gracey J, López-Sobrino T, Massberg S, et al. Venoarterial extracorporeal membrane oxygenation or standard care in patients with cardiogenic shock complicating acute myocardial infarction: the multicentre, randomised EURO SHOCK trial. EuroIntervention. 2023;19(6):482-92.
17. Yannopoulos D, Bartos J, Raveendran G, Walser E, Connett J, Murray TA, et al. Advanced reperfusion strategies for patients with out-of-hospital cardiac arrest and refractory ventricular fibrillation (ARREST): a phase 2, single centre, open-label, randomised controlled trial. Lancet. 2020;396(10265):1807-16.
18. Belohlavek J, Smalcova J, Rob D, Franek O, Smid O, Pokorna M, et al.; Prague OHCA Study Group. Effect of Intra-arrest Transport, Extracorporeal Cardiopulmonary

Resuscitation, and Immediate Invasive Assessment and Treatment on Functional Neurologic Outcome in Refractory Out-of-Hospital Cardiac Arrest: A Randomized Clinical Trial. JAMA. 2022;327(8):737-47.
19. Suverein MM, Delnoij TSR, Lorusso R, Brandon Bravo Bruinsma GJ, Otterspoor L, Elzo Kraemer CV, et al. Early Extracorporeal CPR for Refractory Out-of-Hospital Cardiac Arrest. N Engl J Med. 2023;388(4):299-309.
20. Richardson ASC, Tonna JE, Nanjayya V, Nixon P, Abrams DC, Raman L, et al. Extracorporeal Cardiopulmonary Resuscitation in Adults. Interim Guideline Consensus Statement From the Extracorporeal Life Support Organization. ASAIO J. 2021;67(3):221-8.
21. Van Drumpt AS, Kroon HM, Grüne F, van Thiel R, Spaander MCW, Wijnhoven BPL, et al. Surgery for a large tracheoesophageal fistula using extracorporeal membrane oxygenation. J Thorac Dis. 2017;9(9):E735-8.
22. Zhou R, Liu B, Lin K, Wang R, Qin Z, Liao R, et al. ECMO support for right main bronchial disruption in multiple trauma patient with brain injury—a case report and literature review. Perfusion. 2015;30(5):403-6.
23. Lang G, Ghanim B, Hötzenecker K, Klikovits T, Matilla JR, Aigner C, et al. Extracorporeal membrane oxygenation support for complex tracheo-bronchial procedures†. Eur J Cardiothorac Surg. 2015;47(2):250-6.
24. Kim JJ, Moon SW, Kim YH, Choi SY, Jeong SC. Flexible bronchoscopic excision of a tracheal mass under extracorporeal membrane oxygenation. J Thorac Dis. 2015;7(3):E54-57.
25. Lei J, Su K, Li XF, Zhou YA, Han Y, Huang LJ, et al. Ecmo-assisted carinal resection and reconstruction after left pneumonectomy. J Cardiothorac Surg. 2010;5(1):89.
26. Odish MF, Yang J, Cheng G, Yi C, Golts E, Madani M, et al. Treatment of Bronchopleural and Alveolopleural Fistulas in Acute Respiratory Distress Syndrome With Extracorporeal Membrane Oxygenation, a Case Series and Literature Review. Crit Care Explor. 2021;3(5):e0393.
27. Park AH, Tunkel DE, Park E, Barnhart D, Liu E, Lee J, et al. Management of complicated airway foreign body aspiration using extracorporeal membrane oxygenation (ECMO). Int J Pediatr Otorhinolaryngol. 2014;78(12):2319-21.
28. Ramanathan K, Leow L, Mithiran H. ECMO and adult mediastinal masses. Indian J Thorac Cardiovasc Surg. 2021;37(S2):338-43.
29. Carlson SF, Smith NJ, Joyce LD, Joyce DL, Rossi PJ. Acquired tracheomalacia due to aortic aneurysm managed with venopulmonary extracorporeal membrane oxygenation for perioperative support. J Vasc Surg Cases Innov Tech. 2021;7(4):737-40.
30. Suk P, Šrámek V, Čundrle I Jr. Extracor gery. Membranes (Basel). 2021;11(6):416.
31. Mason DP, Thuita L, Nowicki ER, Murthy SC, Pettersson GB, Blackstone EH. Should lung transplantation be performed for patients on mechanical respiratory support? The US experience. J Thorac Cardiovasc Surg. 2010;139(3):765-773.e1.
32. Rinieri P, Peillon C, Bessou JP, Veber B, Falcoz PE, Melki J, et al. National review of use of extracorporeal membrane oxygenation as respiratory support in thoracic surgery excluding lung transplantation. Eur J Cardiothorac Surg. 2015;47(1):87-94.
33. Dang Van S, Hamy A, Hubert N, Fouquet O. Cardiogenic shock induced by a voluminous phaeochromocytoma rescued by concomitant extracorporeal life support and open left adrenalectomy. Eur J Cardiothorac Surg. 2016;50(4):782-3.
34. Tincrès F, Conil JM, Crognier L, Rouget A, Georges B, Ruiz S. Veno-arterial extracorporeal membrane oxygenation in a case of amniotic fluid embolism with coexisting hemorrhagic shock: lessons learned. Int J Obstet Anesth. 2018;33:99-100.
35. Mikami T, Kamiunten H. Emergent caesarean section under mechanical circulatory support for acute severe peripartum cardiomyopathy. J Cardiol Cases. 2018;17(6):200-3.

36. Vitulo P, Beretta M, Martucci G, Hernandez Baravoglia CM, Romano G, Bertani A, et al. Challenge of Pregnancy in Patients With Pre-Capillary Pulmonary Hypertension: Veno-Arterial Extracorporeal Membrane Oxygenation as an Innovative Support for Delivery. J Cardiothorac Vasc Anesth. 2017;31(6):2152-5.
37. Staudacher DL, Bode C, Wengenmayer T. Severe mitral regurgitation requiring ECMO therapy treated by interventional valve reconstruction using the MitraClip. Catheter Cardiovasc Interv. 2015;85(1):170-5.
38. Mizote I, Schirmer J, Schäfer U. A case of successful Mitraclip implantation in a patient having a large coaptation gap under extracorporeal membrane oxygenation (ECMO). Catheter Cardiovasc Interv. 2018;91(4):827-30.
39. Drews T, Pasic M, Buz S, Dreysse S, Klein C, Kukucka M, et al. Elective use of femoro-femoral cardiopulmonary bypass during transcatheter aortic valve implantation. Eur J Cardiothorac Surg. 2015;47(1):24-30.
40. Baratto F, Pappalardo F, Oloriz T, Bisceglia C, Vergara P, Silberbauer J, et al. Extracorporeal Membrane Oxygenation for Hemodynamic Support of Ventricular Tachycardia Ablation. Circ Arrhythm Electrophysiol. 2016;9(12):e004492.
41. Tarzia V, Bortolussi G, Bianco R, Buratto E, Bejko J, Carrozzini M, et al. Extracorporeal life support in cardiogenic shock: Impact of acute versus chronic etiology on outcome. J Thorac Cardiovasc Surg. 2015;150(2):333-40.
42. Hollenberg SM. Cardiogenic shock. Crit Care Clin. 2001;17(2):391-410.
43. Yeh CF, Wang CH, Tsai PR, Wu CK, Lin YH, Chen YS. Use of Extracorporeal Membrane Oxygenation to Rescue Patients With Refractory Ventricular Arrhythmia in Acute Myocardial Infarction. Medicine (Baltimore). 2015;94(30):e1241.
44. Hsieh CE, Lin HC, Tsui YC, Lin PY, Lin KH, Chang YY, et al. Extracorporeal Membrane Oxygenation Support in Potential Organ Donors for Brain Death Determination. Transplant Proc. 2011;43(7):2495-8.
45. Skerritt C, Carton E. Veno-venous extracorporeal membrane oxygenation in the management of malignant hyperthermia. Br J Anaesth. 2019;122(6):e82-3.
46. Bacon B, Silverton N, Katz M, Heath E, Bull DA, Harig J, et al. Local Anesthetic Systemic Toxicity Induced Cardiac Arrest After Topicalization for Transesophageal Echocardiography and Subsequent Treatment With Extracorporeal Cardiopulmonary Resuscitation. J Cardiothorac Vasc Anesth. 2019;33(1):162-5.
47. Esnault P, Née L, Signouret T, Jaussaud N, Kerbaul F. Reverse Takotsubo cardiomyopathy after iatrogenic epinephrine injection requiring percutaneous extracorporeal membrane oxygenation. Can J Anesth. 2014;61(12):1093-7.
48. Carelli M, Seco M, Forrest P, Wilson MK, Vallely MP, Ramponi F. Extracorporeal membrane oxygenation support in refractory perioperative anaphylactic shock to rocuronium: a report of two cases. Perfusion. 2019;34(8):717-20.
49. Valchanov K, Ercole A, Fowles J, Parmar J, Gopalan D. Veno-Venous Extracorporeal Membrane Oxygenation for Fat Embolism. J Med Cases. 2014;5(9):488-90.
50. Keshavamurthy S, Bazan V, Tribble TA, Baz MA, Zwischenberger JB. Ambulatory extracorporeal membrane oxygenation (ECMO) as a bridge to lung transplantation. Indian J Thorac Cardiovasc Surg. 2021;37(Suppl 3):366-79.
51. Cove ME. Disrupting differential hypoxia in peripheral veno-arterial extracorporeal membrane oxygenation. Crit Care. 2015;19(1):280.
52. Rajagopal K. Left Ventricular Distension in Veno-arterial Extracorporeal Membrane Oxygenation: From Mechanics to Therapies. ASAIO J. 2019;65(1):1-10.
53. Lüsebrink E, Binzenhöfer L, Kellnar A, Müller C, Scherer C, Schrage B, et al. Venting during venoarterial extracorporeal membrane oxygenation. Clin Res Cardiol. 2023;112(4):464-505.

54. Pisani A, Braham W, Brega C, Lajmi M, Provenchere S, Danial P, et al. Right axillary artery cannulation for venoarterial extracorporeal membrane oxygenation: a retrospective single centre observational study. Eur J Cardiothorac Surg. 2021;59(3):601-9.
55. Downey P, Ragalie W, Gudzenko V, Ardehali A. Ambulatory central veno-arterial extracorporeal membrane oxygenation in lung transplant candidates. J Heart Lung Transplant. 2019;38(12):1317-9.
56. Ohira S, Malekan R, Goldberg JB, Lansman SL, Spielvogel D, Kai M, et al. Axillary artery cannulation for veno-arterial extracorporeal membrane oxygenation support in cardiogenic shock. JTCVS Tech. 2021;5:62-71.
57. Danial P, Hajage D, Nguyen LS, Mastroianni C, Demondion P, Schmidt M, et al. Percutaneous versus surgical femoro-femoral veno-arterial ECMO: a propensity score matched study. Intensive Care Med. 2018;44(12):2153-61.
58. Calderon D, El-Banayosy A, Koerner MM, Reed AB, Aziz F. Modified T-Graft for Extracorporeal Membrane Oxygenation in a Patient with Small-Caliber Femoral Arteries. Tex Heart Inst J. 2015;42(6):537-9.
59. Broman LM, Taccone FS, Lorusso R, Malfertheiner MV, Pappalardo F, Di Nardo M, et al. The ELSO Maastricht Treaty for ECLS Nomenclature: abbreviations for cannulation configuration in extracorporeal life support - a position paper of the Extracorporeal Life Support Organization. Crit Care. 2019;23(1):36.
60. Bartlett RH. Physiology of Gas Exchange During ECMO for Respiratory Failure. J Intensive Care Med. 2017;32(4):243-8.
61. Fresiello L, Hermens JAJ, Pladet L, Meuwese CL, Donker DW. The physiology of venoarterial extracorporeal membrane oxygenation—a comprehensive clinical perspective. Perfusion. 2024;39(1_suppl):5S-12S.
62. McMichael ABV, Ryerson LM, Ratano D, Fan E, Faraoni D, Annich GM. 2021 ELSO Adult and Pediatric Anticoagulation Guidelines. ASAIO J. 2022;68(3):303-10.
63. Olson SR, Murphree CR, Zonies D, Meyer AD, Mccarty OJT, Deloughery TG, et al. Thrombosis and Bleeding in Extracorporeal Membrane Oxygenation (ECMO) Without Anticoagulation: A Systematic Review. ASAIO J. 2021;67(3):290-6.
64. Kurihara C, Walter JM, Karim A, Thakkar S, Saine M, Odell DD, et al. Feasibility of Venovenous Extracorporeal Membrane Oxygenation Without Systemic Anticoagulation. Ann Thorac Surg. 2020;110(4):1209-15.
65. Šoltés J, Skribuckij M, Říha H, Lipš M, Michálek P, Balík M, et al. Update on Anticoagulation Strategies in Patients with ECMO—A Narrative Review. J Clin Med. 2023;12(18):6067.
66. Vasques F, Romitti F, Gattinoni L, Camporota L. How I wean patients from veno-venous extra-corporeal membrane oxygenation. Crit Care. 2019;23(1):316.
67. Fried JA, Masoumi A, Takeda K, Brodie D. How I approach weaning from venoarterial ECMO. Crit Care. 2020;24(1):307.
68. Shekar K, Fraser JF, Smith MT, Roberts JA. Pharmacokinetic changes in patients receiving extracorporeal membrane oxygenation. J Crit Care. 2012;27(6):741.e9-18.
69. Shekar K, Roberts JA, Ghassabian S, Mullany DV, Ziegenfuss M, Smith MT, et al. Sedation during extracorporeal membrane oxygenation-why more is less. Anaesth Intensive Care. 2012;40(6):1067-9.
70. Shekar K, Roberts JA, Mcdonald CI, Fisquet S, Barnett AG, Mullany DV, et al. Sequestration of drugs in the circuit may lead to therapeutic failure during extracorporeal membrane oxygenation. Crit Care. 2012;16(5):R194.
71. Shekar K, Roberts JA, Mullany DV, Corley A, Fisquet S, Bull TN, et al. Increased sedation requirements in patients receiving extracorporeal membrane oxygenation for respiratory and cardiorespiratory failure. Anaesth Intensive Care. 2012;40(4):648-55.
72. Nigoghossian CD, Dzierba AL, Etheridge J, Roberts R, Muir J, Brodie D, et al. Effect of Extracorporeal Membrane Oxygenation Use on Sedative Requirements in Patients with Severe Acute Respiratory Distress Syndrome. Pharmacotherapy. 2016;36(6):607-16.

73. Shekar K, Fraser JF, Taccone FS, Welch S, Wallis SC, Mullany DV, et anl.; ASAP ECMO Study Ivestigators. The combined effects of extracorporeal membrane oxygenation and renal replacement therapy on meropenem pharmacokinetics: a matched cohort study. Crit Care. 2014;18(6):565.
74. Donadello K, Antonucci E, Cristallini S, Roberts JA, Beumier M, Scolletta S, et al. β-Lactam pharmacokinetics during extracorporeal membrane oxygenation therapy: a case-control study. Int J Antimicrob Agents. 2015;45(3):278-82.
75. Cheng V, Abdul-Aziz MH, Burrows F, Buscher H, Cho YJ, Corley A, et al. ASAP ECMO Investigators. Population Pharmacokinetics of Vancomycin in Critically Ill Adult Patients Receiving Extracorporeal Membrane Oxygenation (an ASAP ECMO Study). Antimicrob Agents Chemother. 2022;66(1):e0137721.
76. Mulla H, Pooboni S. Population pharmacokinetics of vancomycin in patients receiving extracorporeal membrane oxygenation. Br J Clin Pharmacol. 2005;60(3):265-75.
77. Su Y, Liu K, Zheng JL, Li X, Zhu DM, Zhang Y, et al. Hemodynamic monitoring in patients with venoarterial extracorporeal membrane oxygenation. Ann Transl Med. 2020;8(12):792.
78. Ortoleva JP, Alfadhel A, Dalia AA. Invasive Hemodynamic and Physiologic Considerations in Patients Undergoing Extracorporeal Membrane Oxygenation. J Cardiothorac Vasc Anesth. 2021;35(9):2549-51.
79. Scherer C, Stremmel C, Lüsebrink E, Stocker TJ, Stark K, Schönegger C, et al. Manual Compression versus Suture-Mediated Closure Device Technique for VA-ECMO Decannulation. J Interv Cardiol. 2022;2022:9915247.

# CHAPTER 20

# High-Altitude Medicine: Anesthesiology and Critical Care Challenges

*Shagun Bhatia Shah, Rajiv Chawla, Uma Hariharan*

## ABSTRACT

High-altitude-induced pathophysiological changes pose unique anesthetic challenges. The human body responds to hypobaric hypoxia with increased heart rate, blood pressure, minute ventilation, and erythropoiesis. The spectrum of high-altitude illness (HAI) ranges from headache to pulmonary and cerebral edema. Although rapid descent to lower altitudes is the definitive treatment for HAI, this is only practical in some scenarios where supplemental oxygen, portable hyperbaric bags, and drugs are pivotal. Anesthetic challenges include tackling hypoxia, hypothermia, HAI, and effects on anesthesia vaporizers, gas analyzers, flowmeters, and other equipment. This becomes more daunting in patients with cardiac comorbidity (pulmonary hypertension, left to right shunts, and tachyarrhythmias). Regional anesthesia, ketamine-induced dissociative anesthesia, and total intravenous anesthesia, being relatively unaffected by high altitude, are preferred anesthetic options. Inhalational anesthetic techniques should avoid nitrous oxide. Trapped air pockets in the body/equipment will expand with rapid ascent in the eventuality of aeromedical evacuation.

**Keywords:** Anesthetic challenges; Gas analyzers; High altitude; Hypoxia; Mountain sickness; Vaporizers

## KEY POINTS

- Most pathophysiological changes at high altitudes are attributable to hypobaric hypoxia.
- The spectrum of high-altitude illness (HAI) ranges from headache to pulmonary and cerebral edema to even chronic mountain sickness (pulmonary hypertension and cor pulmonale).
- Anesthetic challenges include hypoxia, hypothermia, HAI, effects on anesthesia vaporizers, flowmeters, and other equipment, and a constrained environment.
- Regional techniques, ketamine-induced dissociative anesthesia, and total intravenous anesthesia, being relatively unaffected by high altitude, are preferred anesthetic options.
- Inhalational anesthesia should be the last resort in this scenario.
- Gases such as oxygen and nitrous oxide have a reduced partial pressure and a lower clinical effect. Nitrous oxide should be avoided, given its insignificant analgesic effect and the expansion of trapped air pockets during aeromedical evacuation.
- The partial pressure of volatile anesthetics and the performance of vaporizers remain the same at high altitudes, except for desflurane.
- Equipment based on gas density, such as flowmeters and gas mixing devices, have an altered function.

# INTRODUCTION

High-altitude medicine presents unique challenges due to the pathophysiological changes induced by high altitudes, mainly hypoxemia due to the reduced inspired oxygen partial pressure with altitudinal gain. Implementing rules for safe acclimatization at altitudes above 2,500 m (ascending at most 300–500 m above sleeping altitude per day; rest day after every 1,000 m altitude gain) is often hampered due to logistics.[1] The Indo-Australian tectonic plate is still moving toward Eurasia, pushing Tibet northward, and hence, the world's highest mountain, the Himalayas, continues to rise by >1 cm annually.[2] India holds 55%, Nepal 30% (including most tall peaks), Bhutan 10%, while Pakistan, Afghanistan, and China share the remainder. It is projected that recreation, adventure, and religious pilgrimage shall attract 250 million tourists to the Indian hill states by 2025 (vs. 100 million prepandemic tourists). Data reveals that 90% of India's earthquakes, landslides, and cloudbursts plague the Himalayas.[3] Our soldiers guard these treacherous borders. The first death of an Agniveer soldier on duty has been attributed to high-altitude illness (HAI).[4] In this scenario, where millions of visiting low landers are susceptible to HAI, and natives require operation theater services routinely, and during natural calamities, the magnitude of the problem is phenomenal. We present some key anesthetic considerations and challenges for anesthesiologists, intensivists, and emergency care physicians.

# CLASSIFICATION OF ALTITUDE REGIONS

Altitude regions are usually defined as high (1,500–3,500 m; ~5,000–11,500 ft), very high (3,500–5,500 m; ~11,500–18,000 ft), and extreme (>5,500 m; >18,000 ft).[1] HAI is known to occur at altitudes above 2,000 m, e.g., Darjeeling (2,050 m), Ooty (2,250 m), and Amarnath (5,100 m).

# PHYSICS AT HIGH ALTITUDE

The partial pressure of inspiratory oxygen ($PiO_2$) is a fixed proportion (21%) of total barometric pressure. The percentage of oxygen in ambient air is 21% at sea level (atmospheric pressure 760 mm Hg), one mile above sea level (Denver; atmospheric pressure 540 mm Hg), and even at the Mount Everest summit. However, the $PiO_2$ falls from 160 mm Hg at sea level to 113 mm Hg at Denver to 50 mm Hg atop Mount Everest, necessitating supplemental oxygen to bolster $FiO_2$.[5]

As per the alveolar gas equation:[6,7]

$$P_AO_2 = FiO_2 (P_B - P_{H_2O}) - PaCO_2/\text{Respiratory quotient}$$

($P_AO_2$ = Partial pressure of oxygen in alveoli; $FiO_2$ = Fraction of inspired oxygen; $P_B$ = Barometric/atmospheric pressure; $P_{H_2O}$ = Water Vapor pressure at body temperature (47 mm Hg); $PaCO_2$ = Partial pressure of carbon dioxide in arterial blood; Respiratory quotient is 0.82).

Partial pressure of oxygen in arterial blood ($PaO_2$) is calculated from $P_AO_2$ by adjusting for the alveolar-arterial (A-a) gradient (5–10 mm Hg for a young adult nonsmoker). The A-a gradient increases with age and is estimated as (age/4) + 4. Hence, the expected A-a gradient in a 40-year-old should be <14. The Severinghaus equation converts $PaO_2$ to $SaO_2$ (oxygen saturation). **Table 1** depicts the variations in $PiO_2$, $P_AO_2$, $PaO_2$, and $SaO_2$ as a function of altitude.[6-9]

**TABLE 1:** Variations in $PiO_2$, $P_AO_2$, $PaO_2$, and $SaO_2$ with altitude.

| Altitude (Feet) | Atmospheric pressure (mm Hg) | Effective $O_2$ Conc. (%) | $PiO_2$ (mm Hg) | $P_AO_2$ (mm Hg) | $PaO_2$ (mm Hg) | $SaO_2$ (%) | Representative place in India |
|---|---|---|---|---|---|---|---|
| Sea level | 760 | 21 | 159 | 101 | 86 | 97 | 30: Kolkata, 46: Mumbai |
| 5,000 | 632 | 17.3 | 133 | 73 | 59 | 91 | 4,990: Shillong, 5,200: Vaishno Devi + Srinagar |
| 10,000 | 522 | 14.3 | 110 | 51 | 37 | 86 | 10,000: Rakcham village |
| 15,000 | 438 | 11.8 | 92 | 32 | 18 | 62 | 14,931: Kunzum pass (Lahaul Spiti) |
| 20,000 | 364 | 9.7 | 76 | 17 | 3 | 24 | 20,000: Stok Kangri peak |
| 29,000 | 253 | 6.9 | 53 | 27 | 26 |  | Mount Everest (Nepal) |

*Note:* Breathing without $O_2$ support is not possible beyond 20,000 ft; Mt. Everest is added for reference only; Absolute $O_2$ concentration is 21% at all altitudes but due to low atmospheric pressure the effective $O_2$ concentration is much lesser.
($PiO_2$: partial pressure of inspiratory oxygen; $PaO_2$: Partial pressure of oxygen in arterial blood; $P_AO_2$: partial pressure of oxygen in alveoli; $SaO_2$: oxygen saturation)

Three main compensatory mechanisms exist that counter this hypoxia, attempting to make the partial pressure of oxygen ($PO_2$) in mixed venous blood at high altitudes the same as at sea level.[10] First is a reduction in tissue metabolism, consequent to decreased oxygen availability. The second mechanism comprises the adjustment of oxygen transport characteristics. Thirdly, in the absence of suppression by central carbon dioxide ($CO_2$) receptors, a lower $PAO_2$ activates the peripheral arterial chemoreceptors, producing hyperventilation. Although the resulting hypocapnia tends to shift the oxygen-hemoglobin dissociation curve (ODC) leftward, it increases the alveolar oxygen tension by 25–30%. Increased red blood corpuscular 2, 3 diphosphoglycerate improves $O_2$ unloading to tissues by shifting the ODC rightward. The oxygen cascade is less steep at high altitudes versus sea levels, and at 1–2 mm Hg $PO_2$ in mitochondria, anaerobic metabolism commences. Hyperventilation-induced respiratory alkalosis shifts the ODC leftward, increasing oxygen uptake by red cells in the pulmonary circulation.

As renal bicarbonate excretion increases to compensate for the hypocapnia-induced respiratory alkalosis from hyperventilation, bicarbonate is also lost from cerebrospinal fluid (CSF) besides blood, leading to decreased buffer capacity. Changes in CSF $CO_2$ levels result in quicker changes in hydrogen ion concentration, leading to heightened $CO_2$ sensitivity. At this stage of acclimatization, ventilatory sensitivity to $CO_2$ is enhanced. After gradual respiratory acclimatization, an increase in the hypoxic ventilatory response (HVR) occurs.

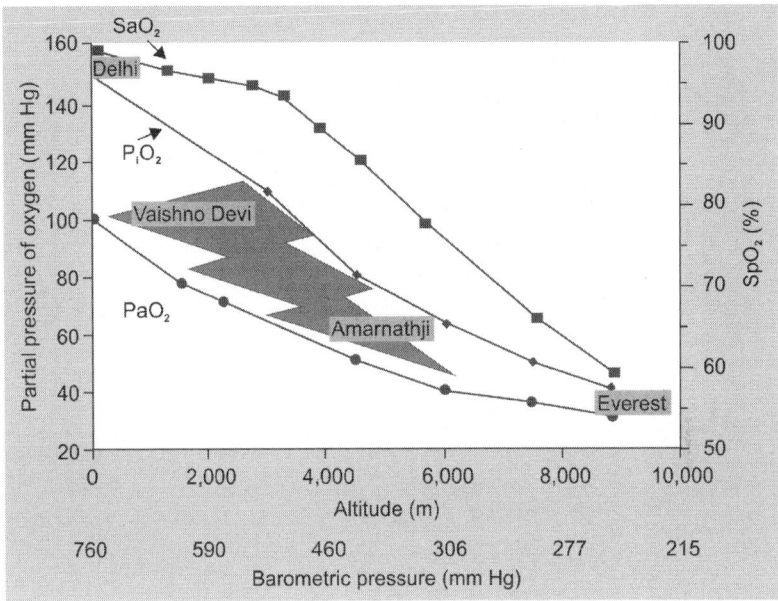

**Fig. 1:** The change in oxygen cascades with altitude.

At high altitudes, the oxygen cascade begins at a lower $PO_2$, and less oxygen is available at each cascade step **(Fig. 1)**. However, compensatory mechanisms (mainly increased cardiac output) strive to keep the mixed venous oxygen tension nearly the same at all altitudes.[11]

## ACCLIMATIZATION

Initiated after 2–3 weeks, physiological adaptation or acclimatization to high altitudes requires months. Hypoxia produces the following physiological adaptive changes **(Table 2)**.[6]

## HIGH-ALTITUDE PATHOPHYSIOLOGY

*Hypoxic ventilatory response:* Atop Mt. Everest (8,848 m), the $PiO_2$ of ambient air is only 50 mm Hg versus 160 mm Hg at sea level. The corresponding $PaO_2$ is only 37.6 mm Hg, lower than the partial pressure of $O_2$ in the mixed venous blood in healthy resting adults at sea level. The estimated minute ventilation (a product of tidal volume and respiratory rate) is roughly 166 L/min, mainly due to severe hypoxic hyperventilation.[12] However, this potent compensatory mechanism is drastically compromised under volatile anesthetics with concentrations below 1 minimum alveolar concentration (MAC) and completely abolished at 1.1 MAC of halothane. It is imperative to note that inhalation of even a subanesthetic concentration (0.1 MAC) of volatile anesthetics profoundly diminishes HVR even in the absence of concurrent opioid administration. The volatile anesthetics aligned in decreasing order of potency of HVR suppression are halothane > sevoflurane > isoflurane > desflurane.[13]

*Periodic breathing (Cheyne Stokes breathing):* This central breathing disorder comprises altitude-induced breathing instability in low landers transferred to a

| TABLE 2: Physiological adaptation to high altitude. ||
|---|---|
| Respiratory and oxygen transport changes | ↑Respiratory rate; ↑Tidal volume |
| | ↓$PaCO_2$ and respiratory alkalosis |
| | 3–4 fold ↑in pulmonary oxygen diffusion capacity |
| | ↑Pulmonary capillary blood flow |
| | ↑Lung volume and ↑surface area of alveolar membrane |
| | ↑Blood supply of upper lobes of lungs |
| Cardiovascular changes | ↑Cardiac output (↑Heart rate due to hypoxia-induced sympathetic stimulation) |
| | Hypertension |
| | ↑Erythropoiesis [Hematocrit ↑from 45 to 65%; ↑hemoglobin (Hb) from 15 to 22 g%] |
| | ↓Plasma volume by 10–20% (fluid shift from vascular to interstitial space) |
| | ↑Oxygen carrying capacity of blood (due to hemoconcentration) |
| | Hyperplastic bone marrow |
| Renal changes | Natriuresis |
| | Diuresis and bicarbonate excretion to offset respiratory alkalosis |
| | ↑Renal erythropoietin production |

high altitude, where ambient hypoxia increases controller gain. Occurring most commonly during sleep, periodic breathing is attributable to loss of cortical control of respiration. It is characterized by hyperventilation followed by spells of apnea spanning 10–15 seconds. Idiopathic central sleep apnea (CSA), relatively uncommon at sea level, occurs more frequently in individuals with an elevated hypercapnic ventilatory response (high controller gain), leading to hypocapnia and respiratory control instability during sleep. Patients with idiopathic CSA tend to have low $PaCO_2$ levels, even while fully awake.[14]

## ■ PREGNANCY AND ALTITUDE

Since the fetus in utero does not derive oxygen directly from the low atmospheric pressure at high altitudes, it appears little affected by acute exposure to altitudes up to 2,500–3,000 m and suffers no adverse effects. Adaptation includes a decrease in villous membrane thickness and increased placental capillary volume. At high altitudes, newborns are abruptly exposed to a hypoxic environment, causing a more gradual transition to adult circulation, with a higher incidence of patent foramen ovale and patent ductus arteriosus. An increased incidence of acute respiratory distress syndrome and pulmonary arterial hypertension potentially necessitate mechanical ventilation.[7]

## ■ HIGH-ALTITUDE ILLNESS

The HAI comprises a spectrum of symptoms ranging from mild headache to pulmonary edema followed by cerebral edema and maybe acute or chronic.

## Acute Mountain Sickness

High-altitude headache (HAH) is the mildest form of acute mountain sickness (AMS). The latter appears 2-12 hours after rapid ascent from low to high altitudes (>2,000 m), often during/after the first night, and resolves within 12-48 hours without further ascent. Headache may occur in isolation or the dominant grievance among a constellation of symptoms (anorexia, nausea, vomiting, insomnia, dizziness, and fatigue). Individual susceptibility to AMS decides the trajectory of severity of symptoms, which increases during the first 6-12 hours at high altitudes.[1] AMS has a higher propensity for females[15] and younger individuals.[16] Improvement with a descent to a 300 m lower altitude is the hallmark of AMS. The differential diagnosis includes alcohol hangover, carbon monoxide poisoning, dehydration, drug intoxication, exhaustion, hyponatremia, and migraine. Pulse oximetry is often within the normal range for the altitude or, occasionally, slightly lower. The Lake Louise score (analyzing headache, gastrointestinal symptoms, fatigue, dizziness, and sleeping difficulty) is used to diagnose AMS.[17]

## High-Altitude Pulmonary Edema

Chest congestion, cough, exaggerated dyspnea on exertion, and reduced exercise capacity herald the onset of high-altitude pulmonary edema (HAPE). Unrecognized/ untreated, HAPE typically progresses to dyspnea at rest and respiratory distress, accompanied by blood-stained pink frothy sputum over 1-2 days. Auscultatory rales and pulse oximetric oxygen saturation levels at least 10 points lower than in healthy people at the same altitude (between 50% and 70%) are observed. Without rapid descent or therapy, HAPE is fatal in roughly 50% of patients. Oxygen (2-4 L/min) via face mask/oxygen canister or utilizing a hyperbaric bag, if available, is recommended. Drug therapy plays a secondary role. If nifedipine is unavailable, nifedipine or a phosphodiesterase inhibitor can help by pulmonary vasodilation.[17]

## High-Altitude Cerebral Edema

High-altitude cerebral edema (HACE) represents "end stage" AMS and occurs secondary to HAPE-induced hypoxemia. HACE is an encephalopathy characterized by altered mental status, ataxia, confusion, and drowsiness, similar to alcohol intoxication. Focal neurologic deficits/seizures are rare. Coma ensues within 12-24 hours of the onset of ataxia in the absence of treatment (supplemental oxygen; portable hyperbaric bag) or descent.[17]

## Chronic Mountain Sickness (Monge Disease)

Excessive erythrocytosis and pulmonary hypertension leading to cor pulmonale progressing to congestive cardiac failure are the hallmarks of chronic mountain sickness. It has attained the stature of a public health problem in the Andes. Symptoms include chronic headache, vertigo, dyspnea, palpitations, focal cyanosis, plantar and palmar burning sensation, vasodilation, myalgia, arthralgia, lack of mental focus, and memory deficits. Although phlebotomy provides transient relief, descent to a lower altitude is the definitive treatment. The Qinghai score assesses the severity of Monge disease.[18,19]

## Prevention of High-altitude Illness

Besides acclimatization and following the rules of ascent (not >300–500 m/day with a rest day after completion of every 1,000 m), prophylactic drug therapy **(Table 3)** helps prevent AMS.

**TABLE 3:** Prophylaxis and drug treatment in high-altitude illness.

| | Drug mechanism of action | Prophylactic dose | Therapeutic dose | Adverse effects |
|---|---|---|---|---|
| AMS/ HAH | Oxygen<br>Major limitation of prophylactic *Strategy:* Logistical restraints + High costs | Low flow (1–2 L/min) applied during sleep via nasal cannula | 4–5 L/min via face mask; Hyperbaric | Nasal dryness |
| | Acetazolamide<br>Inhibits carbonic anhydrase → ↓ Renal bicarbonate reabsorption → Metabolic acidosis compensates for respiratory alkalosis at altitude → Optimizes respiratory drive and adaptation | Oral 125 mg × 12 hourly (24 hours before ascent till 48 hours after reaching maximum altitude) | Oral 250 mg × 12 hourly | ↑ Diuresis dizziness, nausea, vomiting, diarrhea, dysgeusia |
| | Dexamethasone<br>• Potent glucocorticoid with little mineralo-corticoid activity<br>• Anti-inflammatory effect | Oral 4 mg × 12 hourly | Oral/IV/IM 8 mg once, then 4 mg × 6 hourly | Hyperglycemia |
| | Ibuprofen | – | 600 mg × 8 hourly | Gastric irritation |
| | Acetaminophen | | 500 mg × 8 hourly | |
| | Ondansetron | – | 4 mg × 8 hourly | Headache |
| | Ginkgo biloba (Herbal) | Oral | 120 mg twice daily | GI upset Skin rash |
| HAPE | Nifedipine<br>Calcium channel blocker | Oral 30 mg × 12 hourly | Oral 30 mg × 12 hourly | ↓BP, dizziness, headache |
| | Dexamethasone | Oral 4 mg × 12 hourly | NA | Hyperglycemia |
| | Tadalafil/Sildenafil<br>Pulmonary artery vasodilation | Oral 10 mg × 12 hourly/50 mg × 8 hourly | NA | ↓BP, dizziness, headache |
| | Salmeterol<br>↑Alveolar fluid clearance due to stimulated transepithelial sodium transport | Inhalational 120 µg × 12 hourly (Do not use as monotherapy) | NA | Tremors, tachycardia, hypokalemia |

*Contd...*

*Contd...*

| | Drug mechanism of action | Prophylactic dose | Therapeutic dose | Adverse effects |
|---|---|---|---|---|
| HACE | Dexamethasone Protects against ↑permeability of vascular endothelium and blood-brain barrier, Suppression of inflammatory cytokines + reactive oxygen species, sympatholysis | Oral 4 mg × 12 hourly | Oral/IV/IM 8 mg once, then 4 mg × 6 hourly | Hyperglycemia |
| | Acetazolamide | Oral 125 mg × 12 hourly | – | ↑ Diuresis |
| Monge Disease | Acetazolamide Reduces erythropoietin and hematocrit by abolishing HPV | – | Oral 250 mg × 12 hourly for 6 months | ↑ Diuresis, dizziness, nausea |
| | Domeperidone | – | Oral 10 mg 3 times a day | Dry mouth, Tachyarrhythmias |
| | ACE inhibitors (Enalapril) | – | 10 mg/day for 30 days | First dose hypotension |
| | Medroxyprogesterone and Almitrine Respiratory stimulants | – | 20 mg/3 times a day × 10 weeks | Headache, weight gain, spotting |
| | | | 1.5 mg/kg/day × 4 weeks | Headache |
| | Nifedipine (Calcium channel blocker) and Sildenafil (Phosphodiestrase inhibitor) Reduce pulmonary artery pressure | – | 120 mg/day | Postural hypotension |
| | | | Oral 5 or 20 mg × 8 hourly | ↓BP Vertigo priapism, vision issues |

(ACE: angiotensin-converting enzyme; AMS: acute mountain sickness; BP: blood pressure; GI: gastrointestinal; HAH: high-altitude headache; HACE: high-altitude cerebral edema; HAPE: high-altitude pulmonary edema; HPV: hypoxic pulmonary vasoconstriction; IV: intravenous; IM: intramuscular)

## Treatment of High-altitude Illness

The various treatment options are discussed in the following text.

### Oxygen Supplementation

Oxygen (2–4 L/min) is supplemented via a face mask or an oxygen canister.[20]

### Rapid Descent

Rapid descent to a lower altitude may not be possible due to logistic reasons.

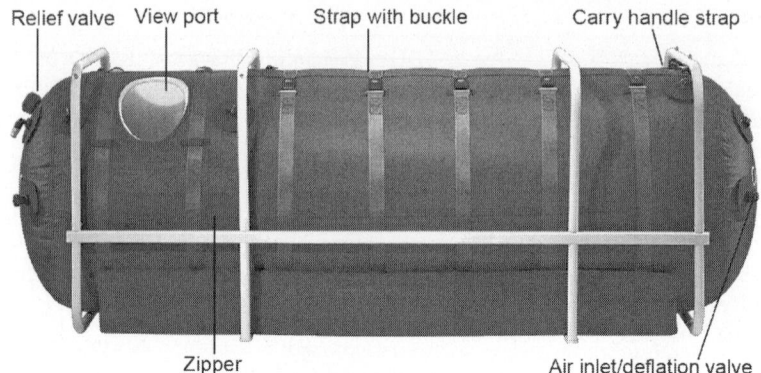

**Fig. 2:** Portable hyperbaric bag.

## *Portable Hyperbaric Bag*

This can be lifesaving when immediate evacuation/descent to lower altitudes is impossible. Gamow bag is the commercially available version fabricated from acoustically transparent, temperature-resistant, nonpermeable, and urethane-coated nylon **(Fig. 2)**. Five encircling nylon web straps provide structural rigidity, limit movement, and tether the Gamow bag. Two view ports allow victim observation and communication and allow ambient light to enter, reducing claustrophobia. A portable, fabric, and lightweight (7 kg) hyperbaric bag capable of withstanding a pressure of 2 psi was utilized by Taber et al., who reported that AMS, HAPE, and HACE patients required time frames of 2, 4, and 6 hours, respectively, for resolution of symptoms without complications. Inflation of the bag to 2 psi after placing the patient in the bag, at 13,920 ft in Nepal, corresponded with a descent to 8,400 ft.[21]

## *Drug Treatment*

Acetaminophen and ibuprofen are suitable for HAH. A combination of calcium channel blockers (nifedipine) and phosphodiesterase inhibitors (sildenafil) should be avoided due to potential severe hypotension. In addition to HAH prevention, acetazolamide ameliorates altitude-related excessive periodic breathing sleep disorder and enhances sleep quality. Dexamethasone is the drug of choice for AMS prophylaxis but only a second-line drug for the treatment of AMS. It proves helpful when acetazolamide is contraindicated (sulfonamide allergy, history of adverse effects) and when an appropriate ascent protocol is not feasible. Reduction in aquaporin-mediated transmembrane water transport, antioxidant, vasodilatory, and anti-inflammatory effects are AMA-specific mechanisms of action of acetazolamide besides producing mild metabolic acidosis. Concerns exist regarding the effectiveness of dexamethasone treatment of severe and life-threatening HACE with preexisting dexamethasone prophylaxis. The drug treatment of HAI[17,19,22,23] is summarized in **Table 3**.

## ■ ANESTHETIC CHALLENGES

These are broadly divided into two categories: those related to high-altitude-induced pathophysiological changes in the human body and those due to high-altitude variations in anesthesia resources and equipment functioning.

## Challenges Due to Pathophysiological Changes

*Hypobaric hypoxia:* The reduced $PO_2$ in high altitudinal ambient air leads to hypoxic hypoxia. Anesthesia and critical care personnel should adjust oxygen supplementation to counter perioperative hypoxemia. Prolonged preoxygenation before anesthetic induction is crucial to augment oxygen reserves. Postoperative oxygen supplementation for a minimum of one hour and opioid-sparing postoperative pain relief with a high index of suspicion for respiratory depression in the postoperative period is essential. Anesthesiologists should be cautious with the administration of sedatives or narcotic analgesics. Both of these blunt the hypoxic ventilatory drive and may precipitate hypoxic symptoms of irritability, confusion, and restlessness, which may be misinterpreted as being due to pain and misguide us.

*Hypothermia:* The higher the altitude, the lower the atmospheric pressure. As any gas rises to lower pressure regions, the gas expands, and the gas particles absorb energy from the surroundings to do so. Hence, the surrounding environment is often cold, compounding the risk of hypothermia during anesthetic procedures. Active patient warming techniques such as forced-air convective warming blankets, warm mattresses, and warmed intravenous fluids should be employed. Hypothermia induces marked irritability of the atrioventricular bundle, potentially leading to atrial and ventricular fibrillation. MAC of agents is lowered in the presence of hypothermia.

*Low humidity:* A heat and moisture exchange (HME) filter should be connected to the breathing circuit.

*Risk of aspiration:* Delayed gastric emptying observed at high altitudes significantly increases the aspiration risk during anesthetic induction.[24]

*Blood loss:* High venous pressure, hypothermia, venous dilatation, and increased capillary density may contribute to increased intraoperative blood loss and oozing of blood from surgical wounds.[25]

*Risk of venous thromboembolism:* An altitude >4,000 ft above sea level is an independent risk factor for postoperative venous thromboembolism after total shoulder arthroplasty.[26]

*Postoperative Urinary Retention:* The risk of postoperative retention of urine is significantly higher at high altitudes.[27]

*Altitude-related illness:* Anesthesiologists and critical care physicians should be familiar with the entire spectrum of HAI, which may present with symptoms such as headache, nausea, vomiting, confusion, dyspnea, and cough. These may compound postoperative nausea and vomiting (PONV), and multimodal PONV prophylaxis using dexamethasone, ondansetron, and metoclopramide concurrently is warranted.

*Cerebral effects:* Increased blood-brain barrier permeability and increased cerebral vascular blood flow secondary to hypoxia may produce delayed awakening from anesthesia.

*Cardiovascular effects:* Hypoxic pulmonary vasoconstriction (HPV) at high altitudes elevates pulmonary artery pressure, especially in older people. The normal pulmonary arterial pressure at sea level is 12 mm Hg, rising to 28 mm Hg at high altitude. Systemic blood pressure also increases upon initial ascent to altitude, owing to sympathetic stimulation, especially in men. Despite acclimatization, respiratory and heart rates, pulmonary and systemic vascular pressures, and sympathetic activity remain elevated. However, stroke volume decreases, bringing cardiac output back to baseline and improving arterial oxygen saturation.[28]

High altitude can exacerbate preexisting cardiovascular comorbidity. Anesthesiologists need to employ advanced cardiac output monitoring devices, if available, and goal-directed fluid therapy. Patients should avoid high altitudes for 2 weeks postacute coronary event, stent placement, or cardiopulmonary bypass surgery. Rapid ascent to high altitude may increase the frequency of supraventricular and ventricular tachyarrhythmias in cardiac patients. Intraoperative continuous electrocardiogram, preservative-free lignocaine, amiodarone, and a defibrillator must be immediately available during surgical procedures for such patients. Right-to-left shunt fraction through a probe patent foramen ovale might be aggravated in hypoxic conditions due to increased pulmonary artery and right heart pressures. Patent foramen ovale is associated with 56% of patients susceptible to HAPE versus 11% of nonsusceptible individuals.[29] Patients with cyanotic congenital heart disease may be at heightened risk at even moderate altitudes. In nine male coronary artery disease patients, clinical/electrocardiographic signs of myocardial ischemia appeared at lower workloads at higher altitudes.[30] The heart rate and rate pressure product at the onset of angina were similar at the two altitudes (3,100 m vs. 1,600 m), suggesting that patients should limit their activity at high altitudes by heart rate control (70-85% of the ischemic threshold rate at sea level) rather than workload control. Extrapolated to surgery, tachycardia must not be allowed under anesthesia.

*Respiratory challenges:* Patients with chronic obstructive pulmonary disease (COPD) may experience exacerbations at high altitudes due to hypobaric hypoxia. Management should focus on optimizing respiratory function and avoiding hypercapnia. Pulmonary hypertension, attributable to vascular remodeling and ongoing HPV, may develop at high altitudes, especially with coexisting chronic hypoxemic lung disease.[31]

*Fluid management:* High-altitude environments can exacerbate dehydration due to increased respiratory (hyperventilation) and renal (compensatory bicarbonate excretion) water losses. At altitudes above 3,500 m, plasma volume rapidly dwindles by 3-5 mL/kg after ascent. This deficit persists for 3 or 4 months before heading toward baseline. Hence, fluid and electrolyte balance need careful monitoring in patients undergoing surgery or critical care management at high altitudes.

*Emergency preparedness:* Emergencies at high altitudes include airway obstruction, cardiac arrest, and altitude-related complications. Access to appropriate equipment, medications, and evacuation resources is essential for ensuring patient safety. Trapped air pockets in the body/equipment will expand rapidly during aeromedical evacuation. Unvented pneumothorax, pneumoperitoneum, pneumocephalus, and bowel gas will expand, possibly to dangerous levels. Air bubbles in intravenous lines and tracheal cuffs should also be monitored. Rapid ascent from sea level to 18,000 feet (ft) will double the volume of trapped gas.

## Challenges Due to the Effect of High Altitude on Anesthesia Resources and Equipment

### Remote Location
The austere high-altitude environments are often resource constrained.

### General Anesthesia
*The first documented case:* Open drop chloroform

Historically, in 1933, the administration of open drop chloroform anesthesia by Dr. Greene to a Tibetan assistant with a clavicular fracture on an expedition to Mt. Everest at 14,000 ft resulted in cardiopulmonary arrest. Open drop induction utilizes the patient's spontaneous ventilation to inhale the anesthetic vapor. Tibetan highlanders have a minute ventilation of 11.5 L/min at 5,000 m instead of 5-7 L/min in adults at sea level. The first school of thought is that an overdose of cardiotoxic chloroform vapors leads to cardiac arrest. As per the second school of thought, arrest resulted from an inadequate depth of anesthesia due to decreased chloroform vaporization in a cold environment, administration of chloroform "sparingly" to avert potential ventilatory depression or lack of depth of anesthesia monitors.[32]

### Modern Inhalational Anesthesia
*Controlled ventilation:* To prevent renal retention of bicarbonate, potentially reducing the ventilatory drive in the postoperative period, patients requiring controlled ventilation should have their $PaCO_2$ maintained at the baseline value rather than in the traditionally normal range. Similarly, maintenance of $PaO_2$ within the sea-level normal range will result in loss of adaptation and difficult readaptation of the patient to breathing room air.

*Effect on floating bobbin flowmeters:* At a simulated altitude of 10,000 ft, nitrous oxide ($N_2O$), and $O_2$ floating-bobbin flowmeters under-read the actual gas flow rate. The error percentage progressively increased up to 4 L/min, at which point both flowmeters were 20% in error. A hazard may arise when a low flow of $O_2$ is mixed with a higher flow of $N_2O$. This can be explained by the fact that spinning bobbin flowmeters rely on gas density, which reduces with altitude. Unless an $O_2$ analyzer is available, the delivered percentage of $O_2$ may be significantly lower than that calculated based on the flowmeter readings.[33]

An equation to derive the correction factor for high altitude is given below.

$$F_1 = F_0 \times \sqrt{(d_0/d_1)}$$

Here, $F_1$ is the gas flow at high altitude, $F_0$ is flow on the scale calibrated at sea level, $d_0$ is the density of gas at sea level, and $d_1$ is the density of gas at high altitude.[7]

*Effect on anesthesia vaporizers:* The partial pressure of an anesthetic gas, an index of its thermodynamic activity, controls its pharmacologic/anesthetic effect. The maximum partial pressure of a volatile anesthetic is its saturated vapor pressure, which is unique to each anesthetic and is directly proportional to its temperature. Although volatile anesthetics and gaseous anesthetics are characterized by a vapor pressure of <1 atm at 20°C, vaporizers (VAs) have a boiling point above 20°C. In contrast, gaseous anesthetics have a boiling point below 20°C. VAs comprise a small fraction of the inspiratory gas mixture. In contrast, gaseous anesthetics ($N_2O$, xenon), because of lower anesthetic potency, comprise a significant fraction of an inspiratory gas mixture, and hence, gaseous anesthetics produce additional effects (concentration effect, second gas effect, and airspace expansion). This partial pressure is expressed as the percentage (or fraction) of the delivered gas mixture at an atmospheric pressure of 760 mm Hg. The same inhaled concentration of an anesthetic gas results in a reduced pharmacologic effect at higher altitudes because the absolute partial pressure of the anesthetic is lower. Anesthetics move from regions of high partial pressure to low partial pressure, unaffected by the other components of the gas mixture, and equilibrium is achieved when the partial pressure of an anesthetic is equal in the different compartments. Correcting these values to absolute partial pressure is essential when ambient atmospheric pressure differs significantly from standard (high altitude, deep sea, and hyperbaric chamber).[13]

The partial pressure (mm Hg), rather than the concentration (%) of an anesthetic, correlates with its anesthetic effects. Modern VAs (isoflurane, sevoflurane) are agent-specific, temperature-compensated, and variable bypass. This design ensures that partial pressures are unaffected by altitude, resulting in unchanged gas delivery. At an altitude with atmospheric pressure half of sea level (380 mm Hg), the same number of anesthetic gas molecules will create a higher concentration of anesthetic gas vapor in the vaporizing chamber. However, the partial pressure remains unchanged. A vaporizer that supplies 2% sevoflurane at sea level supplies 4% at 5,000 ft, but the partial pressure (mm Hg) is the same (2% × 760 mm Hg = 15.2 mm Hg = 4% × 380 mm Hg). Hence, no compensation is required. The dial reading will be inaccurate, but the sevoflurane effect will be preserved as accurate. This was clinically tested by James and White using Fluotec Mark II and Dräger halothane VAs at sea level and high altitudes (5,000 ft and 10,000 ft). At any given setting, the delivered percentage of halothane increased with altitude, but its partial pressure and potency remained constant, regardless of altitude.

*Desflurane:* The Tec 6 vaporizer (Datex-Ohmeda) is not a variable bypass vaporizer and heats desflurane to 39°C, maintaining a vapor pressure of 2 atm. This produces a constant, predictable output concentration of desflurane. With this fixed output volume concentration, any altitudinal decrease in atmospheric pressure will reduce the partial pressure of desflurane. The following calibration formula is employed to achieve the same potency with desflurane at high altitudes as at sea level.

Required dial setting (%) = Desired % × (760 mm Hg/barometric pressure at high altitude in mm Hg).[34]

*Nitrous oxide:* The anesthetic potency of $N_2O$ is directly proportional to barometric pressure and progressively decreases with an increase in altitude. A 50% reduction in the analgesic effect of $N_2O$ is observed at 5,000 ft, dwindling to insignificant analgesia at 10,000 ft. The expansion of trapped-air pockets during aeromedical evacuation is another reason $N_2O$ is best avoided.[34,35]

*Gas analyzers:* Most gas analyzers respond to a physical property of the agent gas (number/activity of molecules) independent of the other gases in the mixture. Although they measure partial pressure and not the concentration of agents, these analyzers are traditionally calibrated in percentages (2% sevoflurane and not 15.2 mm Hg of sevoflurane at sea level). This calibration scale might produce serious errors when specialized equipment is used at high altitudes.

*Oxygen analyzers:* All oxygen analyzers (paramagnetic, fuel cell, and oxygen electrode devices) respond to $PO_2$ alone and alter the total measurement output in volume percentage when atmospheric pressure changes as a function of altitude. An oxygen analyzer calibrated at sea level to measure 21% oxygen in air gives a reading of 17.4% oxygen at 5,000 ft. Hence, the analyzer must be recalibrated at high altitudes to read 21% when air is sampled. If the oxygen activity were to be presented as $PO_2$ (mm Hg), the device would reflect oxygen availability to the patient's lungs at any altitude.

*Carbon dioxide analyzers:* Infrared-absorption-based $CO_2$ analyzers have scales that read in percentages, although the sensitive element responds to the increasing partial pressure of carbon dioxide. Calibrating these analyzers using precise gas mixtures to read exact percentages at any given altitude is possible. An analyzer calibrated at sea level will show decrease in the percentage scale proportional to the barometric pressure at a higher altitude with the same percentage of gas.

*Peak flowmeters:* Hand-held peak flowmeters underestimate peak expiratory flow rate by 6–8% for every 100 mm Hg fall in atmospheric pressure.[34]

*Bispectral index (BIS) guided anesthesia:* Frequency of anesthetic overdose with MAC-guided anesthesia at high altitude may potentially produce complications (delayed recovery, upper respiratory obstruction, postoperative delirium, length of stay, and nausea or vomiting), especially in frail patients. Under dosage potentially increases the risk of intraoperative awareness. A prospective cohort study on 50 patients reported the frequency of anesthetic overdose measured using BIS in Bogotá-Colombia, 2,600 m above sea level.[36] 10 minutes postsurgical incision, BIS, mean alveolar concentration, mean arterial pressure, and $SaO_2$ were recorded. BIS was classified as superficial (60), adequate (40–60), and deep (<40). Mean alveolar concentration was classified as low (<0.8), standard (0.8–1.2), and high (>1.2). Mean values of mean alveolar concentration and BIS were 1.14 and 38.66, respectively. The frequency of anesthetic overdose measured with BIS was 54% against only 20% with mean alveolar concentration. There was no correlation between mean alveolar concentration and BIS (Pearson r = 0.161) or between BIS and mean arterial pressure (Pearson r = 0.367). BIS-guided anesthesia could be helpful in the assessment and prevention of anesthetic overdose at high altitudes.

*Closed-loop anesthesia:* Closed-loop anesthesia delivery systems (CLADS) are a recent advancement in accurate titration of anesthetic drugs, superior to target-controlled infusion or manual titration of drug delivery for maintaining adequate depth of anesthesia even at high altitudes. 20 patients underwent abdominal/orthopedic procedures under general anesthesia at Leh (3,505 m). A patented closed-loop system utilized BIS feedback to titrate the propofol infusion rate. CLADS successfully maintained a BIS within ±10 of the target of 50 for 85% of surgery without any report of awareness under anesthesia. Heart rate and mean arterial pressure were within 25% of baseline values for 91% and 94% of the anesthesia time, respectively. Patients awakened within 3 minutes after cessation of propofol infusion with fitness to recovery room discharge within the next 15 minutes.[37]

## Total Intravenous Anesthesia with Propofol or Ketamine

The outcomes of propofol-based total intravenous anesthesia (TIVA) are superior to intravenous-inhalational anesthesia combination for laparoscopic gynecological surgery.[38] Dissociative anesthesia with ketamine (2 mg/kg), which preserves the hypoxic ventilatory drive and the laryngopharyngeal reflexes, has been successfully used at an altitude of 3,900 m in a resource-constrained setting in Nepal.[39] Supplemental oxygen was helpful in the recovery phase for less acclimatized patients. Emergence delirium was avoided using midazolam as premedication and a quiet recovery area.

### Regional Anesthesia

*Subarachnoid block:* Subarachnoid block, with the most negligible impact on ventilation, should be the anesthetic technique of choice, whenever available, at high altitudes. The onset time of complete sensory and motor blocks is shorter, and the duration of both motor and sensory blocks is longer at sea level compared to moderately high altitudes. More significant anesthetic requirements to achieve the same duration of block and a higher incidence of postdural puncture headache (PDPH) are observed at high altitudes in acclimatized/highlander patients. Possible basis includes chronically elevated CSF pressure, dehydration, and altered central nervous system sensitivity to intracranial pressure changes.

The CSF volume variability is the most critical factor affecting injected local anesthetics' intrathecal spread. Altitude gain increases cerebral arterial blood flow, reduces cardiac output, and swells CSF volume. 140 consecutive patients living at moderately high altitude (Erzurum, 1,890 m) and sea level (Sakarya, 31 m) scheduled for elective lower extremity surgery underwent spinal anesthesia with hyperbaric bupivacaine 0.5 %, 9 mg (1.8 mL).[40] The onset of the block was significantly shorter at the sea level (14.3 minutes) than at moderate altitude (20.4 minutes). Duration of motor block (310 minutes vs. 200 minutes) and sensory block (200 minutes vs. 155 minutes) was prolonged at sea level versus the moderate altitude. The moderate-altitude group had significantly higher mean arterial pressures and a lower heart rate at baseline, during surgery, and the first two postoperative hours than the sea level group. PDPH occurred more frequently (7.14 vs. 2.85%) at moderate altitudes.

*Venturi masks:* Venturi-type gas-mixing devices or high airflow oxygen entrainment masks (HAFOE) are often used to supplement oxygen during regional anesthesia. HAFOE masks tend to deliver higher concentrations of $O_2$ at high altitudes than at sea level. A lower atmospheric pressure reduces the pressure drop across the inlet orifice to reduce room air entrain. At an altitude of 10,000 ft, a venturi mask designed to deliver 35% $O_2$ at sea level gives 41% $O_2$ with less total flow.[34]

## ■ RECENT ADVANCES

A novel method of prehabilitating elderly/sedentary surgical patients by stationing them in a simulated high-altitude environment with reduced oxygen for a week before surgery succeeded in improving hemoglobin levels and treating anemia.[41] Methazolamide, a methylated lipophilic acetazolamide analog, is a new alternative for preventing and treating HAI at lower doses and with fewer fatigue-like side effects. Besides inhibiting carbonic anhydrase, methazolamide directly activates antioxidative nuclear factor-related factor-2 and blocks interleukin-1β release for enhanced effects.[42]

## ■ CONCLUSION

High altitude induces direct detrimental changes in human physiology and activates compensatory mechanisms that cannot be overlooked when administering anesthesia. If recalibrated, anesthetic equipment, including gas analyzers and flowmeters, can be fixed. TIVA and regional anesthesia are the most practical options at high altitudes.

## ■ REFERENCES

1. Burtscher M, Hefti U, Hefti JP. High-altitude illnesses: Old stories and new insights into the pathophysiology, treatment and prevention. Sports Med Health Sci. 2021;3(2):59-69.
2. Constable H. (2022). How tall will Mount Everest get before it stops growing? Available from: https://www.bbc.com/future/article/20220407-how-tall-will-mount-everest-get-before-it-stops-growing. [Last accessed July, 2024].
3. Bhushan C. (2023). Uncontrolled tourism, growth threaten Himalayas. Available from: https://www.deccanherald.com/india/uncontrolled-tourism-growth-threaten-himalayas-2707905. [Last accessed July, 2024].
4. Singh M. (2023). Policy poser after Agniveer's Siachen casualty. Available from: https://www.newindianexpress.com/explainers/2023/Oct/29/policyposer-afteragniveerssiachencasualty-2627926.html. [Last accessed July, 2024].
5. Wani Z, Sharma M. High altitude and anesthesia. J Cardiac Crit Care. 2017;1:30-3.
6. Brown C. High-Altitude Physiology and Anesthesia. In: McIssac J, McQueen K, Kucik C (Eds). Essentials of Disaster Anesthesia, 1st edition. USA: Cambridge University Press; 2020. pp.106-15.
7. Berry JM, Camporesi E. Anesthesia at High Altitude. In: Ehrenwerth J, Eisenkraft JB, Berry JM (Eds). Anesthesia equipment, 3rd edition. Philadelphia PA: WB Saunders; 2021. pp. 468-78.
8. Bryant R. (2017). Altitude adjusted PERC oxygen saturation. Available from: https://rebelem.com/altitude-adjusted-perc-oxygen-saturation/. [Last accessed July, 2024].
9. Hypoxico. (2024). Altitude to oxygen chart. Available from: https://hypoxico.com/pages/altitude-to-oxygen-chart. [Last accessed July, 2024].
10. Mark Dearden. High-Altitude Anesthesia. In: Abd-Elsayed A (Ed). Advanced Anesthesia Review. New York: Oxford University Press; 2023. pp. 39-42.
11. Kim YY, Lee SM. Treatment and prevention of high-altitude illness and mountain sickness. J Korean Med Assoc. 2007;50(11):1005-15.
12. Garrido E, Sibila O, Viscor G. Breathing at extreme altitudes. Scientific projects "EVEREST" (first part). Arch Med Deporte. 2017;34(5):293-7.
13. Forman SA, Ishizawa Y, Gropper MA, Miller RD. Inhaled anesthetic uptake, distribution, metabolism and toxicity. In: Gropper MA, Eriksson LI, Fleisher LA, Wiener-Kronish JP, Cohen NH, Leslie K (Eds). Miller's Anesthesia, 9th edition. Philadelphia, PA: Elsevier; 2020. pp. 509-39.
14. White DP. Sleep medicine. Am J Resp Crit Care Med. 2005;172(11):1363-7.
15. Hou YP, Wu JL, Tan C, Chen Y, Guo R, Luo YJ. Sex-based differences in the prevalence of acute mountain sickness: a meta-analysis. Mil Med Res. 2019;6(1):38-43.
16. Gianfredi V, Albano L, Basnyat B, Ferrara P. Does age have an impact on acute mountain sickness? A systematic review. J Trav Med. 2020;27(6):taz104.
17. Smedley T, Grocott MP. Acute high-altitude illness: a clinically orientated review. Br J Pain. 2013;7(2):85-94.
18. Haddad I, Pearson T, Musa R, Karakattu S, El Minaoui W. Acetazolamide for the treatment of chronic mountain sickness (Monge disease): a systematic review and meta-analysis. Chest. 2020;158(4):A1836.
19. Villafuerte FC, Corante N. Chronic mountain sickness: Clinical aspects, etiology, management, and treatment. High Alt Med Biol. 2016;17(2):61-9.

20. Hackett P, Shlim D. (2024). High Elevation Travel & Altitude Illness. Available from: https://wwwnc.cdc.gov/travel/yellowbook/2024/environmental-hazards-risks/high-elevation-travel-and-altitude-illness. [Last accessed July, 2024].
21. Taber RL. Protocols for the use of a portable hyperbaric chamber for the treatment of high-altitude disorders. J Wilderness Med. 1990;1(3):181-92.
22. Swenson ER. Pharmacology of acute mountain sickness: old drugs and newer thinking. J App Physio. 2016;120(2):204-15.
23. Luks AM, Auerbach PS, Freer L, Grissom CK, Keyes LE, McIntosh SE, et al. Wilderness Medical Society Clinical Practice Guidelines for the prevention and treatment of acute altitude illness: 2019 Update. Wilderness Environ Med. 2019;30(4S):S3-18.
24. Hinninghofen H, Musial F, Kowalski A, Enck P. Gastric emptying effects of dietary fiber during 8 hours at two simulated cabin altitudes. Aviat Space Environ Med. 2006;77(2):121-3.
25. Dickinson JG: Severe acute mountain sickness. Postgrad Med J. 1979;55:454-8.
26. Damodar D, Vakharia R, Vakharia A, Sheu J, Donnally III CJ, Levy JC, et al. A higher altitude is an independent risk factor for venous thromboembolisms following total shoulder arthroplasty. J Orthop. 2018;15(4):1017-21.
27. Al-Sawat A, Fayoumi N, Alosaimi MA, Alhamyani AS, Aljuaid AM, Alnefaie AM. The effect of high altitude on short-term outcomes of post-hemorrhoidectomy. Cureus. 2023;15(1):e33873.
28. Mallet RT, Burtscher J, Richalet JP, Millet GP, Burtscher M. Impact of high altitude on cardiovascular health: Current perspectives. Vasc Health Risk Manag. 2021;17:317-35.
29. Allemann Y, Hutter D, Lipp E, Sartori C, Duplain H, Egli M, et al. Patent foramen ovale and high-altitude pulmonary edema. JAMA. 2006;296(24):2954-8.
30. Alexander JK. Coronary heart disease at altitude. Tex Heart Inst J. 1994;21(4):261-6.
31. Kavanagh BP, Hedenstierna G. Respiratory Physiology and Pathophysiology. In: Gropper MA, Eriksson LI, Fleisher LA, Wiener-Kronish JP, Cohen NH, Leslie K (Eds). Miller's Anesthesia, 9th edition. Philadelphia, PA: Elsevier; 2020. p. 365.
32. Firth PG, Pattinson KTS. Anaesthesia and high altitude: a history. Anaesthesia. 2008;63(6):662-70.
33. James MF, White JF. Anesthetic considerations at moderate altitude. Anesth Analg. 1984;63(12):1097-105.
34. Duncan L. The physics of altitude and anaesthesia. South Afri J Anaesth Analg. 2023;29(5 Suppl 1):S164-6.
35. James MF, Manson ED, Dennett JE. Nitrous oxide analgesia and altitude. Anaesthesia. 1982;37:285-88.
36. Giraldo JC, Acosta C, Giraldo-Grueso M. Frequency of anesthetic overdose with mean alveolar concentration-guided anesthesia at high altitude. Med Gas Res. 2018;8(4):150-3.
37. Puri GD, Jayant A, Tsering M, Dorje M, Tashi M. Closed loop anaesthesia at high altitude (3505 m above sea level): Performance characteristics of an indigenously developed closed loop anaesthesia delivery system. Indian J Anaesth. 2012;56(3):238-42.
38. Xu R, Zhou S, Yang J, Li H, Zhang Q, Zhang G, et al. Total intravenous anesthesia produces outcomes superior to those with combined intravenous–inhalation anesthesia for laparoscopic gynecological surgery at high altitude. J Int Med Res. 2017;45(1):246-53.
39. Bishop RA, Litch JA, Stanton JM. Ketamine anesthesia at high altitude. High Alt Med Bio. 2000;1(2):111-4.
40. Aksoy M, Ince I, Ahıskalıoglu A, Karaca O, Bayar F, Erdem AF. Spinal anaesthesia at low and moderately high altitudes: a comparison of anaesthetic parameters and hemodynamic changes. BMC Anesthesiol. 2015;15:123.
41. McClure P. (2023). High altitude 'prehab' may reduce surgical complications in older patients. Available from: https://newatlas.com/medical/pre-op-altitude-treatment-improves-hemoglobin-in-older-patients/. [Last accessed July, 2024].
42. Lu H, Zhang H, Jiang Y. Methazolamide in high-altitude illnesses. Eur J Pharmaceut Sci. 2020;148:105326.

# CHAPTER 21

# Epidemiology and Management of Burnout among Anesthesiologists

Marycarmen Flores, Ricardo Lopez-Betancourt, Anoushka M Afonso

## ABSTRACT

Recent studies on professional burnout among physicians highlight its alarming prevalence, particularly among frontline physicians, anesthesiologists, and critical care intensivists. Anesthesiologists who transitioned to frontline roles during the recent COVID-19 pandemic experienced heightened burnout risk. This increased risk is strongly associated with workplace factors such as support and culture and increased hours amid staffing shortages. To effectively combat burnout among healthcare providers, it is crucial that organizations implement tailored interventions that specifically address these workplace characteristics and improve overall workplace culture.

**Keywords:** Burnout; Anesthesiologists; Workplace interventions

## KEY POINTS

- Burnout is experienced across various occupations, with US physicians experiencing a higher prevalence, especially frontline physicians.
- Physician burnout negatively affects physicians and patients, including wellness, personal relationships, professional performance, healthcare outcomes, and patient safety.
- Burnout is prevalent and imposes significant risk among anesthesiologist attendings, trainees, and staff across the US and internationally. Burnout has since been worsened across the globe following the COVID-19 pandemic.
- Workplace factors, including lack of support and staffing shortages, strongly correlate with increased burnout.
- Organizations must accordingly implement interventions to improve the workplace culture and environment to alleviate burnout in their healthcare providers.

## ■ INTRODUCTION

Professional burnout has been described as behavioral and physical symptoms that arise due to a person's occupation.[1,2] In 1974, Herbert Freudenberger first used the term to describe the emotional and physical stressors experienced by healthcare providers working in free clinics that cared for patients from marginalized communities.[2] Freudenberger argued that the most dedicated healthcare providers were the most vulnerable to burnout as the disproportionate professional commitment created excessive amounts of pressure to meet the needs of patients and hospital administrators. Consequently, healthcare providers often increase their working hours and devote more energy to the workplace despite the negative cost to their well-being. Freudenberger further discussed that what begins as personal neglect of the healthcare provider ultimately transforms into withdrawal, social isolation, and other adverse behavioral changes that may eventually lead to depersonalization and burnout.[2,3]

In 1981, the Maslach Burnout Inventory (MBI) was developed, which defined burnout as "emotional exhaustion and cynicism".[4] The World Health Organization (WHO) defines burnout syndrome as workplace stress characterized by emotional exhaustion, depersonalization, and reduced sense of personal accomplishment.[5,6] These three components of burnout are effectively assessed as a continuum using the MBI Human Services Survey. This highly validated and widely accepted 22-question survey has become the leading method to evaluate physician burnout.[7-10]

## ■ PHYSICIAN BURNOUT

Individuals in any occupation can experience burnout, yet extensive studies found a significantly higher prevalence among US physicians than other workers.[8,11,12] In 2012, using the MBI, Shanafelt et al. reported that 45.8% of US physicians had at least one symptom of burnout.[8] Additionally, they found significantly poor rates in all three dimensions of burnout, reporting increased emotional exhaustion and depersonalization and decreased sense of personal accomplishment in 37.9%, 29.4%, and 12.4% of US physicians, respectively.[8] Follow-up studies in 2015 and 2019 reported widespread burnout among US physicians.[11,12] Some studies even suggest that the prevalence of burnout among US physicians may now exceed 50%.[13] However, burnout may only affect some medical specialties evenly. Studies show a significant difference in the prevalence of burnout between different medical fields, with frontline physicians having the highest risk of burnout.[8]

Physician burnout has been associated with problematic personal relationships, suicidal ideation, and alcohol abuse, leading to severe personal ramifications and adverse effects on their well-being and quality of life.[14-17] It is reasonable to assume that the negative impact of burnout on physicians' well-being likely contributes to poorer healthcare outcomes. Indeed, recent studies show that burnout is linked to significantly decreased patient safety, clinical quality of care, physician professionalism, and patient satisfaction.[18,19] A study that included >7,900 US surgeons reported the degree of burnout among surgeons was strongly associated with significant medical errors.[18] Additionally, data indicates that each of the three domains of burnout was significantly associated with medical errors.[18]

## ■ BURNOUT AMONG ANESTHESIOLOGISTS

Anesthesiology is a very rewarding field of medicine that allows one to work in diverse medical settings and assume leadership roles. However, with increased workplace responsibilities, anesthesiology can become one of the most stressful specialties in medicine.[20] Many characteristics that make anesthesiology a unique and exciting career, such as leading various medical teams and managing life-threatening situations, are also the source of increased stress in the workplace.

Despite the well-documented significance of burnout among physicians, only recently have extensive studies investigated the prevalence of burnout, specifically among anesthesiologists. As US physicians experience burnout at more excellent rates than other occupations, detailed data has shown that US anesthesiologists are at an even higher risk of burnout (48%) when compared to the average physician.[8] A systematic review including 15 studies found a high prevalence of burnout among anesthesiologists, reporting that up to 59% are at least at moderate risk of burnout.[20] Additionally, a 2021 national survey among 3,898 US. anesthesiologists attending physicians found that 59.2% of respondents were at high risk for burnout.[6] Furthermore, all three dimensions of burnout were elevated among respondents (53.3% emotional exhaustion, 37.2% depersonalization, and 25.9% low sense of personal accomplishment).[6] A granular evaluation of the data in the study demonstrates that workplace characteristics such as lack of support at work were significantly associated with increased burnout.[6]

Most recently, the findings of a 2024 national survey including over 2,600 US attending anesthesiologists were even more troubling, with 67.7% of respondents at high risk for burnout and 18.9% with burnout syndrome.[21] Once again, the data showed that workplace aspects such as lack of support and staffing shortages were leading factors strongly associated with increased burnout. Equally troubling, the study found that more than one-third of US anesthesiologists were likely to leave their current jobs within two years, which could further worsen staffing shortages and burnout rates in anesthesiology.[21]

A recent study about burnout included over 1,300 subspecialty anesthesiologists, including pediatric, cardiac, and acute and chronic pain management. Like previous studies, Hyman et al. reported overall elevated burnout rates among all subspecialties (43.4%), with chronic pain specialists having significantly worse burnout scores (depersonalization, emotional exhaustion) than control groups and the remaining three subspecialties.[22] Conversely, pediatric anesthesiologists had lower scores in depersonalization, emotional exhaustion, and lack of personal accomplishments than control.[22]

Unfortunately, the increased rates of burnout within anesthesiology are not exclusively found among attending anesthesiologists. As early in the career as anesthesiology training, studies have found a high prevalence of burnout, with one study including over 1,500 US anesthesiology trainees reporting that 41% were at high risk of burnout.[23] Another recent study that included >5,200 US anesthesiology trainees reported an even more disturbing burnout rate of 51%.[24] While a recent smaller national survey that included 384 anesthesiology residents reported lower rates of burnout, it still found that a concerning 24% of the respondents were at high risk of burnout.[25] More specifically, it also found that those anesthesiology residents who worked >70 hours per week and more than seven overnight calls per month had significantly increased odds of burnout.[25] Additionally, a recent systematic review that included 12 studies from multiple countries found that the prevalence of burnout among anesthesiology trainees has been reported as high as 67% in a survey conducted in Australia.[26] Yet, this systematic review also exposed an extensive range in the reported rates of burnout (2.7- 67%) across different populations due, at least in part, to the methodological heterogeneity utilized in measuring burnout.[26]

The high prevalence of burnout among anesthesiology trainees and attending physicians has also been reported internationally. An Italian national survey, which included over 850 physicians, found that almost 80% of anesthesiologists and intensive care physicians had moderate burnout.[27] Additionally, a recent study of over 650 anesthesia care providers in Switzerland reported that 59% of physicians were at high risk of burnout.[28] These high rates of burnout were also reported in smaller studies among Greek, French, Irish, Polish, and Dutch anesthesiologists.[29-33] Recent studies of burnout among anesthesiologists in Africa and Asia have also reported significantly high rates of burnout.[34-38]

## CORONAVIRUS DISEASE-2019 EFFECTS ON BURNOUT AMONG ANESTHESIOLOGISTS

The pandemic created a ripple effect worldwide, especially within the healthcare community. Many studies have since emerged, showing the negative impact of the pandemic and the ensuing increased rates of burnout among healthcare professionals. The coronavirus disease-2019 (COVID-19) pandemic placed anesthesiologists on the frontlines, further augmenting pre-pandemic workplace demands and stress. As frontline healthcare workers during this global crisis, anesthesiologists were exposed to larger volumes of critically ill patients and longer and more fluctuating working hours. Furthermore, some measures directed at curtailing the spread of the virus had unintended consequences that negatively affected physicians by limiting access to various support systems and resources.

For instance, a Malaysian study reported that both burnout and depression were associated with worry regarding COVID-19.[39] Additionally, a large study in China that included over 6,300 anesthesiologists who were surveyed after the peak of the COVID-19 pandemic reported that 52.7% of their respondents met the criteria for burnout.[40] A smaller study in Brazil, including over 200 anesthesiology residents during the second wave of the COVID-19 pandemic, reported that a staggering 73.2% were at risk of developing burnout. In contrast, 57.1% were at high risk.[41] A study of 300 critical care anesthesiologists demonstrated an increased sense of burnout from working as an intensivist during COVID-19, with 73% female and 58% male respondents reporting burnout.[42]

A national survey among US anesthesiologists showed concerning results demonstrating that the elevated pre-pandemic rates of high-risk burnout and burnout syndrome had further increased by 14.4% and 37%, respectively. Ultimately, this large study found that more than two out of every three anesthesiologists in the US were at high risk of burnout. Additionally, this study alarmingly found that 77% of US critical care intensivists were at high risk of burnout among the subspecialties.[21] In line with the pre-pandemic findings, this post-pandemic study found that workplace factors such as lack of support and staffing shortages were most strongly associated with burnout rather than personal or demographical characteristics.[6,21] Despite the strong association of lack of workplace support with burnout, another post-pandemic study reported that 75% of respondents felt that the wellness resources available at their institution could have been more helpful.[42]

## INTERVENTIONS FOR BURNOUT

Recent evidence demonstrates the importance of identifying factors that increase the risk of burnout and properly implementing interventions that prevent and alleviate burnout among physicians. While Freudenberger's original explanation for burnout focused on the individual characteristics of healthcare providers, recent studies have pivoted to more significant predictors of burnout—workplace characteristics and culture.

Lack of support and other workplace factors has been reported to be strongly associated with burnout among US anesthesiologists.[6,21] In a recent national study, over half of 2,600 US anesthesiologists reported the need for adequate staffing, improved support from leadership, improved workplace morale/culture, reduced weekly hours, and increased compensation for necessary interventions as measures needed to alleviate the effects of burnout.[21] Consequently, there has been a greater focus on implementing interventions addressing workplace environment changes to mitigate burnout's effects.[43] Fortunately, a systematic review and meta-analysis, including 15 randomized control trials and 37 cohort studies with almost 3,000 physicians, demonstrated that effective interventions can mitigate burnout's effects.[44] This study reported that the overall burnout rate decreased by 10% after implementing personal and organizational interventions.[44]

Furthermore, a small study in Detroit of 44 anesthesiologists developed and analyzed the effect of a physician well-being initiative. This initiative aimed to promote social support in the workplace, a positive view of leadership, physician wellness, flexibility and control of time, and a sense of autonomy. The effects were analyzed using the Well-Being Index (score 0–7), which evaluates professional stress and distress in the medical field.[45] Significantly, the study reported a 0.05 improvement in the sum score for every month spent in the physician well-being initiative.[45] This further demonstrates the importance of longitudinal interventions to improve well-being and mitigate the effects of burnout. A systematic review also found that protected rest time and restricted work hours effectively prevented burnout.[26]

Harry et al. study on Physician Task Load (PTL) and burnout also suggested multiple potential structural and organizational changes that could lessen burnout among physicians—to increase standardization and decrease split attention and redundancy. These workplace modifications may reduce cognitive load and, thus, PTL and burnout. This also supports the importance of protected academic development time and continuing medical education (CME) to improve expertise and decrease cognitive load.[46] Additionally, at least two systematic reviews and meta-analyses have reported that mentorship and peer-to-peer programs may significantly reduce burnout if implemented by organizations.[44,47]

Many potential interventions are suggested in the literature to determine the effects of burnout. A small study reported no improvement in burnout after 4 months of using a meditation application utilized by anesthesia trainees.[48] This suggests the need for continuous interventions based on factors strongly associated with burnout (i.e., changes in the workplace environment). Consequently, the National Academy of Medicine's Action Collaborative on Clinician Well-being and Resilience plays a pivotal role in the strive for change at a higher level as they advocate for systemic and organizational changes.[49]

Through the plethora of data continuing to indicate the significance of workplace characteristics on physician burnout, organizations are now tasked with implementing interventions proven to prevent and reduce burnout through a focus on workplace culture and institutional leadership. Creating a more supportive work environment requires removing barriers to attaining mental and physical health assistance. Consequently, this will require a workplace environment and culture to be effective in reducing the stigmatization of mental healthcare. This may be accomplished with leadership support and feedback to continuously improve strategic interventions based on the current needs of healthcare workers.

The creation of this psychological safety is pivotal to organizational sustainability. As we continue to face the adverse effects of the COVID-19 pandemic with staffing shortages, interventions tasked with decreasing burnout may help alleviate burnout and aid employee retention and recruitment. The current demand for improvement in work culture and environments is a call to action for institutions and policymakers to implement actionable interventions to alleviate burnout among physicians.

## ■ CONCLUSION

Physician burnout has been affected by inadequate support systems and demanding workloads. Although research has identified potential interventions at the organization and individual levels, efficacy has varied. Physician burnout needs to be addressed by a comprehensive approach that involves systemic reform. By optimizing the health and well-being of anesthesiologists, we aim to optimize patient care, ensure high-quality healthcare, and preserve the health of our workforce.

## ■ REFERENCES

1. Maslach C, Leiter MP. How to Measure Burnout Accurately and Ethically. Harvard Business Review Digital Articles; 2021. pp. 1-8.
2. Freudenberger HJ. Staff Burn-Out. J Soc issues. 1974;30(1):159-65.
3. Freudenberger HJ. The staff burn-out syndrome in alternative institutions. Psychotherapy (Chicago, Ill.). 1975;12(1):73-82.
4. Maslach C, Jackson SE. The measurement of experienced burnout. J Organ Behav. 1981;2(2):99-113.
5. World Health Organization. Burn-out an "occupational phenomenon": International Classification of Diseases. 2019.
6. Afonso AM, Cadwell JB, Staffa SJ, Zurakowski D, Vinson AE. Burnout rate and risk factors among anesthesiologists in the United States. Anesthesiology (Philadelphia), 2021134(5):683-96.
7. Maslach C, Jackson SE, Leiter MP. Maslach Burnout Inventory. 3rd edition. In: Zalaquett CP, Wood RJ (Eds). Evaluating Stress: A Book of Resources. Scarecrow Education: Lanham, MD; 1997. pp. 191-218.
8. Shanafelt TD, Boone S, Tan L, Dyrbye LN, Sotile W, Satele D, et al. Burnout and satisfaction with work-life balance among US physicians relative to the general US Population. Arch Intern Med. 2012;172(18):1377-85.
9. Rotenstein LS, Torre M, Ramos MA, Rosales RC, Guille C, Sen S, et al. Prevalence of burnout among physicians: a systematic review. JAMA. 2018;320(11):1131-50.
10. Hyman SA, Shotwell MS, Michaels DR, Han X, Card EB, Morse JL, et al. A survey evaluating burnout, health status, depression, reported alcohol and substance use, and social support of anesthesiologists. Anesth Analg. 2017;125(6):2009-18.
11. Shanafelt TD, Hasan O, Dyrbye LN, Sinsky C, Satele D, Sloan J, et al. Changes in burnout and satisfaction with work-life balance in physicians and the general US working population between 2011 and 2014. Mayo Clin Proc. 2015;90(12):1600-13.
12. Shanafelt TD, West CP, Sinsky C, Trockel M, Tutty M, Satele DV, et al. Changes in burnout and satisfaction with work-life integration in physicians and the general US working population between 2011 and 2017. Mayo Clin Proc. 2019;94(9):1681-1694.
13. Rothenberger DA. Physician burnout and well-being: a systematic review and framework for action. Diseases of the colon & rectum, 2017;60(6):567-76.
14. Lacy BE, Chan JL. Physician burnout: the hidden health care Crisis. Clin Gastroenterol Hepatol. 2018;16(3):311-7.
15. Warde CM, Moonesinghe K, Allen W, Gelberg L. Marital and parental satisfaction of married physicians with children. J Gen Intern Med. 1999;14(3):157-65.

16. Shanafelt TD, Balch CM, Dyrbye L, Bechamps G, Russell T, Satele D, et al. Special report: suicidal ideation among American surgeons. Arch Surg. 2011;146(1):54-62.
17. Oreskovich MR, Kaups KL, Balch CM, Hanks JB, Satele D, Sloan J, et al. Prevalence of alcohol use disorders among american surgeons. A Arch Surg. 2012;147(2):168-74.
18. Shanafelt TD, Balch CM, Bechamps G, Russell T, Dyrbye L, Satele D, et al. Burnout and medical errors among American surgeons. Ann Surg. 2010;251(6):995-1000
19. Salyers MP, Bonfils KA, Luther L, Firmin RL, White DA, Adams EL, et al. The relationship between professional burnout and quality and safety in healthcare: A Meta-Analysis. Gen Intern Med. 2017;32(4):475-482.
20. Sanfilippo F, Noto A, Foresta G, Santonocito C, Palumbo GJ, Arcadipane A, et al. Incidence and factors associated with burnout in anesthesiology: a systematic review. Biomed Res Int. 2017;2017:8648925.
21. Afonso AM, Cadwell JB, Staffa SJ, Sinskey JL, Vinson AE. U.S. Attending anesthesiologist burnout in the postpandemic Era. Anesthesiology. 2024;140(1):38-51.
22. Hyman SA, Card EB, De Leon-Casasola O, Shotwell MS, Shi Y, Weinger MB. Prevalence of burnout and its relationship to health status and social support in more than 1000 subspecialty anesthesiologists. Reg Anesth Pain Med. 2021;46(5):381-387.
23. de Oliveira GS Jr, Chang R, Fitzgerald PC, Almeida MD, Castro-Alves LS, Ahmad S, et al. The prevalence of burnout and depression and their association with adherence to safety and practice standards: a survey of United States anesthesiology trainees. Anesth Analg. 2013;117(1):182-93.
24. Sun H, Warner DO, Macario A, Zhou Y, Culley DJ, Keegan MT. Repeated cross-sectional surveys of burnout, distress, and depression among anesthesiology residents and first-year graduates. Anesthesiology. 2019;131(3):668-77.
25. Bui D, Winegarner A, Kendall MC, Almeida M, Apruzzese P, De Oliveira G. Burnout and depression among anesthesiology trainees in the United States: An updated National Survey. J Clin Anesth. 2023;84:110990.
26. Chong MYF, Lin SHX, Lim WY, Ong J, Kam PCA, Ong SGK. Burnout in anaesthesiology residents: a systematic review of its prevalence and stressors. Eur J Anaesthesiol. 2022;39(4):368-77.
27. Vargas M, Spinelli G, Buonanno P, Iacovazzo C, Servillo G, De Simone S. Burnout Among Anesthesiologists and Intensive Care Physicians: Results From an Italian National Survey. Inquiry. 2020;57:46958020919263.
28. Gasciauskaite G, Lunkiewicz J, Braun J, Kolbe M, Seelandt J, Spahn DR, et al. Burnout and its determinants among anaesthesia care providers in Switzerland: a multicentre cross-sectional study. Anaesthesia. 2024;79(2):168-77.
29. van der Wal RA, Bucx MJ, Hendriks JC, Scheffer GJ, Prins JB. Psychological distress, burnout and personality traits in Dutch anaesthesiologists: a survey. Eur J Anaesthesiol. 2016;33(3):179-86.
30. Mion G, Libert N, Journois D. Burnout-associated factors in anesthesia and intensive care medicine. 2009 survey of the French Society of anesthesiology and intensive care. Ann Fr Anesth Reanim. 2013;32(3):175-88.
31. Walsh AM, McCarthy D, Ghori K. Anesthesiology resident burnout-an Irish perspective. Anesth Analg. 2014;118(2):482-83.
32. Ntalouka MP, Karakosta A, Aretha D, Papaioannou A, Nyktari V, Chloropoulou P, et al. GReek Anaesthesiologists's Burnout EPidemic within the COVID-19 pandemic (GRABEP study) a multicenter study on burn out prevalence among Greek anesthesiologists and association with personality traits. Psychiatriki. 20232;34(3):193-203.
33. Podhorodecka K, Radkowski P, Boniecka P, Wojtkiewicz J. Psychological Distress after the COVID-19 Pandemic among Anesthesiologists in Poland-An Observational Study. Int J Environ Res Public Health. 2022;19(15):9328.

34. Li H, Zuo M, Gelb AW, Zhang B, Zhao X, Yao D, et al. Chinese anesthesiologists have high burnout and low job satisfaction: a cross-sectional Survey. Anesth Analg. 2018;126(3):1004-12.
35. Shams T, El-Masry R. Job Stress and Burnout among Academic Career Anaesthesiologists at an Egyptian University Hospital. Sultan Qaboos Univ Med J. 2013;13(2):287-95.
36. Kasemy ZA, Sharif AF, Bahgat NM, Abdelsattar S, Abdel Latif AA. Emotional intelligence, workplace conflict and job burn-out among critical care physicians: a mediation analysis with a cross-sectional study design in Egypt. BMJ Open. 2023;13(10):e074645.
37. Lwiza AF, Lugazia ER. Burnout and associated factors among healthcare workers in acute care settings at a tertiary teaching hospital in Tanzania: An analytical cross-sectional study. Health Sci Rep. 2023;6(5):e1256.
38. Nazeema A, Lowton K, Tenea Z, Anic A, Jayrajh P. Study of burnout and depressive symptoms in doctors at a central level, state hospital. S Afr J Psychiatr. 2023;29:1866.
39. Tsan SEH, Kamalanathan A, Lee CK, Zakaria SA, Wang CY. A survey on burnout and depression risk among anaesthetists during COVID-19: the tip of an iceberg? Anaesthesia. 2021;76 Suppl 3(Suppl 3):8-10.
40. Che L, Ma S, Zhang YL, Huang Y. Burnout among Chinese anesthesiologists after the COVID-19 pandemic peak: a national survey. Anesth Analg. 2023;137(2):392-8.
41. Pietroski Dos Santos N, Biseo Henriques LE, Pivovar De Camargo Rosa R, Midory Marques Monteiro R, Vicente Sanches Gonçalves R, Canga JC, Callegari DC, et al. Burnout risk among anesthesiology residents in Brazil during the second wave of COVID-19: a cross-sectional survey. Braz J Anesthesiol. 2023;73(1):120-22.
42. Siddiqui S, Tung A, Kelly L, Nurok M, Khanna AK, Ben-Jacob T, et al. Anxiety, worry, and job satisfaction: effects of COVID-19 care on critical care anesthesiologists. Can J Anaesth. 2022 Apr;69(4):552-4.
43. Khan A, Vinson AE. Physician well-being in practice. Anesth Analg. 2020;131(5):1359-69.
44. West CP, Dyrbye LN, Erwin PJ, Shanafelt TD. Interventions to prevent and reduce physician burnout: a systematic review and meta-analysis. Lancet. 2016;388(10057):2272-81.
45. Zador L, Nowak K, Sitarik A, MacLean L, Han X, Kalsi M, et al. The burnout epidemic within a viral pandemic: impact of a wellness initiative. Perioper Care Oper Room Manag. 2022;27:100251.
46. Harry E, Sinsky C, Dyrbye LN, Makowski MS, Trockel M, Tutty M, et al. Physician task load and the risk of burnout among US physicians in a national survey. Jt Comm J Qual Patient Saf. 2021;47(2):76-85.
47. Panagioti M, Panagopoulou E, Bower P, Lewith G, Kontopantelis E, Chew-Graham C, et al. Controlled interventions to reduce burnout in physicians: a systematic review and meta-analysis. JAMA Intern Med. 2017;177(2):195-205.
48. Carullo PC, Ungerman EA, Metro DG, Adams PS. The impact of a smartphone meditation application on anesthesia trainee well-being. J Clin Anesth. 2021;75:110525.
49. Abda R, Pietrzyk G, Scott PW, Fennimore L. Taking action against clinician burnout through reducing the documentation burden with an operating room supply scanning approach. Comput Inform Nurs. 2024;42(1):14-20.

# CHAPTER 22

# Mentoring Anesthesiologists

*Mukul Chandra Kapoor*

## ABSTRACT

Excellence in the medical profession cannot be achieved with just knowledge. Multiple nuances and skills can only be acquired through good guidance and handholding. Mentoring plays a crucial role in the development and success of healthcare professionals. Mentorship is essential for training and career advancement in academic medicine today. Anesthesiology is a specialized field that requires a high level of skill, knowledge, and expertise. Mentoring junior doctors is vital for transitioning from medical school to clinical practice. Mentoring works beyond the curriculum content and conveys nonclinical aspects of training such as professionalism, networking, values, clinical judgment, and other soft skills that need to be taught in a structured curriculum format. Effective mentoring can help them navigate the complexities of the specialty, develop clinical competencies, and excel in their careers.

**Keywords:** Mentoring; Anesthesiologists; Mentor; Mentee; Training

## KEY POINTS

- Mentoring plays a crucial role in the development and success of healthcare professionals.
- Mentoring junior anesthesiologists is vital for transitioning from medical school to clinical practice.
- A mentor must be a teacher, elder, sponsor, advisor, agent, role model, coach, and confidante of the mentee.
- Mentoring in anesthesiology can provide benefits such as job satisfaction, clinical skill development, professional growth, career guidance, well-being and resilience, enhanced research, networking, faculty retention, inspiration to excel, and improved patient care.
- Mentoring is needed at different times of an individual's career, especially during career growth.
- Mentorship programs must be monitored to ensure that their objectives are achieved.
- Communication with all participants must be constantly maintained, and feedback must be solicited.

## ■ INTRODUCTION

The medical profession is an amalgam of science and art. Excellence in the profession cannot be achieved with just knowledge. Multiple nuances and skills can only be acquired through good guidance and handholding. Mentoring plays a crucial role in the development and success of healthcare professionals. Mentorship is essential for training and career advancement in academic medicine today.[1] There is a significant variation in the prevalence of mentorship in the medical field, and it has been reported to vary from 19 to 93%, depending on the medical discipline.[2] The General Medical Council of the United Kingdom recommends regular mentoring of doctors, particularly during changes in their career roles.[3]

The Standing Committee on Postgraduate Medical and Dental Education of the United Kingdom recommended mentoring as part of the residents 'stress support system. However, a survey in the United Kingdom found that only 20% of anesthesia trainees knew who their mentor was; of them, only 38% had met with their mentor.[4] Anesthesiology is a specialized field that requires a high level of skill, knowledge, and expertise. Mentoring junior doctors is vital for transitioning from medical school to clinical practice. Mentoring young anesthesiologists is essential for their professional growth and development. Effective mentoring can help them navigate the complexities of the specialty, develop clinical competencies, and excel in their careers. Mentorship benefits include better education, better pay, faster climbing the ladder, and more career satisfaction.[5]

**What is mentorship?**
The Oxford Dictionary defines a mentor as "an experienced person who advises and helps somebody with less experience over time" and a mentee as "a person who is advised, trained, or counseled by a mentor". The concept of mentorship has been practiced through the ages, and we find its mention in ancient literature worldwide. Ancient Indian literature used the term "guru-shishya" while Western literature referred to it as "chaperoning", "fostering", and "godfathering". A classic example of mentorship followed in the early 20th century was sending girls to "finishing schools" or assigning them a companion to instruct them on household management, social skills, and social grace. Mentorship is a mutually beneficial relationship between a mentor and a mentee.

## ▪ ATTRIBUTES OF A MENTOR

A mentor must be a teacher, elder, sponsor, advisor, agent, role model, coach, and confidante of the mentee. Essential attributes of a mentor include seniority, compassion, amiability, motivation, accessibility, patience, and honesty.[6,7] The qualities of a good mentor[8] have been defined as follows:
- Relevant expertise, skill, and knowledge
- Enthusiasm for sharing expertise
- Respectful attitude
- Eagerness to invest in the development of others
- Ability to give honest and direct feedback
- Reflective listening and empathy
- Willingness to be a sponsor

## ▪ NEED FOR MENTORSHIP

Postgraduate medical education is a period of intense learning and growth during which doctors transition from students to independent practitioners. Over the last few decades, postgraduate teaching programs have moved from an intimate guide-student relationship to a more scientific knowledge-sharing and knowledge-acquiring program. In India, the number of doctoral students assigned to a senior guide also increased, reducing the time that could be allocated to mentor them. A disconnect between the postgraduate guide and the student became quite evident. There is an inescapable requirement to foster these students, as effective mentoring during this phase can significantly impact the future careers of these doctors. Increased use of mentorship is critical to developing the next generation of leaders in medicine.[9] Following a mentorship culture is essential for a center's success and should be treated as a strategic priority.[9]

The education process and the evaluation of knowledge and competence in Anesthesiology and its subspecialties are constantly changing. The emergence of training and the conduct of assessments on cadavers, computers, or simulators has changed in anesthesiology. Technology, medications, and procedures, once considered not very important, have evolved. Ultrasound, fluoroscopy-guided pain procedures, and transesophageal echocardiography have significantly changed how we practice anesthesia. Elaborate ultrasound-guided regional anesthesia techniques in all patient populations, transesophageal real-time views of the heart in cardiovascular surgery, and the development of electronic medical records and computer technology have dramatically changed our practices.

## ■ BENEFITS OF MENTORSHIP

Mentorship benefits the mentor, mentee, organization, specialty, patients, and the nation. The mentee benefits from job satisfaction, improved personalized academic training, career advancement, and enhanced research opportunities and publications. The mentor benefits through personal fulfillment, development, leadership and coaching skills, and career advancements.[10] The institution benefits from improved work performance and output, professional development of employees, and accelerated training. The specialty benefits from improved standards of care and research. The patients benefit by receiving compassionate care from dedicated, competent, and righteous professionals—the nation benefits by achieving high healthcare standards. Mentorship extends the faculty's legacies and ensures the next-generation physicians' professional longevity.[9]

### Benefits of Mentoring in Anesthesia Programs

Some benefits of mentoring in anesthesia post-graduate programs are as follows:
- *Clinical skill development:* Anesthesia residents require guidance and support to develop proficiency in administering anesthesia, managing perioperative care, and handling critical situations. An accomplished mentor can guide the mentee to follow the proper steps and teach them to be meticulous. Mentoring helps residents acquire the necessary skills and knowledge to deliver safe and effective patient anesthesia care.
- *Professional growth:* Mentors play a crucial role in shaping the professional identity of anesthesia residents, instilling values of professionalism, ethics, and patient-centered care. Professional identity plays a significant role in clinicians' social and professional standing. Mentoring provides residents with guidance on career pathways, opportunities for specialization, and networking connections

within anesthesiology. Mentoring facilitates professional growth by offering insights, advice, and opportunities for development.

- *Career guidance:* Mentors provide valuable insights into anesthesiology career pathways, subspecialization opportunities, and career advancement strategies. They educate residents about the benefits and pitfalls of different career options and can help them choose the path best suited for them. Mentors play a crucial role in shaping the professional identity of residents, instilling values of compassion, integrity, and excellence in practice.
- *Well-being and resilience:* The demanding nature of anesthesia practice can affect residents' physical, social, and mental well-being. Mentors offer emotional support and stress management strategies and promote work-life balance. They make the mentees work hard to learn and look after their personal and social interests. Mentors support residents in building resilience to cope with the demands of anesthesia practice.
- *Research and scholarly activity:* Mentoring can foster residents' interest in research, quality improvement projects, and scholarly activities, enhancing their academic profile. Mentors are the best guides for teaching the methodology of a research project and writing projects to seek grants.[11]
- *Networking:* Professional networking is vital in research and attaining social standing. Mentoring often leads to interactions within the medical community, opening doors to research collaborations, job opportunities, and professional growth.[12]
- *Faculty retention:* Academic faculty retention increases with the implementation of faculty mentorship programs. One study showed that the quality of mentoring influences the probability of continuing an academic career.[13]
- *Inspire to excel:* A mentor with exceptional achievements is a source of inspiration for the mentee. He always remains an icon for the mentee, and mentees tend to follow the mentor's path to success.
- *Improved patient care:* Mentored doctors are better equipped to provide high-quality patient care, as the mentoring program aims to guide and support them in enhancing their professional development and facilitating a successful transition to independent practice.

## Strategies for Effective Mentoring in Anesthesia Programs

- *Clear goals:* Clear learning objectives and goals for the mentoring relationship must be defined to ensure the mentor and mentee are aligned on expectations.
- *Individualized learning plans:* Every mentee is different, including their competence and interests. Mentoring experiences must be tailored to each anesthesia resident's needs and goals. Individualized learning plans tailored for a mentee need to be developed to address areas of strength and areas for improvement.
- *Clinical preceptorship:* A mentor will have expertise in specific clinical skills—the mentee gains from observing and learning the skill from the mentor. Mentoring helps anesthesiologists develop the clinical skills, knowledge, and competencies required for their specialty. Apart from clinical skills, they also need to develop communication and leadership skills for their professional growth. Mentorship provides hands-on clinical preceptorship where residents work closely with

experienced anesthesiologists to gain practical skills and exposure to diverse clinical challenges.
- *Case-based learning:* In anesthesia practice, case-based discussions enhance residents' clinical reasoning, decision-making, and critical thinking abilities. Mentors should make mentees present cases that are challenging to manage so that they develop critical and analytical patient management skills. Mentees must maintain a journal of their activities.
- *Creating a supportive environment:* Creating an environment that is supportive and inclusive, where juniors feel comfortable seeking guidance and asking questions. A culture of collaboration with the team must be encouraged to enhance their professional development.
- *Emotional support:* Medical training can be challenging and stressful. There have been multiple cases of resident doctors developing mental diseases and even committing suicide. Mentors offer emotional support and encouragement to help doctors navigate through difficult times.
- *Lead by example:* Mentors must demonstrate professionalism, integrity, and dedication to inspire their junior colleagues. Mentors must serve as role models, demonstrating professionalism, ethical behavior, and excellence in patient care. They should perform like icons whom the mentee emulates.
- *Personal touch:* The mentor and the mentee must connect personally. The mentor must see the mentee's qualities and flaws appropriate to their training level. A mentor needs to be emotionally engaged in the mentee's success. The mentor-mentee association is of two individuals who share a common goal, which can ultimately lead to success. The relationship must extend to the personal and family levels and include social interaction.
- *Simulation training:* Teaching management of challenging situations takes a lot of work. The advent of high-fidelity simulators has been a boon to practical teaching. Simulation training sessions must be incorporated to allow residents to practice anesthesia techniques, crisis management, and teamwork skills in a controlled environment. The mentor must guide the mentee during simulation sessions to teach the best practices.
- *Encourage continuous learning:* Mentees must be encouraged to pursue continuous learning opportunities, such as workshops, conferences, and further education. They must be coached to deliver talks/presentations. Along with the mentors, they must be actively involved in writing review articles, journal articles, and tutorials, and their contributions must be acknowledged.
- *Reflection:* Reflection is a powerful tool for learning and growth. Mentors must be encouraged to reflect on their experiences, challenges, and successes. There should also be mutual respect and clear expectations from both parties.
- *Evaluation and monitoring:* The mentoring program should be evaluated periodically to assess effectiveness and identify areas for improvement. The mentees' progress must be monitored, and feedback must be provided to ensure that mentoring relationships are beneficial and supportive.
- *Feedback:* A culture of feedback must be followed in which mentors provide timely, constructive, and honest feedback on mentees' performance. Mentors must encourage mentees to reflect on their experiences and identify areas for growth.

## ■ MENTORING NEEDS CHANGE WITH TIME

Mentoring needs differ at different phases of life and career. A mentee's developmental needs and processes vary according to an individual's life-career season. Most successful mentees need more than one mentor. They scan the horizon for leaders who embody their values or value their strengths throughout their careers. Mentorship during postgraduate training has different objectives from that during subspecialization.

Similarly, mentorship during the budding phase of a job should focus on career building. Once competent in their chosen field, mentees need guidance to take higher responsibility, status, and rewards. Midcareer mentorship trains someone to step up the ladder and become a leader. During your career's growth phase, you need someone guiding you and keeping you on the right course.[14]

## ■ THE MENTORSHIP JOURNEY

Identifying a mentor and working under their tutelage is just the beginning. The relationship must be consistently nurtured and periodically refreshed. Successful protégés understand that sustaining sponsorship looks a lot like earning it. They also find ways to support a mentor's passion or help build their legacy outside the organization. A mentor must be personally connected and emotionally engaged in the mentee's success. The best mentorships are more like the relationship between a parent and a child than between a boss and an employee. Mutual respect, trust, shared values, and good communication characterize them. A mentor gains stature and eminence if they successfully mentor someone. A person successfully mentored makes a good mentor later in life. Mentors derive personal satisfaction from knowing they are contributing to the growth and success of a fellow professional. The mentoring relationship echoes the relationship between a lawyer and a client and involves positive regard, setting boundaries, active listening, and ethical behavior.

### Remote Mentoring

With technological advancements, distance, and remote mentoring have become increasingly prevalent in healthcare settings. The advent of distance and remote mentoring has expanded and opened new avenues for learning and collaboration in healthcare settings. Distance mentoring sessions can be facilitated with telemedicine and virtual communication tools such as video conferencing, messaging applications, etc. Regular communication can be established by scheduling regular virtual meetings to maintain communication and provide ongoing support and guidance. Active participation and engagement are needed to maximize the benefits of distance mentoring. Remote mentoring helps share educational resources, best practices, and teaching tools to support their professional development. Mentees can engage in virtual workshops and online learning activities to gain expert knowledge and expertise from pioneers and established practitioners. However, a survey found that almost 80% of mentees undertaking long-distance mentoring felt it was less effective than onsite mentoring.[15]

### Speed Mentoring

In some cultures, speed dating has been successful in traditional matchmaking. The same method has also been tried to facilitate matching mentors and mentees. A mentee spends about 10 minutes talking with each rotation mentor during speed mentoring. In a study, mentees felt that the event helped them expand their network and identify needed resources. Both mentees and mentors thought that this short interaction benefitted them.[16] Speed mentoring ensures that the expertise of a mentor benefits multiple mentees, and if the mentees need further help, they can interact again. Speed mentoring is a low-resource intervention requiring minimal time commitment for mentees and mentors. It has been successfully used to mentor women anesthesiology trainees.[17]

## Reverse Mentorship

The current generation is very comfortable with information technology and is skilled at managing the hospital's electronic medical records. This enables cross-generational mentorship to introduce the concept of "reverse mentorship". Reverse mentorship may also help overcome gender-specific and ethnic barriers. Female physicians-in-training could mentor their faculty members in modern challenges specific to females. Reverse mentorship was particularly relevant to postgraduate medical education during the coronavirus disease 2019 (COVID-19) pandemic.[18] Junior anesthesiologists can also provide new perspectives on clinician management. They can help change the workplace culture and promote learning.[19]

## ■ PHASES OF A MENTORING PROGRAM

- *Matching phase:* Potential mentees search for experienced, successful people they perceive as good role models. The program's proposed volunteer mentors/mentees are initially matched. Based on common goals/objectives, specialty interests, career goals, and personality compatibility, mentors are paired with mentees.
- *Initiation phase:* An introductory meeting is conducted to understand and establish goals, expectations, and communication preferences.
- *Cultivation phase:* This is the primary stage of learning and development. Periodic meetings between mentors and mentees are scheduled to discuss progress, challenges, and growth opportunities. The mentor shares lessons from the mentor's experience and expertise, new technologies, new methodologies, and emerging issues in the field with the mentee. Psychosocial mentoring begins after the mentor and mentee have established an interpersonal bond.
- *Feedback phase:* A feedback mechanism for mentors and mentees is established to provide input on the effectiveness of the mentoring relationship.
- *Separation phase:* The mentoring relationship may continue unless something is left to learn, or the mentee wants to establish an independent identity. It generally describes the end of a mentoring relationship.
- *Redefinition stage:* After the mentoring relationship is completed, both mentor and mentee recognize that their relationship can continue as a collegial or social friendship, no longer focusing on the mentee's career development.[20]

The suggested schedule for a 20-week mentoring program for anesthesiologists is discussed in **Table 1**.

## ■ SELECTION PROCESS FOR MENTORSHIP PROGRAM

- Publicize the mentor program through newsletters of professional and academic bodies, meeting announcements, letters to members of the associations, and personal contacts.

**TABLE 1:** Suggested schedule for mentoring in a 20-week anesthesia program.

| Week | |
|---|---|
| Week 1–2 | *Orientation:*<br>• Introduce mentees to the program<br>• Discuss expectations, goals, and objectives<br>• Preinduction assessment to identify areas for development |
| Week 3–6 | *Clinical preceptorship:*<br>• Pair mentees with mentors for hands-on clinical experience<br>• Rotate through different subspecialties to gain diverse clinical exposure<br>• Debrief after clinical sessions to discuss cases, challenges, and learning points |
| Week 7–10 | *Case-based learning:*<br>• Facilitate case-based discussions on complex anesthesia scenarios<br>• Analyze case studies to enhance clinical reasoning and decision-making skills<br>• Encourage mentees to present cases and participate in group discussions |
| Week 11–14 | *Simulation training:*<br>• Organize simulation sessions to practice anesthesia techniques and crisis management<br>• Conduct debriefing sessions to review performance, provide feedback, and identify areas for improvement<br>• Emphasize teamwork, communication skills, and leadership in simulated sessions |
| Week 15–18 | *Research and scholarly activities:*<br>• Support mentees in identifying research projects or quality improvement initiatives<br>• Provide guidance on literature review, study design, data analysis, and manuscript preparation<br>• Encourage mentees to present their work at conferences or publish in peer-reviewed journals |
| Week 19–20 | *Reflection and goal setting:*<br>• Reflect on the mentoring experience and discuss achievements, challenges, and lessons learned<br>• Set goals for future professional development and career advancement<br>• Evaluate the effectiveness of the mentoring program and provide feedback for improvement |

- Potential mentors must submit an enrollment form to indicate their interest in being a mentor.
- Senior practitioners who have trained students for other activities, such as fellowships or internships, must be approached and offered the opportunity to become mentors.
- Potential mentees must be provided with application forms.
- A system must be designed to match mentors and mentees based on professional interests and potential pairs identified.
- Interviews and meetings are held to clarify participants' areas of interest and commitment levels.

- Provide mentors and mentees with a brief biography of their potential mentor or mentee.
- If the participants accept joining the program and provisionally accept being mentors and mentees, a meeting of the two must be fixed.
- The mentorship program details must be scheduled after the final acceptance in the physical or a virtual platform-based face-to-face meeting between the mentor and the mentee.

## ■ MONITORING OF THE PROGRAM

The mentorship program must be monitored to ensure that its objectives are achieved. Communication with all participants must be constantly maintained, and feedback must be solicited on its efficacy. A written summary of the mentorship experience from all participants must be taken. Group meetings or socials must be regularly conducted to evaluate the program and to suggest ways to improve it. All participants must complete a program evaluation form at the end of the program. The proceedings of these meetings and the participants' feedback will help suggest improving the mentor program for future mentors and mentees. The standard parameters to evaluate mentees attending the mentoring program are discussed in **Box 1**, and the parameters for assessing mentors are discussed in **Box 2**.

## ■ BARRIERS TO SUCCESSFUL MENTORING

Mentoring learning experiences usually occur outside the mentors' and mentees' working hours. Time constraints in busy clinical practice are a significant barrier

**BOX 1:** Evaluation of the mentee—standard parameters to evaluate a mentee.[21]

- Publishing in peer-reviewed journals
- Receiving research-related internal/external awards or honors
- Preparing and securing extramural research grants
- Participating as a facilitator in a seminar series
- Achieving a position on an appropriate journal editorial board
- Participating in grant writing development workshops
- Leading session of national meetings
- Receiving an invitation to speak at an institution or conference

**BOX 2:** Assessment of the mentor by the mentee—standard parameters to evaluate a mentor.[21]

- Was your mentor available to you when needed?
- Did your mentor respond to you in a timely fashion?
- Did your mentor address your concerns?
- Was your mentor flexible?
- Was your mentor generous?
- Was your mentor respectful?
- Was your mentor well organized?
- Was your mentor well prepared?
- Did your mentor realistically devise the mentoring experience?
- Did your mentor advise appropriate reading material?
- Did your mentor advise you to meet relevant professionals?
- Did your mentor advise you to attend relevant workshops?
- Do you have a positive learning experience?

to successful mentoring. Many medical mentorship schemes fail, lack visibility, or cannot be maintained.[22] Mentorship schemes are resource-intensive and require substantial investment, which makes them difficult to sustain.[23]

## ■ MENTORSHIP MALPRACTICE

Mentorship malpractice can be active or passive. Some examples of active mentorship malpractice are the mentor hijacking a mentee's idea, project, or grant for self-gain, the mentor acting like an exploiter who destroys a mentee's success by burdening them with low-yield activities, and the mentor dominating the mentee across various areas of collaboration. Some examples of passive mentorship malpractice are: The mentor is preoccupied with his priorities and does not have the time or the desire to attend to mentees, the mentor evades conflict and avoids difficult but necessary conversations, the mentor spends little time or effort on mentoring and instead exploits the mentee for self-promotion, and the mentor discourages mentees from seeking other mentors as it stokes the mentor's ego.[24]

## ■ CONCLUSION

Mentorship is the partnership between a mentor, who acts as a guide, and a mentee, who acts as a learner. It works beyond the curriculum content and conveys nonclinical aspects of training such as professionalism, networking, values, clinical judgment, and other soft skills that need to be taught in a structured curriculum format. Mentoring is essential for personal and professional trainee growth. Mentoring enhances individual practice, well-being, and professional development of mentees and mentors and benefits patients' care. It is precious during change and when taking on new roles, such as for newly appointed consultants. It enhances job satisfaction, well-being, working relationships with patients and colleagues, confidence, problem-solving abilities, collegiality, organizational commitment, and job performance.

## ■ REFERENCES

1. Flexman AM, Gelb AW. Mentorship in anesthesia. Curr Opin Anaesthesiol. 2011;24(6):676-81.
2. Sambunjak D, Straus SE, Marusic A. Mentoring in academic medicine: a systematic review. JAMA. 2006;296(9):1103-15.
3. McCrossan R, Swan L, Redfern N. Mentoring for doctors in the UK: what it can do for you, your colleagues, and your patients. BJA Educ. 2020;20(12):404-10.
4. Gould G. Mentor system for anaesthesia trainees. Anaesthesia. 2004;59(4):411.
5. Roch GR. Much ado about mentors. Harv Bus Rev. 1979;57(1):14-20.
6. Tobin MJ. Mentoring: seven roles and some specifics. Am J Respir Crit Care Med. 2004;170(2):114-7.
7. Straus SE, Chatur F, Taylor M. Issues in the mentor-mentee relationship in academic medicine: a qualitative study. Acad Med. 2009;84(1):135-9.
8. Maguire A. (2020). 7 Qualities That Make a Good Mentor (and How to Find Someone Who Has Them All). Available from: https://www.themuse.com/advice/how-to-find-qualities-good-mentor [Last accessed, July 2024].
9. Choi AMK, Moon JE, Steinecke A, Prescott JE. Developing a Culture of Mentorship to Strengthen Academic Medical Centers. Acad Med. 2019;94(5):630-3.
10. Bin Ghali KN, Al Subaie AT, Nawab AA. Mentorship in anesthesia: a perspective survey among anesthesia residents in Riyadh, Saudi Arabia. Saudi J Anaesth 2021;15(2):144-8.

11. Orandi BJ, Blackburn S, Henke PK. Surgical mentors' and mentees' productivity from 1993 to 2006. Am J Surg. 2011;201(2):260-5.
12. Keyser DJ, Lakoski JM, Lara-Cinisomo S, Schultz DJ, Williams VL, Zellers DF, et al. Advancing institutional efforts to support research mentorship: a conceptual framework and self-assessment tool. Acad Med. 2008;83(3):217-25.
13. Weinert CR, Billings J, Ryan R, Ingbar DH. Academic and career development of pulmonary and critical care physician-scientists. Am J Respir Crit Care Med. 2006;173(1):23-31.
14. ADEDIRAN, Bewley LW, Shewchuk RM. (2016). Mentorship mediated by life-career seasons: an analysis of a multi-dimensional model of mentoring among career groups of United States army officers. Available at https://journalofbusiness.org/index.php/GJMBR/article/view/2009/4-Mentorship-Mediated-by-Life-Career_html [Last accessed, July 2024].
15. Luckhaupt SE, Chin MH, Mangione CM, Phillips RS, Bell D, Leonard AC, et al. Mentorship in academic general internal medicine. Results of a survey of mentors. J Gen Intern Med. 2005;20(11):1014-8.
16. Cook DA, Bahn RS, Menaker R. Speed mentoring: an innovative method to facilitate mentoring relationships. Med Teach. 2010;32(8):692-4.
17. Pollard EM, Sharpe EE, Gali B, Moeschler SM. Closing the Mentorship Gap: Implementation of Speed Mentoring Events for Women Faculty and Trainees in Anesthesiology. Womens Health Rep (New Rochelle). 2021;2(1):32-6.
18. Clarke AJ, Burgess A, van Diggele C, Mellis C. The role of reverse mentoring in medical education: current insights. Adv Med Educ Pract. 2019;10:693-701.
19. Robinson A. Sixty seconds on ... reverse mentoring. Br Med J. 2018;363:k4887.
20. American Psychological Association. (2012). Introduction to Mentoring: A Guide for Mentors and Mentees. Available from: https://www.apa.org/education-career/grad/mentoring [Last accessed, July 2024].
21. Studypool. Mentoring Plan MHDI. Available from: https://www.studypool.com/documents/28965169/mentoring-plan-mhdi [Last accessed, July 2024].
22. Ehrich L, Hansford B, Tennant L. Formal mentoring programs in education and other professions: A review of the literature. Educ Admin Q. 2004;40(4):518-40.
23. Taherian K, Shekarchian M. Mentoring for doctors. Do its benefits outweigh its disadvantages? Med Teach. 2008;30(4):e95-9.
24. Chopra V, Edelson DP, Saint S. A piece of my mind. Mentorship Malpractice. JAMA. 2016;315(14):1453-4.

# CHAPTER 23

# Safety in Anesthesia—Global Perspective

*Carolina Haylock-Loor*

## ABSTRACT

Patient safety and anesthesia is a universal concern that requires a global approach. The key factors include provider training, access to essential equipment and medication standardized protocols, and collaboration among anesthesia providers worldwide. Proper education, certification, and ongoing professional development are crucial for anesthesia providers. Standardized guidelines and protocols help standardize care delivery and reduce the risk of errors. Collaboration and knowledge-sharing initiatives among organizations like the World Federation of Societies of Anaesthesiologists (WFSA), and other partners can continuously improve safety outcomes. By prioritizing safety, investing in education and resources, and fostering a culture of excellence, the global anesthesia community can work together to enhance patient outcomes and uphold the highest standard of care globally.

**Keywords:** Patient safety; Training; Education; Aesthesia standards

## KEY POINTS

- *Standardized protocols and guidelines:* Establishing and adhering to best practices for anesthetic assessment, intraoperative monitoring, and postanesthesia care. Adapting international standards to local context while maintaining safety and quality.
- *Well-trained and resilient workforce:* Provider training and competency—the importance of proper education, certification, and ongoing professional development for anesthesia providers. Addressing challenges in access to specialized training programs, especially in low-resource settings. Collaboration and knowledge sharing. Facilitating platforms for sharing best practices, research findings, and innovative approaches. Promoting international conferences, training programs, and online forums for continuous improvement.
- *Access to essential equipment and medication:* Ensuring availability of critical monitoring devices, capnography pulse oximetry, and emergency education. Addressing disparities in resources between high-income and low-resource settings.
- *Multifaceted approach to safety culture:* Combining training, resources, protocols, and collaboration to enhance patient outcomes. Fostering a culture of continuous improvement and excellence in anesthesia care globally.

# INTRODUCTION

Anesthesia is a cornerstone of modern medical practice, allowing for painless procedures and surgeries while ensuring patient comfort and safety. However, the administration of anesthesia also carries inherent risks that must be carefully managed to safeguard patients' well-being. From high-income countries (HIC) to low-resource settings, ensuring safety in anesthesia is a universal concern that transcends borders, requiring a global perspective to address diverse challenges and disparities.

This topic explores the critical elements of anesthesia safety, including provider training, access to essential equipment, standardized protocols, and international collaboration. By examining these key areas, we can better understand how to enhance patient safety and improve outcomes in anesthesia care worldwide.

## ANESTHESIOLOGY, ANESTHESIOLOGISTS, AND SAFE ANESTHESIA

The World Federation of Societies of Anaesthesiologists (WFSA) is the foremost global alliance of anesthesiologists, the specialist physicians dedicated to the comprehensive care of patients before, during, and after surgery. The WFSA represents 150,000 anesthesiologists and comprises 141 society members from over 150 countries, making it the utmost global organization in the field. The WFSA's vision is to achieve universal access to safe anesthesia, underscoring its commitment to enhancing patient safety and improving anesthesia care worldwide.[1] Through its extensive network and collaborative efforts, the WFSA plays a pivotal role in advancing global standards and safe practices of anesthesia.

The WFSA has established three foundational pillars that steer its advocacy efforts. Access, safety, and unity are the three pillars instrumental in fulfilling the organization's overarching mission of enhancing patient care and ensuring access to safe anesthesia.[2] By uniting anesthesiologists worldwide, these guiding principles help the WFSA drive significant improvements in anesthesia practices and patient outcomes globally.

Anesthesia and surgical care are central to a well-functioning health system and, therefore, essential to realize "universal health coverage (UHC)". WHA resolution 68.153 highlights this.[3]

The WFSA's position on UHC emphasizes the intricate and potentially risky nature of anesthesia, highlighting the critical role of anesthesiologists in delivering optimal patient care.[4] The organization acknowledges the essential nature of effective teamwork in ensuring patient safety within anesthesia, underscoring the importance of collaborative efforts in enhancing healthcare outcomes.

The WFSA describes in the UHC statement that:
- *Anesthesiology* is the medical science and practice of anesthesia. It includes anesthesia for surgical, obstetric, and trauma care, and areas of practice, such as perioperative medicine, pain medicine, resuscitation, and intensive care medicine.
- An *anesthesiologist* is a qualified physician who has completed a nationally recognized specialist training program in anesthesiology. In some countries, the term anesthetist is used instead of anesthesiologist".
- "*Anesthesia* is complex, and potentially hazardous, and optimal patient care depends on anesthesia being provided, led, or overseen by an anesthesiologist.

The WFSA recognizes that effective teamwork is a vital component of patient safety".[4]

In 2008, the World Health Organization (WHO) launched the "Safe Surgery Saves Lives" campaign. This was the first international endeavor to critically review surgical and anesthesia care safety in low and middle income countries (LMICs). This move by WHO made safe perioperative care a public health priority. The initiative formed the WHO's Second Global Patient Safety Challenge.[5] WHO asked a panel of experts to review four key areas of perioperative care, which are (1) safe anesthesia delivery, (2) prevention of surgical-site infection, (3) safe surgical teams, and (4) yardsticks for surgical services.[5]

The committee's work culminated in 2009 with 10 critical objectives for safe surgery.[6] After observing the results of a multisite pilot study that significantly reduced perioperative complications and mortality rates following implementation, the committee advocated for the global adoption of the WHO surgical checklist, which is as follows:

- *Objective 1:* The correct patient at the correct site will be operated.
- *Objective 2:* The team will use methods known to prevent harm from administering anesthetics while protecting the patient from pain.
- *Objective 3:* Recognition and effective preparation for life-threatening loss of airway or respiratory function.
- *Objective 4:* Recognition and effective preparation for the risk of high blood loss.
- *Objective 5:* Avoid inducing an allergic or adverse drug reaction for which the patient is known to be at significant risk.
- *Objective 6:* Consistently use methods known to minimize the risk of surgical site infection.
- *Objective 7:* Prevent inadvertent retention of instruments and sponges in surgical wounds.
- *Objective 8:* Secure and accurately identify all surgical specimens.
- *Objective 9:* Effectively communicate and exchange critical information for the safe conduct of the operation.
- *Objective 10:* Routine monitoring of surgical capacity, volume, and results by hospitals and public health systems.

In 2015, the Lancet Commission on Global Surgery published the six core Indicators to monitor the realization of universal access to safe, affordable surgical and anesthesia care when needed (access to timely essential surgery, workforce density, perioperative mortality, surgical volume, protection against impoverishing expenditures for surgical care, and protection against catastrophic expenditures for surgical care).[7] Meara et al. outlined five key messages[7] that had to be addressed: (1) 5 billion people of the world's 7 billion lack access to safe, affordable surgical and anesthesia care when needed; (2) 143 million additional surgical procedures are required each year to save lives and prevent disability; (3) 33 million individuals face catastrophic health expenditure due to payment for surgery and anesthesia each year; (4) investment in surgical and anesthesia services is affordable, saves lives, and promotes economic growth; and (5) surgery is an indivisible, indispensable part of health care. The 10 needs and their recommendations to provide safe surgical and anesthesia care include:[7]

1. Qualified surgical provider.
2. Qualified anesthesia provider.

3. Infrastructure, equipment, and supplies necessary to perform safe general anesthesia, locoregional anesthesia, laparotomy, cesarean delivery, and treatment of open fracture [including, for example, personal protective equipment for staff, basic laboratories, human immunodeficiency virus (HIV)-testing capabilities, and electricity and water].
4. Facility to decontaminate and sterilize.
5. Provision for safe and affordable blood supply (screened and cross-matched blood).
6. Drugs, including anesthetics, antibiotics, and pain medicines (from the WHO model list of essential medicines).
7. Nursing care, including a record of appropriate physiological observations.
8. 24-hour surgical cover with the ability to review and respond to a deteriorating patient.
9. Quality-improvement processes, including audit of surgical mortality.
10. Risk assessment and operation planning for the planned surgery.

Surgical care is crucial to managing 30% of the global disease burden.[8] Over 300 million surgeries are performed annually worldwide. Only 6% occur in LMICs.[9] Deaths from surgically amenable diseases exceed the combined deaths from HIV/acquired immunodeficiency syndrome (AIDS), malaria, and tuberculosis (TB).[10,11] For instance, perioperative deaths in sub-Saharan Africa are *double* those in HIC. Still, the patients are *half the age* of those in HIC.[12] While in HIC, more patients die from poor quality care than from a *failure to seek care*: medication errors are twice as frequent in low-income countries (LIC).[13]

The adoption by the World Health Assembly in 2023 of Resolution WHA76.2, on integrated emergency, critical, and operative care (ECO) for UHC and protection from health emergencies (the ECO resolution)[14,15] was a noteworthy step taken for underserved communities. It brought essential services such as anesthesia and surgery closer to the people in need of them and when they need them. Resolution 76.2 was on UHC, 68.15 was on strengthening emergency and essential surgical care and anesthesia, 72.16 was on emergency care systems, and 74.7 was strengthening WHO preparedness to respond to health emergencies. The WFSA welcomed the introduction of a uniform strategy and action plan for integrated ECO and resolved to help contribute to implementing the plan. Patient outcomes suffer when vital services such as anesthesia and surgery are ignored by incoherent healthcare planning. The WFSA emphasizes integrating these services as a primary component of the basic approach to achieving UHC.[14,15]

## ■ STANDARDIZED PROTOCOLS AND GUIDELINES

Standardized protocols and guidelines for anesthesia practice play a crucial role in ensuring safety on a global scale. Establishing best practices for pre-anesthetic assessment, intraoperative monitoring, and post-anesthesia care helps standardize care delivery and reduce the risk of errors or adverse events. These guidelines should be adaptable to the local context while upholding international safety and quality standards.

In 2018, WFSA, in collaboration with the WHO, developed the International Standards for the Safe Practice of Anesthesia,[16] categorized based on hospital type and case complexity. Many places have embraced these safe practice standards, although some recommendations are considered aspirational in some contexts.

However, engaging National Anesthesia Societies and governments to adopt them in low-resource settings remains a significant challenge.[16]

This highlights the need for increased advocacy, support, and resources to implement these essential safety measures, ultimately improving patient outcomes and healthcare quality in these regions. Documenting the current capacity for safe anesthesia is critical to enhancing patient safety. For this purpose, the International Standards have been converted into a checklist—Anaesthesia Facility Assessment Tool (AFAT).[2,17]

## ■ WELL-TRAINED AND RESILIENT WORKFORCE

The workforce is an aspect of patient safety that is only sometimes acknowledged. However, a workforce of appropriate size and education is fundamental.

The Lancet Commission on Global Surgery advised a minimum density of 20 specialist surgeons, anesthesiologists, and obstetricians per 100,000 individuals.[7] The crucial threshold for specialist anesthesiologists, linked to maternal mortality rates, is approximately 5/100,000 population. Below this threshold, there is a significant and escalating rise in this mortality.[7]

Davies et al. report that a minimum of 4 specialist anesthesiologists per 100,000 population is necessary to achieve a reasonable standard of healthcare.[18] Although this is a modest target, many countries must enhance doctor training programs to produce more specialist anesthesiologists. Considering this target when developing national workforce plans is crucial, even if a phased approach to workforce planning is adopted.

There is a sizeable deficit of anesthesia providers across the world. A survey was conducted by the WFSA in 2016 to count the number of anesthesia providers worldwide.[19] The WFSA updated this count of anesthesia providers between 2021 and 2023 by an electronic survey. Tyler Law et al. received responses from 172 of 193 United Nations (UN) member countries.[20] With around 500,000 specialist anesthesiologists, the global anesthesia provider density was reported to be 8.8 [physician anesthesia provider (PAP) 6.6 nonphysician anesthesia provider (NPAP) 2.3]. 76 countries had a PAP density <5, whereas 66 countries had a total provider density <5. PAP density has increased everywhere except for HIC and LIC and the African region. The number of anesthesia providers worldwide has increased over time. However, most countries still need more anesthesia providers, meaning that significant work remains despite extensive efforts to increase the number of anesthesia providers.[20]

One key aspect of anesthesia safety is the *training and competency* of anesthesia providers. Proper education, certification, and ongoing professional development are essential to ensure that anesthesiologists have the knowledge and skills to deliver safe anesthesia care. This is particularly crucial in regions where resources may be limited and access to specialized training programs is challenging.

*Collaboration and knowledge—sharing* among anesthesia providers worldwide are essential for advancing patient safety in anesthesia. Platforms for sharing best practices, research findings, and innovative approaches to anesthesia care can help raise the standard of care globally and drive continuous improvement in safety outcomes. Initiatives such as international conferences, training programs, and online forums can facilitate this exchange of knowledge and expertise.

While not downplaying the importance of the initiatives mentioned above, the WFSA collaborates with its Member Societies to ensure a *resilient anesthesia workforce*, prioritizing their well-being,[21] directly impacting patient safety outcomes.

Another form of multiprofessional collaboration is the Utstein modification of the Lancet Commission on Global Surgery Metrics, a WFSA-led project, which suggests five metrics for global and national reporting that cover the entire spectrum of patient surgical care: (1) Geospatial access, (2) workforce, (3) volume, (4) perioperative mortality rate (POMR), and (5) financial risk protection (FRP).[22]

One of the more challenging indicators is National surgical volumes,[22] which is crucial to determine the country's surgical capacity and to develop national plans to increase it. The higher GDP per capita had higher surgical volumes.[23] Patil et al. looked into data to determine whether LMICs are achieving the Lancet Commission Global Benchmark for Surgical Volumes, marked as 5,000 surgeries per 100,000 population.[7] They reported that none of the LMICs met the benchmark and remarked that:[23]

- With increased gross domestic product (GDP) per capita, the surgical volume increased while the proportions of hernia and cesarean sections reduced.
- *Definitions of what constitutes surgery:* Many essential surgeries, such as chest tubes and tracheostomies, are not counted as surgeries.
- The publications left out "open fracture" fixation as an index surgery despite its status as a bellwether procedure. The cesarean section remained the most researched and measured indicator of surgical volume.
- The surgical volume indicator is challenging to collect and interpret. They reported that in LMICs, some high-volume surgeries are commonly performed in camp settings (not in the regular hospital registries).

## ESSENTIAL EQUIPMENT AND MEDICATIONS

In addition to provider training, the availability of essential equipment and medications is vital for safe anesthesia delivery. From monitoring devices such as capnography and pulse oximetry to emergency medication for resuscitation, ensuring that anesthesia providers have access to the necessary tools is fundamental to patient safety. Disparities between HIC and low-resource settings can significantly impact outcomes.

### Patient Monitoring

The WHO-WFSA International Standards for the Safe Practice of Anesthesia (2018) included pulse oximetry and capnography.[16]

Pulse oximetry was the first monitor to introduce essential anesthesia monitoring equipment in LIC due to its ease of use and broad applicability. The WHO's Global Pulse Oximetry Project (2008)[24] led to increased availability of pulse oximeters[25] with Lifebox running training workshops on the WHO surgical safety checklist and pulse oximetry in many LMICs.[26]

While pulse oximetry is included in the WHO surgical safety checklist, capnography is not and is often lacking in LIC and LMICs.[24] The coronavirus disease 2019 (COVID-19) pandemic has accelerated the availability of pulse oximetry but not capnography.

In 2016, the Global Capnography Project (GCAP) was established to investigate the feasibility and sustainability of introducing capnography as a standard of care in LIC and LMICs.[27]

The WHO-WFSA International Standards for the Safe Practice of Anesthesia (2018) states.[16] "If a tracheal tube is used, correct placement must be verified by auscultation" (highly recommended).

Confirmation of correct placement by carbon dioxide detection (i.e., nonwaveform capnography or colorimetry) is also *highly recommended*.

Continuous waveform capnography will be *highly recommended* when appropriately robust and suitably priced devices are available. Equipment manufacturers are encouraged to urgently address this deficiency.

The WFSA published the Minimum Capnometer Specifications 2021, which defines the minimum requirements for capnometers[28] based on the International Organization for Standardization (ISO) capnometer specifications. Gelb et al. call for the industry to reduce costs and to achieve a win-win situation by designing and delivering readily available and inexpensive capnometer technology with high durability and simple maintenance, as well as an affordable and straightforward supply of consumables.[28]

Making capnography more widely available is essential to closing the gap, including price, robustness, and supply chain.[29,30]

In a significant effort to enhance the safety of millions of surgical patients annually, Smile Train partnered with Lifebox. It launched the Smile Train-Lifebox Capnograph in 2023, an affordable, user-friendly, high-quality device with sturdy construction and long battery life. It fulfills stringent pediatric patient monitoring specifications and is suitable for low-resource environments.[30,31] Both organizations are working to equip this crucial device in operating rooms within settings that have limited resources.[31,32]

The WFSA, Smile Train, and Lifebox are urging health care systems and equipment standard guidelines, including those set by the WHO globally, to include a capnograph as an essential anesthesia monitor for safer surgery.[32]

## ■ SAFETY CULTURE

After all, ensuring patient safety in anesthesia requires a multifaceted approach that addresses training resources, protocols, and collaborations on a global scale. By prioritizing safety, investing in education and equipment, and fostering a culture of continuous improvement, anesthesia providers worldwide can work together to enhance patient outcomes and uphold the highest standard of care. With a shared commitment to safety and excellence, the global anesthesia community can make significant strides toward ensuring safe and effective anesthesia care for all patients, regardless of their location or resources available.

A simple overarching concept to keep in mind for implementing a safety culture and to continue moving forward with National Surgical, Obstetric, and Anesthesia Plans (NSOAPs) are the three failures.[7,33]

1. *Failure to provide timely access to surgical and anesthesia services:* Multiple factors contribute to delayed definitive treatment of surgical disease, as described in the three-delay model. Perioperative outcomes are significantly impacted, as 40% of patients waited over 24 hours for emergency surgery.
2. *Failure to deliver safe surgical and anesthesia care:* Factors that contribute to inadequate adoption of secure, best practices in perioperative care.
3. *Failure to rescue postoperatively:* Factors that contribute to poor recognition and response to a postoperative complication and failure to deliver time-sensitive care.

Santhirapala V, et al., propose high-quality peri-operative care through high-quality health systems.[33] In high-income nations, perioperative care has advanced and is centered on better diagnostics, risk-scoring systems, and the adoption of modern technologies. However, for most of the world, these advances do not meet the needs of local populations. Significant research, policy, and investment gaps exist in LMIC surgical and anesthesia care, resulting in unsafe, low-quality care. Although the inequities are substantial, there are tangible opportunities for anesthesia and surgical academia, under LMIC leadership, to contribute to human, societal, and economic well-being. Therefore, it is hoped that peri-operative medicine in the 21st century begins to look beyond geographical borders and develop solutions to deliver high-quality perioperative care equitably. After consensus, a driver diagram, a recognized logic tool for communicating quality improvement strategy, was utilized to present the interventions and theory of change relating to their primary aim, the reduction of avoidable perioperative mortality,[33] thus requiring validation with research and evaluation.

To establish or improve safety culture, it is essential to tackle the top-10 anesthesia patient safety issues worldwide:[34]

*Note:* Based on reports from anesthesia leaders of different countries on the current state of anesthesia patient safety. The issues listed are not listed in order of importance.
- Sustained efforts to support the training of appropriate numbers and distribution of PAPs.
- A national-level support system to provide access to appropriate anesthesia-related equipment and drugs.
- Develop and implement databases to track patient and safety outcomes.
- Patient safety initiatives to extend from intraoperative to perioperative care.
- Implementation and use of surgical/anesthesia safety checklists.
- Measures to detect and prevent death from perioperative deterioration.
- Establish cultures of intraoperative and perioperative care, safety, and teamwork.
- No punitive outcomes and criminalization of medical errors.
- Nonoperating room anesthesia practices to be allocated safety research and resources.

Finally, the crucial understanding that "one size does not fit all" is essential in tackling the identified issues.[21] As anesthesiologists and members of the WFSA, we persistently strive for advancements in patient care by promoting safe anesthesia through education, collaboration, and advocacy in the field.[21]

## ■ CONCLUSION

In conclusion, ensuring patient safety and anesthesia requires a comprehensive and collaborative effort globally. By prioritizing provider training, access to essential equipment, adherence to standardized protocols, and fostering collaboration among anesthesia providers worldwide, we can enhance patient outcomes and uphold the highest standards of care. It is imperative to address challenges in education, resource availability, and protocol adherence to mitigate risks and improve safety in anesthesia practice. Through a shared commitment to excellence, continuous improvement, and knowledge sharing, the global anesthesia community can work together to create a safer environment for patients undergoing anesthesia procedures, regardless of their location or resources available. Patient safety must remain at the forefront of anesthesia practice to deliver optimal care and ensure positive outcomes for all individuals receiving anesthesia services.

## ■ REFERENCES

1. World Federation of Societies of Anaesthesiologists. Available from: https://wfsahq.org [Last accessed, July 2024].
2. World Federation of Societies of Anaesthesiologists. WFSA's Guiding Pillars. Available from: https://wfsahq.org/our-work/advocacy/3-pillars/ [Last accessed, July 2024].
3. Sixty-eighth World Health Assembly. (2015). Strengthening emergency and essential surgical care and anaesthesia as a component of universal health coverage. Available from: https://apps.who.int/gb/ebwha/pdf_files/WHA68/A68_R15-en.pdf [Last accessed, July 2024].
4. World Federation of Societies of Anaesthesiologists. WFSA Position statement on Anaesthesiology and Universal Health Coverage. Available from: https://wfsahq.org/wp-content/uploads/UHC_Position_Statement_Final.pdf [Last accessed, July 2024].
5. World Health Organization. The second global patient safety challenge: safe surgery saves lives. https://iris.who.int/handle/10665/70080. Last accessed 01 Jul 2024.
6. World Health Organization. (2009). WHO guidelines for safe surgery: safe surgery saves lives. Available from: https://www.who.int/patientsafety/safesurgery/tools_resources/9789241598552/en/ [Last accessed, July 2024].
7. Meara JG, Leather AM, Hagander L, Alkire BC, Alonso N, Ameh EA, et al. Global Surgery 2030: evidence and solutions for achieving health, welfare, and economic development. Lancet. 2015;386(9993):569-624.
8. Shrime MG, Bickler SW, Alkire BC, Mock C. Global burden of surgical disease: an estimation from the provider perspective. Lancet Glob Health. 2015;3(Suppl 2):S8-9.
9. Rosero EB, Eslava-Schmalbach J, Garzón-Orjuela N, Buitrago G, Joshi GP. Failure to Rescue and Mortality Differences After Appendectomy in a Low-Middle-Income Country and the United States. Anesth Analg. 2023;136(6):1030-8.
10. Ozgediz D, Jamison D, Cherian M, McQueen K. The burden of surgical conditions and access to surgical care in low- and middle-income countries. Bull World Health Organ. 2008;86(8):646-7.
11. GBD 2016 Causes of Death Collaborators. Global, regional, and national age-sex specific mortality for 264 causes of death, 1980-2016: a systematic analysis for the Global Burden of Disease Study 2016. Lancet. 2017;390(10100):1151-210.
12. Biccard B, Madiba T, Kluyts H, Munlemvo DM, Madzimbamuto FD, Basenero A, et al. Perioperative patient outcomes in the African Surgical Outcomes Study: a 7-day prospective observational cohort study. Lancet. 2018;391(10130):1589-98.
13. Nepogodiev D, Martin J, Biccard B, Makupe A, Bhangu A; National Institute for Health Research Global Health Research Unit on Global Surgery. Global burden of postoperative death. Lancet. 2019;393(10170):401.
14. World Federation of Societies of Anaesthesiologists (WFSA), (2024). WHA77 Statement – WFSA constituency statement welcomes the proposed Emergency, Critical & Operative Care implementation plan. Available from: https://wfsahq.org/news/wha77-statement-wfsa-constituency-statement-welcomes-the-proposed-emergency-critical-operative-care-implementation-plan/ [Last accessed, July 2024].
15. Seventy-sixth World Health Assembly. (2023). Integrated emergency, critical and operative care for universal health coverage and protection from health emergencies. Available from: https://apps.who.int/gb/ebwha/pdf_files/WHA76/A76_R2-en.pdf [Last accessed, July 2024].
16. Gelb AW, Morriss W, Johnson W, Merry AF; International Standards for a Safe Practice of Anesthesia Workgroup. World Health Organization-World Federation of Societies of Anaesthesiologists (WHO-WFSA) International Standards for a Safe Practice of Anesthesia. Can J Anaesth. 2018;65(6):698-708.
17. World Federation of Societies of Anaesthesiologists. Introduction. Available from: https://uk.surveymonkey.com/r/HBP6F26 [Last accessed, July 2024].

18. Davies JI, Vreede E, Onajin-Obembe B, Morriss WW. What is the minimum number of specialist anesthetists needed in low-income and middle-income countries? BMJ Glob Health. 2018;3(6):e001005.
19. World Federation of Societies of Anaesthesiologists. World Anaesthesiology Workforce Map. Available from: https://wfsahq.org/resources/workforce-map/ [Last accessed, July 2024].
20. Law TJ, Lipnick MS, Morriss W, Gelb AW, Mellin-Olsen J, Filipescu D, et al. The Global Anesthesia Workforce Survey: Updates and Trends in the Anesthesia Workforce. Anesth Analg. 2024;139(1):15-24.
21. World Federation of Societies of Anaesthesiologists. WFSA Strategy 2023-28. Available from: https://wfsahq.org/wp-content/uploads/WFSA-Strategy-2023-28_final.pdf [Last accessed, July 2024].
22. Davies JI, Gelb AW, Gore-Booth J, Martin J, Mellin-Olsen J, Åkerman C, et al. Global surgery, obstetric, and anaesthesia indicator definitions and reporting: An Utstein consensus report. PLoS Med. 2021;18(8):e1003749
23. Patil P, Nathani P, Bakker JM, van Duinen AJ, Bhushan P, Shukla M, et al. Are LMICs Achieving the Lancet Commission Global Benchmark for Surgical Volumes? A Systematic Review. World J Surg 2023;47(8):1930-9.
24. World Health Organization. Why safe surgery is important? Available from: https://www.who.int/teams/integrated-health-services/patient-safety/research/safe-surgery [Last accessed, July 2024].
25. Funk LM, Weiser TG, Berry WR, Lipsitz SR, Merry AF, Enright AC, et al. Global operating theatre distribution and pulse oximetry supply: an estimation from reported data. Lancet. 2010;376(9746):1055-61.
26. Lifebox Foundation. The Lifebox Pulse Oximeter. Available from: https://www.lifebox.org/our-work/pulse-oximetry/ [Last accessed, July 2024].
27. Jooste R, Roberts F, Mndolo S, Mabedi D, Chikumbanje S, Whitaker DK, et al. Global Capnography Project (GCAP): implementation of capnography in Malawi - an international anaesthesia quality improvement project. Anaesthesia. 2019;74(2):158-166.
28. Gelb AW, McDougall RJ, Gore-Booth J, Mainland PA; WFSA Ad Hoc Capnometry Workgroup. The World Federation of Societies of Anaesthesiologists Minimum Capnometer Specifications 2021-A Guide for Health Care Decision Makers. Anesth Analg. 2021;133(5):1132-7.
29. Wollner E, Nourian MM, Booth W, Conover S, Law T, Lilaonitkul M, et al. Impact of capnography on patient safety in high- and low-income settings: a scoping review. Br J Anaesth. 2020;125(1):e88-103.
30. Evans FM, Turc R, Echeto-Cerrato MA, Gathuya ZN, Enright A. The capnography project. Anesth Analg. 2023;137(5):922-8.
31. Smile Train. Global Health Organizations Rally to Close Critical Gap in Surgical Safety. Available from: https://www.smiletrain.org/news/global-health-organizations-rally-close-critical-gap-surgical-safety. [Last accessed, July 2024].
32. World Federation of Societies of Anaesthesiologists. (2024). CapnoWeek: Closing the Global Capnography Gap. Available from: https://wfsahq.org/news/capno-week-closing-the-global-capnography-gap/. [Last accessed, July 2024].
33. Santhirapala V, Peden CJ, Meara JG, Biccard BM, Gelb AW, Johnson WD, et al. Towards high-quality peri-operative care: a global perspective. Anaesthesia. 2020;75(Suppl 1):e18-e27.
34. Warner MA, Arnal D, Cole DJ, Hammoud R, Haylock-Loor C, Ibarra P, et al. Anesthesia Patient Safety: Next Steps to Improve Worldwide Perioperative Safety by 2030. Anesth Analg. 2022;135(1):6-19.

# CHAPTER 24

# Role of Anesthesiologist in Perioperative Patient Safety

*Shashi Kiran, Neha Aeron, Kate Boothroyd*

## ABSTRACT

Patient safety, particularly in the perioperative period, is of paramount importance. While it is the shared responsibility of all medical and paramedical personnel to ensure smooth patient care and prevent any iatrogenic harm, the role of an anesthesiologist often needs to be determined. Lack of awareness and education gaps at the level of both patients and doctors are common contributing factors. Acknowledgment and careful analysis of critical incidents help prevent patient-related accidents. Adopting a blame-free culture that is open to every viewpoint and addresses patient grievances is essential. Using checklists and systematic risk analysis methodologies enables healthcare organizations to identify potential risks and implement preventive measures. Anesthesiologists play a vital role in preventing medication errors, ensuring safe patient transfers, and providing patient safety and care in perioperative and critical care settings. Recent advancements such as artificial intelligence technology have significantly enhanced patient care and ensured patient safety.

**Keywords:** Patient safety; Medication errors; Surgical checklists; Protocols; Artificial intelligence

## KEY POINTS

- Anesthesiologists, as members of a multidisciplinary team, significantly impact perioperative patient safety.
- Bridging education gaps and following safety checklist protocols go a long way in ensuring patient safety.
- Developing a blame-free culture and a careful root cause analysis is valuable.
- Avoiding medication errors, maintaining hand hygiene, and preventing healthcare-associated infections are paramount.
- Recent advancements, such as artificial intelligence technology, have proven to be milestones in enhancing patient care and assuring patient safety.

## ■ INTRODUCTION

The role of an anesthesiologist is fundamental to patient safety during the perioperative period. Beyond the administration of anesthesia, anesthesiologist plays a crucial role in mitigating risks, ensuring optimal patient outcomes, and fostering a culture of safety within the perioperative setting. From preoperative assessments to postoperative care, responsibility encompasses a spectrum of tasks, including preventing medication errors, managing airway complications, and contributing to the broader aspect of perioperative care. The anesthesiologist's expertise and vigilance are indispensable in navigating the intricacies of patient care during surgery, embodying a commitment to safeguarding the well-being of individuals undergoing medical interventions.

The perioperative period is a critical phase where the risks associated with anesthesia are intertwined with broader perioperative and peri-interventional risks. There is a notable divergence in perspectives on adverse events between clinicians and patients in patient safety, particularly within the perioperative setting. Anesthesiologists play increasingly significant roles in the operative setting and nonoperative contexts such as intensive care units (ICUs). Their involvement spans preoperative assessments, intraoperative management, and postoperative care, highlighting the need for effective teamwork and communication between healthcare professionals. Anesthesia-specific risks are inherent in medical procedures and involve the administration of drugs to induce a reversible state of unconsciousness, muscle relaxation, and analgesia. These risks, including physiological responses to anesthesia, complications related to drug errors, and airway management, contribute to the complexity of the perioperative setting. Collaboration between surgeons and anesthesiologists is paramount in ensuring patient safety during perioperative.

The definition of patient safety, as provided by Charles Vincent, while emphasizing the importance of proactivity within the healthcare process, states that it goes beyond addressing the underlying pathology and focuses on preventing, avoiding, and ameliorating adverse outcomes that may arise during medical or surgical procedures or medication administration.[1]

Adverse events are detrimental and unfavorable outcomes are often experienced by patients undergoing healthcare interventions.[2] These events contribute significantly to undue hospital admissions, with a notable percentage being preventable. The World Health Organization (WHO) highlights a concerning statistic that 1 in every 10 patients experiences harm that could have been avoided.[3] This results in a significant number of deaths, with an annual figure of over 100,000 attributed to the care patients receive.[4] There is a vast global disparity in these statistics, with lower-income countries reporting higher rates of adverse events. Within these countries, specific populations, such as children and older people, are disproportionately affected, further exacerbating healthcare inequalities. Moreover, the impact of adverse events is not uniform across different demographic groups. Black patients, for instance, experience higher rates of adverse events, reflecting systemic disparities in healthcare.[5] These can be rooted in various factors, including access to quality healthcare, cultural competence, and systemic biases within healthcare systems.

The mortality rate associated with adverse events has been estimated at around 8%, but it is crucial to recognize that this figure underestimates the true prevalence. Inadequate recordkeeping and a reluctance to engage in voluntary reporting contribute to the underrepresentation of adverse events in official data.[6] This points to a significant challenge in accurately assessing the scale of the problem, making it essential to improve reporting mechanisms and foster a culture of transparency within healthcare systems.

Patient safety is a complex issue that extends beyond the clinical setting; the lack of education in specific communities predisposes them to a higher burden of chronic disease. This lack of awareness and education can contribute to delayed or inadequate healthcare-seeking behavior, leading to more severe health issues.

To enhance patient safety, a comprehensive approach is necessary, encompassing improvements within healthcare systems and broader societal changes to promote health equity and education.[7]

Adverse events can manifest in various forms, spanning a range of healthcare domains. Issues related to surgical specialties may include complications arising during or after surgical procedures, while medication administration can involve errors in dosage, prescription, or drug interactions. Problems with fluid management might lead to imbalances that can negatively impact a patient's health and healthcare-associated infections (HAIs) pose an additional risk.[6] Addressing these challenges comprehensively is imperative for enhancing patient safety across healthcare settings. This involves implementing measures to improve the accuracy and completeness of recordkeeping, encouraging healthcare providers to report adverse events without fear of reprisal and fostering a culture of continuous improvement. Additionally, enhancing communication and collaboration among healthcare teams, implementing standardized protocols and checklists, and investing in training and education can contribute to preventing and mitigating adverse events.[8]

Despite advancements that have made anesthesia safer over the years, persistent challenges remain, such as a shortage of educated healthcare personnel, medication errors, challenges in maintaining intraoperative hemodynamics, organ injuries, infections, respiratory and airway complications, issues in the transition of care, and the impact of fatigue and stress on healthcare providers.

Patient safety encompasses various categories of issues, each posing unique challenges and requiring targeted interventions, including surgical events, product/device-related concerns, equipment malfunctions, patient protection events, care management issues, environmental factors, and criminal events.[9] Another challenge is the variability in individual patient responses to anesthesia, which is influenced by factors such as age, comorbidities, and the nature of the surgical procedure. Surgical events involve a specific category of patient safety issues, encompassing complications and errors related to surgical procedures.

## ■ TO ERR IS HUMAN

Patient safety is a complex and multifaceted concept comprising three essential components: Guiding principles, a body of knowledge, and a collection of tools.[10] The guiding principles underscore the recognition that errors are inherent in any complex system and are part of a natural process. Rather than assigning blame for errors, these principles advocate for a culture of continuous improvement. This shift in perspective encourages healthcare professionals to view errors as opportunities to identify weaknesses in the system and implement changes to enhance safety. Emphasizing improvement over blame helps foster a more open and proactive approach to addressing issues that may compromise patient safety.[11]

## ■ PATIENT SAFETY—A SHARED RESPONSIBILITY!

The shared responsibility for perioperative safety between surgeons and anesthesiologists is crucial in preventing severe and preventable adverse surgical events. Prospective risk assessment involves a proactive approach to identify and mitigate potential risks before they manifest as adverse events. As part of this method, direct observation allows healthcare professionals to assess and analyze the workflow, communication patterns, and adherence to safety protocols during surgical procedures. This observational approach provides valuable insights into areas where improvements can be made to enhance perioperative safety, facilitating targeted interventions and continuous quality improvement.[12]

Applying knowledge from diverse safety-critical industries, such as mass transportation and nuclear power, allows healthcare professionals to benefit from proven strategies and methodologies for enhancing safety in high-stakes environments. Lessons learned from these fields provide valuable perspectives on accident prevention, risk management, and system resilience.

Initiatives to address imperfections and implement various interventions to improve outcomes include safe system design, development of standardized protocols, promotion of interdisciplinary collaboration, and integration of technological advancements to enhance monitoring and safety during anesthesia administration. The collection of tools utilized in these initiatives is diverse:

- Critical incident reporting systems encourage healthcare workers to report adverse events or near misses, contributing to a culture of transparency and learning.
- Checklists are practical tools to ensure essential steps are followed consistently in complex procedures.
- Safe system design involves creating environments that minimize the impact of human error and provide safeguards against adverse events.
- Communication protocols enhance teamwork and information exchange, reducing the risk of miscommunication.
- Systematic risk analysis methodologies, such as Failure Mode and Effects Analysis (FMEA) or Root Cause Analysis (RCA), enable healthcare organizations to identify potential risks and implement preventive measures proactively.

By combining these tools, healthcare systems can create a robust framework for improving patient safety across various clinical settings.[13,14]

Central to patient safety is analyzing errors and critical incidents and acknowledging the interconnectedness of humans, machines, and equipment within a system. This approach recognizes that errors rarely result from a single cause but often involve a combination of factors. Analyzing incidents comprehensively allows healthcare organizations to identify systemic issues, human factors, and technological contributions to errors. By understanding the complex interactions within the healthcare system, institutions can implement targeted interventions to reduce the likelihood of similar incidents occurring in the future.

Accurate assessment and reporting, particularly in the context of surgical procedures, play a pivotal role in optimizing patient safety and overall outcomes. Developing a positive culture for adverse event reporting encourages healthcare professionals to report incidents without fear of reprisal, facilitating a more comprehensive understanding of safety issues. Collaboration among surgical teams, for example, adherence to guidelines such as the WHO surgical safety checklist, contributes significantly to harm prevention **(Table 1)**.

Accidents are an inherent risk in the healthcare environment, emphasizing the critical importance of proper incident reporting and teamwork for prevention and effective management. Recognizing that errors can occur is foundational to building a safer healthcare system. Establishing a blame-free culture is paramount in creating an environment where individuals feel comfortable acknowledging mistakes,

**TABLE 1:** The World Health Organization surgical checklist.

| Before induction of anaesthesia→ (with at least nurse and anaesthetist) | Before skin incision→ (with nurse, anaesthetist and surgeon) | Before patient leaves operating room (with nurse, anaesthetist and surgeon) |
|---|---|---|
| Has the patient confirmed his/her identity, site, procedure, and consent?<br>☐ Yes | ☐ Confirm all team members have introduced themselves by name and role | Nurse verbally confirms:<br>☐ The name of the procedure<br>☐ Completion of instrument, sponge and needle counts<br>☐ Specimen labelling (read specimen labels aloud, including patient name)<br>☐ Whether there are any equipment problems to be addressed |
| Is the site marked?<br>☐ Yes<br>☐ Not applicable | ☐ Confirm the patient's name, procedure, and where the incision will be made | |
| Is the anaesthesia machine and medication check complete?<br>☐ Yes | Has antibiotic prophylaxis been given within the last 60 minutes?<br>☐ Yes<br>☐ Not applicable | |
| Is the pulse oximeter on the patient and functioning?<br>☐ Yes | Anticipated critical events<br>to surgeon:<br>☐ What are the critical or non-routine steps?<br>☐ How long will the case take?<br>☐ What is the anticipated blood loss?<br>To Anaesthetist:<br>☐ Are there any patient-specific concerns?<br>To Nursing Team:<br>☐ Has sterility (including indicator results) been confirmed?<br>☐ Are there equipment issues or any concerns? | To surgeon, anaesthetist and nurse:<br>☐ What are the key concerns for recovery and management of this patient? |
| Does the patient have a:<br>Known allergy?<br>☐ No<br>☐ Yes<br>Difficult airway or aspiration risk?<br>☐ No<br>☐ Yes, and equipment/assistance available<br>Risk of >500 mL blood loss (7 mL/kg in children)?<br>☐ No<br>☐ Yes, and two IVs/central access and fluids planned | Is essential imaging displayed?<br>☐ Yes<br>☐ Not applicable | |

*Note:* This checklist is not intended to be comprehensive. Additions and modifications to fit local practice are encouraged.
*Source:* WHO. (2009). Surgical Safety Checklist. Available from: https://iris.who.int/bitstream/handle/10665/44186/9789241598590_eng_Checklist.pdf?sequence=2&is Allowed=y [Last accessed July, 2024].

seeking help and improving patient safety. It promotes transparency and encourages healthcare professionals to report incidents without fear of reprisal. This openness is crucial for identifying system weaknesses, understanding the root causes of errors, and implementing corrective measures to prevent similar incidents. It shifts the focus from assigning blame to fostering a culture of continuous learning and improvement.

## CONTINUOUS EDUCATION AND PROFESSIONAL DEVELOPMENT

Continuous education and professional development contribute to maintaining crucial knowledge, aligning perspectives on adverse events, and promoting patient safety. This involves staying abreast of technological advancements, adopting evidence-based practices and participating in ongoing education and training. Simulation training, for instance, allows healthcare providers to practice and refine their skills in a controlled environment, improving their ability to respond to unexpected events during anesthesia administration. There is a pressing need for global efforts to improve infrastructure, education, and access to resources in underdeveloped regions where basic patient safety standards may be lacking.[15] Initiatives that promote the dissemination of best practices, training programs, and the establishment of basic safety standards can contribute significantly to mitigating risks in perioperative care.

## PATIENT COMMUNICATION AND CONSENT

Furthermore, open communication and a transparent approach to informed consent are crucial for aligning perspectives on adverse events between clinicians and patients. Patients should be adequately informed about the potential risks associated with anesthesia, enabling them to participate actively in decision-making processes and setting realistic expectations about their perioperative experience.

## PATIENT PROTECTION EVENTS

Patient protection events involve patient falls, medication errors, or HAIs. Care management issues encompass a broad range of challenges, including communication breakdowns, inadequate handovers, and mistakes in diagnosis or treatment. Addressing these issues involves improving communication among healthcare professionals, implementing standardized protocols and enhancing care coordination.[16,17]

Environmental factors, such as issues with healthcare facilities' physical environment, also contribute to patient safety concerns. These may include problems with sanitation, inadequate infrastructure, or issues related to the availability of essential resources. Creating a safe and conducive environment for patient care is critical for preventing environmental-related patient safety events.

Criminal events involve intentional harm to patients, often perpetrated by individuals within the healthcare system. This can include physical assault, abuse, or other criminal activities. Implementing stringent security measures and fostering a culture of accountability is critical for preventing criminal events and ensuring patient safety.

## ■ CHILD AND ADULT SAFEGUARDING

As healthcare professionals, safeguarding patients and colleagues is our moral and fundamental responsibility. It involves taking additional positive measures to ensure the safety and well-being of individuals prone to abuse or harm, like children, disabled individuals, older people, women, and those from poor socioeconomic backgrounds. The guiding principles for safeguarding work include supporting and encouraging patients to make their own decisions through informed consent, acting before any harm occurs, using appropriate responses to the presented risk, providing support and representation for those in need, and ensuring transparency and accountability. Royal College of Anesthesiologists, UK, recommends level 2 or 3 training for anesthesiologists for child safeguarding. It involves the ability to identify, report, and refer child abuse or neglect as well as assisting in the assessment, planning, and evaluation of requirements of a child or young individual as and when the need for safety arises.[18,19]

## ■ TEAMWORK

The operation theater team is a dynamic group composed of individuals from diverse multidisciplinary professional backgrounds, each bringing their unique biases and stereotypes into the collaborative environment. While this diversity enriches the team's skill set, it can also result in communication gaps due to differing perspectives and information coding.

The multifaceted nature of the team demands effective communication, coordination, and teamwork to ensure seamless collaboration. Diverse professional perspectives can lead to misunderstandings or assumptions, emphasizing the importance of clear and concise communication within the team. Bridging these communication gaps is crucial for identifying and addressing errors, adapting to evolving situations during surgical procedures, and ultimately enhancing patient safety.[20]

Encouraging open communication channels, where team members feel comfortable expressing concerns or seeking clarification, can help overcome biases and stereotypes. Regular team-building activities and training sessions can further strengthen interpersonal relationships and enhance the overall teamwork culture.[21]

Another critical aspect of patient safety is verifying all medical procedures and ensuring patients understand their treatment plans.[22] This process reduces the gap between best practice and the actual delivery of care. Verifying procedures involves cross-checking and confirming each step to minimize the risk of errors. Patient involvement and comprehension of their treatment plans empower them in their healthcare journey and contribute to a safer and more informed healthcare environment.

## ■ PATIENT TRANSFERS

Patient transfers represent a common source of potential harm in healthcare settings and their safe execution requires meticulous attention to detail. This is particularly evident in intrahospital transfers, where patients move between departments or units. Anesthesiologists play a pivotal role in many patient transfers and the coordination and handover from anesthesiologists are crucial elements in ensuring safe transitions.

Safe patient transfers involve using appropriate equipment, such as safe slides or transfer devices, to minimize the risk of injury during the transfer process. Proper coordination among healthcare professionals, including anesthesiologists, is essential to orchestrate a seamless transfer and to ensure that all necessary information about the patient's condition, anesthesia administration, and any potential risks are communicated effectively.[23] Standardized handover protocols and checklists can assist in ensuring that crucial information is noticed and that all team members are on the same page. By prioritizing transparency, teamwork, and effective communication, healthcare organizations can significantly contribute to preventing and managing incidents, ultimately enhancing patient safety and overall healthcare outcomes.[24]

## ■ MEDICATION ERRORS

Perioperative medication management is critical to ensuring patient safety during surgical procedures. Medication errors have many contributory factors, such as human error, system flaws, and communication breakdowns. Despite increased awareness and efforts to improve safety, human factors contribute to medication errors within the perioperative context. Issues such as the need for standardized labels and drug shortages can create confusion, increasing the risk of medication preparation and administration errors.[25] The unique challenges within the perioperative setting, including the absence of standard safety checks during medication administration, demand specific attention to enhance safety protocols.

The anesthesia culture historically emphasizes autonomy and individual responsibility and can pose challenges in improving medication safety. The culture's focus on personal decision-making may hinder the implementation of standardized practices and collaborative approaches to medication management. Overcoming these cultural barriers requires a shift toward a more team-oriented mindset that recognizes the collective responsibility for patient safety. Various strategies have been implemented to mitigate medication errors in the perioperative setting. Standardized medication labels and employing clear and consistent language help reduce confusion and enhance accuracy during medication preparation and administration.

Digital health technologies, encompassing computerized systems and artificial intelligence (AI), have emerged as promising tools to enhance medication safety and reduce errors in healthcare settings. Barcode technology is a valuable tool that allows real-time verification of medication details and patient information before administration.[26]

Integrating electronic health records (EHRs) significantly advances perioperative medication safety. Electronic records provide a comprehensive and accessible platform for healthcare professionals to access patient medication histories, allergies, and other critical information. This facilitates informed decision-making and helps prevent errors related to incomplete or inaccurate medication information.

Further benefits of digitalization include the potential to optimize the physical workspace where medications are prepared and administered, minimizing distraction and providing a safer environment.[27]

Despite the potential benefits of digital health technologies, the deeply ingrained culture of autonomy in anesthesia challenges their widespread adoption and implementation. A cultural shift is required to embrace the integration of digital tools and maximize the impact of technological advancements. A comprehensive and collaborative approach that considers both systemic and cultural factors is essential further to advance patient safety in perioperative medication management.[12]

## ■ AIRWAY COMPLICATIONS

Addressing airway complications is of paramount importance in anesthesia. Despite advancements in airway management, major airway complications remain a concern. The anesthetists' role in predicting airway difficulty and tailoring management accordingly significantly improves outcomes.

Dedicated airway management techniques, such as video laryngoscopy and awake tracheal intubation, are recommended for predicted difficult airways. Video laryngoscopy provides a visual advantage for better visualization of the airway structures and awake tracheal intubation allows for a controlled approach in a spontaneously breathing patient, reducing the risk of complications. Despite their proven benefits, these techniques often need to be more utilized, highlighting the need for increased awareness and education within the anesthesia community.

Advancements in predicting and managing airway complications can significantly improve patient outcomes, emphasizing the importance of embracing evidence-based techniques and fostering a culture of continuous learning and adaptation within the healthcare community.[28]

## ■ HEALTHCARE-ASSOCIATED INFECTIONS

Healthcare-associated infections are a significant concern within the broader context of patient safety. The definition of HAIs includes infections that occur between 48 hours and 30 days after a patient is hospitalized or receives medical care.[29] In the United States, HAIs contribute substantially to morbidity and mortality, impacting 4–10% of all hospitalized patients and resulting in over 700,000 infections and approximately 99,000 deaths annually.[30-33] Inhospital mortality doubles when patients develop multidrug-resistant (MDR) infections, with *Klebsiella pneumoniae* and *Escherichia coli* being the most common in 70% of all ICU HAIs and up to 40% of all ICU deaths.[33]

The coronavirus disease 2019 (COVID-19) pandemic had a notable influence on the landscape of HAIs when a reduction in the development of MDR organism infections was noted in hospitalized patients. This decline could be attributed to the heightened focus on infection prevention measures associated with COVID-19, including increased adherence to hand hygiene (HH), the widespread use of personal protective equipment (PPE), and the practice of social distancing. The increased awareness and implementation of infection control measures, driven by the urgent need to mitigate the spread of COVID-19, have positively impacted overall infection rates.[34-36] This highlights the interconnected nature of HAIs and the potential for broader improvements in infection prevention strategies to yield positive outcomes beyond the immediate context.

## ■ HAND HYGIENE

Anesthesia providers' responsibility in combating HAIs extends beyond timely antibiotic administration. Efforts should focus on protecting patients from environmental bacterial exposure within the operating room (OR) and preventing anesthesia providers from becoming vectors for intraoperative bacterial transmission. The WHO and Centers for Disease Control and Prevention (CDC) have recognized

**TABLE 2:** Principles for team training program.

| Principle | Description |
|---|---|
| Identify critical competencies | Utilize these as a focus for training content |
| Teamwork | Emphasize teamwork over task work, design for teamwork to improve team processes |
| To each its own | Allow team-based learning outcomes desired and organizational resources to guide the process |
| Task exposure is not enough | Provide guided, hands-on practice |
| Simulation | Ensure training relevance to transfer environment |
| Constructive feedback | It must be descriptive, timely, and relevant |
| Go beyond reaction data | Evaluate clinical outcomes, learning, and behaviors on the job |
| Reinforce desired teamwork behaviors | Sustain through coaching and performance evaluation |

HH as a primary prevention strategy.[31,37] Healthcare workers and anesthesia providers demonstrate inadequate HH compliance, with rates below 50% and 23%, respectively.[38]

Research indicates rapid and widespread contamination of the anesthesia work area. For instance, after a simulated intubation sequence, contamination was demonstrated by fluorescent dye on intravenous (IV) hubs, medication syringes, keyboards, and door handles. Contamination during general anesthesia administration increases bacterial contamination, leading to IV stopcock contamination, postoperative sepsis, and increased mortality. Approximately, 16% of 30-day postoperative infections result from bacterial transmission from the anesthesia work area.[30]

A multimodal, evidence-based anesthesia work area infection control program is essential for minimizing pathogen transmission and subsequent infection development. This program includes HH, environmental cleaning, vascular care, and patient decolonization strategies. Intraoperative HH should involve at least 8-hourly hand decontamination events according to the WHO's five moments of HH. While not a panacea, HH remains a critical component of multimodal, evidence-based strategies that, if successfully implemented, can significantly reduce surgical site infections (SSIs) and pathogen transmission events.[39] Team training is designed to equip team members with the competencies to optimize teamwork. Salas et al. proposed eight evidence-based principles for effective planning, implementation, and evaluation of team training programs specific to healthcare[40] **(Table 2)**.

# ■ CONCLUSION

The role of the anesthesiologist in patient safety is pivotal and multifaceted. Beyond the administration of anesthesia, anesthesiologists contribute significantly to the overall safety of patients by managing perioperative risks, coordinating with other healthcare professionals, and fostering a culture of continuous improvement. Their responsibilities extend from preoperative assessments to postoperative care and they play a crucial role in addressing challenges such as medication errors, airway complications, and the broader perioperative environment. Embracing advancements in technology, collaboration, and standardized practices, anesthesiologists are at the forefront of initiatives to enhance patient safety, ensuring that surgical procedures are conducted with the utmost care and precision and a relentless commitment to minimizing risks and optimizing patient outcomes.

## ■ REFERENCES

1. Vincent C. Patient safety, 2nd edition. Oxford: BMJ Books; 2010.
2. Boulanger J, Keohane C, Yeats A. Role of Patient Safety Organizations in Improving Patient Safety. Obstet Gynecol Clin North Am. 2019;46(2):257-67.
3. Slawomirski L, Klazinga N. The economics of patient safety: from analysis to action. Paris: Organisation for Economic Co-operation and Development; 2020.
4. Stewart K, Choudry MI, Buckingham R. Learning from hospital mortality. Clin Med (Lond). 2016;16(6):530-4.
5. Metersky ML, Hunt DR, Kliman R, Wang Y, Curry M, Verzier N, et al. Racial disparities in the frequency of patient safety events: results from the National Medicare Patient Safety Monitoring System. MedCare. 2011;49(5):504-10.
6. Schwendimann R, Blatter C, Dhaini S, Simon M, Ausserhofer D. The occurrence, types, consequences and preventability of in-hospital adverse events - a scoping review. BMC Health Serv Res. 2018;18(1):521.
7. Warner MA, Arnal D, Cole DJ, Hammoud R, Haylock-Loor C, Ibarra P, et al. Anesthesia Patient Safety: Next Steps to Improve Worldwide Perioperative Safety by 2030. Anesth Analg. 2022;135(1):6-19.
8. Kelly FE, Frerk C, Bailey CR, Cook TM, Ferguson K, Flin R, et al. Implementing human factors in anaesthesia: guidance for clinicians, departments and hospitals: Guidelines from the Difficult Airway Society and the Association of Anaesthetists. Anaesthesia. 2023;78:458-78.
9. Kizer KW, Stegun MB. Serious Reportable Adverse Events in Health Care. In: Henriksen K, Battles JB, Marks ES, Lewin DI (Eds). Advances in Patient Safety: From Research to Implementation (Volume 4: Programs, Tools, and Products). Rockville (MD): Agency for Healthcare Research and Quality (US); 2005.
10. Smith AF. Patient safety: people, systems and techniques. Acta Anaesthesiol Scand. 2007;51(Suppl 1):51-3.
11. Mellin-Olsen J, Staender S, Whitaker DK, Smith AF. Helsinki Declaration on Patient Safety in Anaesthesiology. Eur J Anaesthesiol. 2010;27(7):592-7.
12. Jelacic S, Bowdle A, Nair BG, Kusulos D, Bower L, Togashi K. A system for anesthesia drug administration using barcode technology: the Codonics Safe Label System and smart anesthesia manager. Anesth Analg. 2015;121(2):410-21.
13. Winters BD, Gurses AP, Lehmann H, Sexton JB, Rampersad CJ, Pronovost PJ. Clinical review: checklists – translating evidence into practice. Crit Care. 2009;13:210.
14. Vincent C, Taylor-Adams S, Chapman EJ, Hewett D, Prior S, Strange P, et al. How to investigate and analyse clinical incidents: clinical risk unit and association of litigation and risk management protocol. BMJ. 2000;320:777-81.
15. Weinger MB. Time out! rethinking surgical safety: more than just a checklist. BMJ Qual Saf. 2021;30(8):613-7.
16. Thomassen O, Storesund A, Softeland E, Brattebo G. The effects of safety checklists in medicine: a systematic review. Acta Anaesthesiol Scand. 2014;58:5-18.
17. Lyons VE, Popejoy LL. Meta-analysis of surgical safety checklist effects on teamwork, communication, morbidity, mortality, and safety. West J Nurs Res. 2014;36:245-61.
18. Melarkode K, Kathy Wilkinson K. Child protection issues and the anaesthetist. Cont Educ Anaesth Crit Care Pain. 2012;12(3):123-27.
19. Royal College of Anaesthetists. Safeguarding. Available from: https://rcoa.ac.uk/documents/safeguarding [Last accessed July, 2024].

20. Weller J. Shedding new light on tribalism in health care. Med Educ. 2012;46:134-6.
21. Attri JP, Sandhu GK, Mohan B, Bala N, Sandhu KS, Bansal L. Conflicts in operating room: Focus on causes and resolution. Saudi J Anaesth. 2015;9(4):457-63.
22. Toole J, Kohansieh M, Khan U, Romero S, Ghali M, Zeltser R, et al. Does Your Patient Understand Their Treatment Plan? Factors Affecting Patient Understanding of Their Medical Care Treatment Plan in the Inpatient Setting. J Patient Exp. 2020;7(6):1151-7.
23. Robertson ER, Morgan L, Bird S, Catchpole K, McCulloch P. Interventions employed to improve intrahospital handover: a systematic review. BMJ Qual Saf. 2014;23:600-7.
24. Redley B, Bucknall TK, Evans S, Botti M. Inter-professional clinical handover in post-anaesthetic care units: tools to improve quality and safety. Int J Qual Health Care. 2016;28(5):573-9.
25. Cooper R, Fogarty-Mack P, Kroll HR, Barach P. Medication safety in anesthesia: epidemiology, causes, and lessons learned in achieving reliable patient outcomes. Int Anesthesiol Clin. 2019;57(3):78-95.
26. Ye J. Patient Safety of Perioperative Medication Through the Lens of Digital Health and Artificial Intelligence. JMIR Perioper Med. 2023;6:e34453.
27. Ye J, Wang Z, Hai J. Social networking service, patient-generated health data, and population health informatics: national cross-sectional study of patterns and implications of leveraging digital technologies to support mental health and well-being. J Med Internet Res. 2022;24(4):e30898.
28. Myatra SN, Dhawan I, D'Souza SA, Elakkumanan LB, Jain D, Natarajan P. Recent advances in airway management. Indian J Anaesth. 2023;67(1):48-55.
29. Revelas A. Healthcare-associated infections: a public health problem. Niger Med J. 2012;53(2):59-64.
30. Loftus RW, Koff MD, Birnbach DJ. The dynamics and implications of bacterial transmission events arising from the anesthesia work area. Anesth Analg. 2015; 120(4):853-60.
31. Centers for Disease Control and Prevention. Guideline for hand hygiene in health-care settings. MMWR. 2002;51:1-44.
32. Centers for Disease Control and Prevention. (2016). 2014 National and State Healthcare-Associated Infections Progress Report. Available from: https://archive.cdc.gov/www_cdc_gov/hai/data/archive/2016-HAI-progress-report.html [Last accessed July, 2024].
33. Wacker J, Staender S. The role of the anesthesiologist in perioperative patient safety. Curr Opin Anaesthesiol. 2014;27(6):649-56.
34. Wee LEI, Conceicao EP, Tan JY, Magesparan KD, Amin IBM, Ismail BBS, et al. Unintended consequences of infection prevention and control measures during COVID-19 pandemic. Am J Infect Control. 2021;49(4):469-77.
35. Cole J, Barnard E. The impact of the COVID-19 pandemic on healthcare acquired infections with multidrug resistant organisms. Am J Infect Control. 2021;49(5):653-4.
36. Bentivegna E, Luciani M, Arcari L, Santino I, Simmaco M, Martelletti P. Reduction of multidrug-resistant (MDR) bacterial infections during the COVID-19 pandemic: a retrospective study. Int J Environ Res Public Health. 2021;18(3):1003.
37. World Health Organization. WHO guidelines on hand hygiene in health care. Geneva, Switzerland: World Health Organization and WHO Patient Safety; 2009.
38. Pittet D, Simon A, Hugonnet S, Pessoa-Silva CL, Sauvan V, Perneger TV. Hand hygiene among physicians: performance, beliefs, and perceptions. Ann Intern Med. 2004;141(1):1-8.
39. Simmons CG, Hennigan AW, Loyd JM, Loftus RW, Sharma A. Patient Safety in Anesthesia: Hand Hygiene and Perioperative Infection Control. Curr Anesthesiol Rep. 2022;12(4):493-500.
40. Salas E, DiazGranados D, Weaver SJ, King H. Does team training work? Principles for health care. Acad Emerg Med. 2008;15(11):1002-9.

# Index

Page numbers followed by *b* refer to box, *f* refer to figure, *fc* refer to flowchart, and *t* refer to table.

## A

Abdomen
  left upper quadrant of 237*f*
  right upper quadrant of 237*f*
Acclimatization 279
Acetazolamide 284
Acidosis
  respiratory 119
  situations of 118
Acute asthma exacerbations 209
Acute care surgery
  classification of 28, 29*b*
  new timing of 29*b*
Acute hypercapnic chronic obstructive
      pulmonary disease 208
Acute kidney injury 29, 172, 173, 247
Acute respiratory distress syndrome 172, 173,
      197, 204, 207, 246, 258, 267
Adrenaline 249
Advanced cardiovascular life support 55
Advanced trauma life support 30
  classification 30*t*
Airway
  assessment 41, 43, 91
  complications 100, 330
  device, malposition of 113
  management 40, 46, 48, 50, 56, 77, 79, 92, 152
    applications in 230
    techniques 330
  masses, resection of 259
  obstruction, risk of 259
  pressure release ventilation 149
  related severe complications 41
  resistance 106
  structures 42
  ultrasound 189
  virtual endoscopic evaluation of 42
Albumin, theoretical advantage of 247
Alcohol hangover 281
Alfentanil 157*f*
Alkalosis, respiratory 119
Altitude 278, 279*f*
Alveolar hypoxia 117
Alveolar-arterial oxygen gradient 36
Ambulatory anesthesia 18
Ambulatory surgery 13, 17
  center 1-5, 9, 9*f*, 11*t*, 12, 17

American College of Surgeons National Surgical
      Quality Improvement Program 21
American Geriatric Society 169, 175*t*
American Heart Association 258
American Society of Anesthesiologists 2, 32,
      94, 174
  Physical Status classification 33, 33*t*, 34
American Society of Clinical Oncology 170
American Society of Echocardiography 186
American Society of Regional Anesthesia and
      Pain Medicine guidelines 126
Amiodarone 56
Amniotic fluid embolism 54, 60
Analgesia 123, 265
  intrapleural 82
  multimodal 82
  patient-controlled 180
  postoperative 82
  thoracic epidural 124
Anastomosis leakage 82
Anechoic fluid collection 224
Anesthesia 144, 161, 265, 313, 319
  administration, landscape of 89
  care 9, 318
  competency of 316
  deeper level of 8
  general 45, 287
  induction of 94, 152, 161
  inhalational 276, 287
  intravenous 163, 289
  machine 92, 97
  maintenance of 94, 161
  neuraxial 63
  pediatric 163
  plan of 91
  regional 19, 93, 96, 290
  services 4
  spinal 290
  techniques 93
  total intravenous 163, 276, 289
  training of 316
  vaporizers 287
Anesthesiology 276, 294, 313
Anesthetic
  agents 95*t*
  challenges 276, 284
  complications 62
  considerations 144

gas, inhaled concentration of 288
management 70, 77
  goals for 150
  technique 19
Angiotensin 139, 249
Angiotensin-converting enzyme 175, 283
  inhibitors 170
Angiotensin-receptor
  blocker 175
  neprilysin inhibitor 175
Anorexia 281
  cachexia syndrome 177
Anterior pulmonary window 239$f$
Antibiotics 243
Anticoagulation 263, 267
  protocols 258
Anti-inflammatory properties 250
Antioxidant 284
Appropriate fluid prescription 199$f$
Aquaporin-mediated transmembrane water
  transport 284
Argatroban 264
Arrhythmia, cardiac 29
Arterial blood 277, 278
  gases 267
  pressure 141$f$
Arteriotomy, pulmonary 140
Artery, pulmonary 268, 286
Arthralgia 281
Artificial intelligence 37, 40, 41, 49$f$, 322, 329
  role of 37, 40, 47
  use of 41
Aspiration
  pneumonia 75, 79
  pulmonary 151
Asthma 150, 209
Atmospheric pressure 278
Atresia 74
Atrial septal defect 74, 98
Atrial septostomy catheters 83
Attenuation 217
  artifact 218
Augment oxygen reserves 285
Automated infusion devices 166
Automatic implantable cardioverter-defibrillator
  128
Autonomic nervous system 180
Awake fiberoptic intubation 78, 164
Azathioprine 179

## B

Baclofen 175
Balloon 76
  migration 113
Barcode sign 223, 224$f$, 238, 239$f$
Basal metabolic rate 174
Basic anesthetic monitoring 6
Basic extracorporeal membrane oxygenation
  circuit 262$f$

Batwing sign 238$f$
Bedside lung ultrasound 223
Beers criteria 169
Beta-adrenergic agonism 63
Bezold-Jarisch reflex 62, 63
Bicarbonate 278
Bilevel positive airway pressure 205
Biodegradable drug carriers 167
Biopsy 5
Birth weight, low 81
Bispectral index 169, 289
Blame-free culture 322
Bleeding, targeted management of 60
Blood
  brain barrier 149, 150$f$
  lactate concentrations 249
  loss 285
  pressure 283
    cuffs 18
    diastolic 248
    noninvasive 77, 153
    pulmonary 141$f$
    systolic 31, 60, 179
  purification techniques 243, 252
Body
  composition 172
  mass index 7, 17, 20, 34
  surface area 175
Bone marrow 5
Bowel ischemia, laparotomy for 265
Boyle's law 105
Bradyarrhythmia 62
Bradycardia 130
  severe 165
Brain 244
  injury, secondary 144
Breast cancer surgery 176
Breathing, periodic 279
Brisk neck movements 82
British Consensus guidelines 195
British Thoracic Society 209
Bronchial blocker 108, 109, 110$f$, 111$f$, 114$f$
  insertion of 83
Bronchopleural fistula, large 259
Bronchoscopic visualization 113
Bronchoscopy, role of 77
Burnout
  high prevalence of 295
  interventions for 296
  syndrome 293-295

## C

Cancer
  incidence of 170
  prevention of 181
  surgery 170
Capillary refill time 248
Capnography 317
  pulse oximetry 312

# Index

Carbon dioxide
    analyzers 289
    daytime partial pressure of 209
    embolism 84
Carbon monoxide poisoning 281
Cardiac arrest 29, 63, 65
    causes of 64
    management of 61
    nonpregnant 55
    reversible causes of 61
Cardiac contraction 207
    evidence of 187
    lack of 187
Cardiac failure 256
Cardiac function 206
Cardiac output 197, 270
    Fick's estimate of 268
    monitoring 268
Cardiac tamponade 227, 269
Cardiac ultrasound 215, 226
    protocols 240
Cardiogenic pulmonary edema 225
Cardiomyopathy, peripartum 65
Cardiopulmonary arrest 287
Cardiopulmonary bypass 137, 139, 140
    surgery 286
Cardiopulmonary exercise testing 176
Cardiovascular collapse 61
Cardiovascular disease 65, 165
Cardiovascular disorders 179
Carotid artery 221$f$
Cartilaginous rib cage 118
Catalase 149
Cell death 149
Cellular metabolism abnormalities 244
Centers for Disease Control and Prevention 330
Central nervous system 158, 172-175
    depression 64
Central venous access 220
    placement 3
Central venous catheter 269
Central venous pressure 139, 245, 267, 270
Cephalosporins 266
Cerebral autoregulation 147
Cerebral blood flow 147
Cerebral edema 149, 276
Cerebral metabolism 148
Cerebral perfusion 144
    management 145
Cerebrovascular accident 34
Cervical spine 152$f$
    injury 151
Cesarean sections 164
Charlson comorbidity index 35, 169
Chemical
    properties 157
    structure 157
Chemoreflex dysfunction 22

Chest
    compressions 56
    imaging evaluation 107
    wall
        anatomy 125
        deformity 210
    X-ray 73$f$
Cheyne Stokes breathing 279
Chloroform anesthesia 287
Cholangitis 29
Cholecystectomy, laparoscopic 19
Chromosomal disorder 74
Chronic obstructive pulmonary disease 34, 208, 286
    exacerbations of 204
Chronic pain 182
    management 295
Chronic thromboembolic pulmonary hypertension 136
Ciprofloxacin 175
Clamshell incisions 137
Closed-loop anesthesia delivery systems 289
Codeine 180
Cognitive neuropsychological functioning 180
Colloids 196, 243
    balanced 196
Color Doppler mode 219
Comet tail artifact 218$f$
Common femoral
    artery 222$f$
    vein 222$f$, 236$f$
Communication 91
    breakdowns 329
    protocols 325
Compensatory bicarbonate excretions 286
Complete blood count 151
Complex percutaneous coronary intervention 263
Comprehensive geriatric assessment 169, 181
Compression technique 235
Computed tomography 6$f$
Concomitant drug therapy, effects of 150
Concurrent medical disease 150
Congenital anomalies 70, 74
Conscious sedation 164
Contemporary care, process of 252
Continuous paravertebral block 82
Continuous positive airway pressure 114, 204, 205, 208
    application of 84
Continuous renal replacement therapy 269
Continuous wave Doppler 219
Continuous waveform capnography 318
Contusions 151$f$
Cor pulmonale 276
Cormack-Lehane grade 47
Coronary artery disease 34, 286

# Index

Coronavirus disease 2019 (COVID-19) 207, 296, 317, 330
   pandemic 207, 293
Cortex 220
Corticosteroids 139, 243, 250
Cotrimoxazole 175
Cranial cavity 145
Cricoid cartilage 232*f*
Cricothyroid membrane 233*f*
Critical care
   challenges 276
   physicians 270
   practice 256
   specialists 57
Critical incident reporting systems 325
Crystalloids 196, 243, 247
   balanced 196
   large volumes of 247
Curvilinear probe 217, 217*f*
Cyanosis, focal 281
Cytokines, removal of 251

## D

Dabigatran 175
Damage-associated molecular patterns 150*f*
Decision support systems 42
Deep hypothermic circulatory arrest 136, 137
Deep learning 41
Deep vein thrombosis 180, 235
   ultrasound technique for 235
Defibrillation 56
Dehydration 91, 281
Delirium 169, 170
   emergence of 179
   postoperative 179
Delivery 163
Deoxyribonucleic acid break 149
Depressed fracture 148*f*
Depression, myocardial 248
Depth 219
Desaturation, causes of 80
Descending pulmonary arteries 138
Dexamethasone 20
Dexmedetomidine 11, 95, 266
Dextropropoxyphene 180
Diabetes mellitus 34
Diaphragm 225
   normal 225*f*
   paralyzed 225*f*
Diaphragmatic movement 225*f*
   assessment of 225
Diaphragmatic ultrasound 189
Diazepam 179
Difficult airway 40, 43, 44, 63, 150
   equipment 22
Difficult facemask score 45
Difficult intubations 42
Difficult mask ventilation 40, 42

Diffuse axonal injury 147*f*
Digital health technologies 329
Digital subtraction angiography 138
Diligent antibiotic stewardship 243
Direct oral anticoagulants 138
Disseminated intravascular coagulation 34, 61
Distal perfusion cannula 260
Distensibility index 230*f*
Dopamine antagonist 20
Double lumen tube 104, 109, 115
Double tract sign 233*f*
Drug 175, 196
   intoxication 281–283
   treatment 284
Duchenne muscular dystrophy 128
Dynamic hemodynamic parameters 197*t*
Dynamic needle tip positioning 221*f*
Dyspnea 281

## E

Early goal-directed therapy 243
Echocardiography, transesophageal 59
Echogenicity 235
Edema
   pulmonary 65, 208, 225, 225*f*, 261
   vasogenic 149
Ejection fraction 34, 226, 226*f*
   low 227*f*
   measures 226
Electrical energy 216*f*
Electrocardiogram 153
   continuous 97
Electroencephalogram, level of 178
Electronic records 329
Elevated hypercapnic ventilatory response 280
Elevated left atrial pressure 119
Embolism, pulmonary 58*f*, 64, 65
Embryology 73
Emergency 28
   education 312
   general anesthetics, risk of 63
   medication 317
   physician 200
   preparedness 286
   procedures 90
   surgery 27, 32
      acuity score 37
Emotional exhaustion 294, 295
Emotional support 305
Employ advanced cardiac output monitoring devices 286
Endarterectomy, pulmonary 136
End-expiratory occlusion test 246
Endogenous antioxidant system 149
Endoscopy 98
Endotoxin
   activity assay 251
   removal of 251

Endotracheal tube 78, 80, 105, 109, 109b, 110f, 111f, 118f, 230
   placement 43
      confirmation of 230
      shortening of 113f
      transverse view of 233f
End-tidal carbon dioxide 77, 197
Enhanced recovery after surgery 123, 125, 179
   protocols 19
Enoxaparin 175
Epidemiology 55, 137
Epinephrine 56, 61
Erector spinae plane 127f, 129
   blocks 123, 129
Erythrocytosis, excessive 281
*Escherichia coli* 330
Esophageal atresia 71, 71t, 74t
   classification of 71
   repair 82
   types of 72f
Esophageal surgery 106
Esophagus 233f
Establish crisis response systems 55
European Respiratory Society 207
European Society of Cardiology 208
Excitotoxic injury 149
Excretion 159
Exhaled carbon dioxide, sampling of 96
Exhaustion 281
Extracorporeal blood purification 250
   techniques 250
Extracorporeal cardiopulmonary resuscitation 260
Extracorporeal membrane oxygenation 34, 59, 141, 256, 257, 262, 266t
   cannulation 258
   circuit 261
   decannulation 268
   fundamentals 257
   implantation 188
   initiation 264
   machine, modern 257f
   management 266
   modalities 258
   periprocedural 263
   specific monitoring 268
   support, perioperative 256
   troubleshooting 268
   venoarterial 259t, 260, 266, 267
   venovenous 266, 267
Extraluminal approach technique 110
Extraluminal bronchial blocker 111f

## F

Face scans 43
Facial analysis techniques, artificial intelligence-based 45, 46
Fallot tetralogy 74, 75
Female pelvis, ultrasound scan of 237f
Femoral vein 222
   cannulation 222f
Fentanyl 82, 95, 157f, 159, 159t, 162, 266
Fiberoptic bronchoscope 47, 111f, 112f, 114f, 115f
Fibreoptic visualizing devices 47
Fick's method 268
Fistula, types of 71
Flexible fiberoptic bronchoscope 107, 109
Fluid
   administration 196
   coloading 63
   management 80, 286
   overload 194
   removal 198
   responsiveness 194, 215, 229f-231f
      assessment of 246
   resuscitation benefits 245
   selection 247
   stewardship 194, 195, 201
      serves 195
      team 199
   tolerance 194
   types of 202
Focal neurologic deficits 281
Focus assessed transthoracic echocardiography 58
Focused cardiac ultrasound 185, 186
Focused intraoperative transesophageal echocardiography 187
Fondaparinux 175
Forced expiratory volume 172, 173
Forgarty embolectomy catheter 83
Functional objective test 176
Fundamental ultrasound movements 218
Fungal infections, increased risk of 245

## G

Gamow bag 284
Gas
   analyzers 276, 288
   failure 269
   mixture, components of 288
Gastric
   distention 84
   ultrasound 189
Gastroesophageal reflux 82
Gastrointestinal interventions 97
General surgery 162
Generalized muscle atrophy 179
Genital hypoplasia 75
Geriatric
   cancer
      patients, anesthesia for 169
      rates 170
   oncology 170, 181
   pharmacology 170
   population 169

Glasgow Coma Scale 30, 35, 146
Global capnography project 317
Glomerular filtration rate 175
Glutathione 149
    peroxidase 149
    reductase 149
    S-transferase 149
Gross domestic product 317
Growth differentiation factor 172, 173

## H

Haloperidol 180
Hand hygiene 330
Harlequin syndrome 268
Headache 276, 281
Health 324
Healthcare
    facility resources 3
    industry 48
    teams 324
Heart 219, 244
    chambers 228*f*
    disease
        congenital 79
        cyanotic congenital 286
        ischemic 150, 181
    failure 58*f*, 65
    rate 31
Hemadsorption techniques 250, 251
Hematocrit 36
Hematoma
    extradural 146, 146*f*
    intracranial 146
    subdural 146, 146*f*
Hemodiafiltration 250
Hemodialysis, continuous 250
Hemodynamic 266
    compromise, assessment of 227
    instability 83, 252
    intraoperative 324
    monitoring 188
    principles 57
    pulmonary 270
    stabilization 243
    status, clinical assessment of 202
Hemofiltration, high-volume 250, 251
Hemoglobin 35
Hemorrhage 60, 61
    intracerebral 147*f*
    intracranial 235
    intraperitoneal 58*f*
    obstetric 60
    postpartum 54, 60
    pulmonary 106, 141
Hemorrhagic shock, physiological classification of 30*t*
Hepatic blood flow 170
Hepatic endothelium 170

High partial pressure, regions of 288
High post-membrane pressure 269
High pre-membrane pressure 269
High-altitude 280*t*, 286
    cerebral edema 281, 283
    environments 286
    headache 281, 283
    illness 277, 280, 282*t*
        ranges, spectrum of 276
        prevention of 282
        treatment of 283
    medicine 276, 277
    pathophysiology 279
    pulmonary edema 281, 283
High-dependency unit 38, 100
Higher parasympathetic tone 207
High-flow nasal oxygen 211
    devices 205
Hormone 248
Host response, modulation of 243, 250
Human immunodeficiency virus 315
Humidification functions 205
Humidity, low 285
Hybrid courses, completion of 190
Hydrocephalus 235
Hydroxocobalamin 139
Hyomental distance 45
Hyperalgesia 165
Hypercapnia 119
    enhance pulmonary vasoconstriction 118
Hypercapnic respiratory failure 210, 212
Hypercarbia
    benign prostatic 174
    episodes of 138
Hypertension 34, 150
    intracranial 148
    pulmonary 276, 281
        arterial 83, 280
Hyperthermia 119
    malignant 260
Hyperventilation 278, 286
Hypervolemia 196
Hypocapnia 119
Hypoglycemia 91, 100
Hypometabolism, period of 148
Hyponatremia 281
Hypoplastic left heart syndrome 74
Hypotension 130, 144, 248
    potential severe 284
Hypothermia 100, 119, 276, 285
Hypovolemia 196, 245, 269
Hypoxemia 61, 104, 119
    diagnosis of 120
    episodes of 138
    main reasons for 80*b*
    treatment of 120
Hypoxia 65, 79, 144, 276
Hypoxic pulmonary vasoconstriction 117, 119, 283

Hypoxic ventilatory response 279
Hysterotomy
    extension 60
    resuscitative 54, 57

## I

Ideal body weight 267
Idiopathic central sleep apnea 280
Iliocostalis 129
Immature metabolic pathways 82
Immune system 172
Indo-Australian tectonic plate 277
Infarction, indicators of 226
Infections
    healthcare-associated 324, 330
    multidrug-resistant 330
Inferior vena cava 197, 229, 247
    assessment 229
    collapsibility index 229
    diameter of 229$f$, 230
    distensibility index 229
    inspiratory collapse 230
Inflammatory mediators
    production of 244
    simultaneous removal of 251
Inotropes 243
    infusions of 138
Inotropic properties 61
Insomnia 281
Inspiratory oxygen, partial pressure of 277, 278
Inspiratory positive airway pressure 206
Inspired oxygen, fraction of 36, 205, 262$f$, 267
Integrating electronic health records 329
Intensive care 161
    unit 124, 150, 157, 176, 204, 323
Intercostal blocks 82
Interleukin 172, 173
Internal jugular vein 220, 221$f$
International Society of Geriatric Oncology 170
Interstitial lung disease 205
    management of 209
Interventional cardiology 260, 264
Interventional radiology 1, 5, 6$f$, 9$f$, 12, 264
    anesthesia for 1
    procedures 3
    suite design 1, 4
Intra-abdominal compartments 145
Intra-abdominal pressure 145, 197
Intracranial disorder, primary 146
Intracranial pressure 144, 145
Intraluminal approach technique 112
Intraluminal bronchial blocker 112$f$
Intraoperative continuous electrocardiogram 286
Intrapleural pressure 206
Intrathoracic pressure 145, 149
Intravenous catheters 91
Intravenous fluid therapy 195
Intravenous pulmonary vasodilators 61
Intubation 47
Invasive blood pressure monitoring 61
Invasive mechanical ventilation 205
Ischemia 144
    indicators of 226
Ischemic damage 245
Isoflurane 288

## J

Jugular venous oxygen saturation 153

## K

Kepler intubation robot system 48
Ketamine 95, 289
    induced dissociative anesthesia 276
Ketofol 95
Kidney 220
*Klebsiella pneumoniae* 330
Knobology 215, 219

## L

Labor 163
Large-bore intravenous access 61
Laryngotracheal tube 74
Latissimus dorsi 125
Left ventricle 267
    end-diastolic area 227, 228$f$
Left ventricular
    assist device implantation 130
    distension 261
    ejection fraction 176
    failure 61
    function 226
        assessment of 226
    outflow tract 270
        velocity time integral variation 230
    venous return 206
Lethal arrhythmia 65
Lidocaine 56
Life-saving maneuver 61
Limb ischemia, possibility of 265
Linear probe 217, 217$f$
Lipopolysaccharide 251
Liver
    failure 29
    mass 170
Local anesthetic systemic toxicity 54, 64, 96
Low partial pressure 288
Lower extremity
    pulse oximeter monitoring 77
    venous system of 235$f$
Lower functional residual capacity 118
Lung 219, 236
    examination 236
    injury, self-induced 207
    isolation 83
        loss of 113
        technique 107, 108

342 Index

normal ultrasound of 238*f*
retraction 81
sliding 223
　absence of 238
ultrasound 188, 215, 223, 223*fc*, 224*f*, 239*f*
　protocols 240
ventilation strategies 120

## M

Machine learning 40, 41, 49*f*
Magnesium
　supranormal 66
　toxicity 61, 66
Magnetic resonance imaging 98
Main pulmonary arteries 138
Male pelvis, ultrasound scan of 238*f*
Mallampati score, modified 47
Maslach burnout inventory 294
Masses 43
Massive pulmonary embolism 260
Massive transfusion protocol activation 61
Maternal cardiac arrest 54, 67
　causes of 59
　incidence of 55
　management 55
　　general principles of 55, 56*t*
Mean arterial blood pressure 267
Mechanical circulatory support 265
Mediastinal surgery 106
Mediator delivery hypothesis 250
Medication errors 322, 324
Medium molecular substances 251
Medulla 220
Memory deficits 281
Mental focus, lack of 281
Mentee, evaluation of 309*b*
Mentorship 302
　benefits of 303
　malpractice 310
　program 309
　　selection process for 307
　schemes 310
Metabolite 159
Methylene blue 139, 249
Microcirculatory flow 245
Midazolam 11, 95, 179, 266
Migraine 281
Milrinone 61
Mini nutritional assessment 178
Minimal cardiorespiratory depression 94
Minimally invasive
　nature 10
　surgery 70, 166
Minimum alveolar concentration 152, 279
Mitochondrial respiration 149
Mixed venous oxygen saturation 267, 270
Modern surgical techniques 166
Modified early warning scoring system 31*t*

Moisture exchangers 206
Monge disease 281
Monitoring breath sounds 84
Morphine 162
Mortality rate 323
　perioperative 317
Mountain sickness 276
　acute 281, 283
　chronic 281
Multi-organ
　dysfunction 244
　failure 252
Multiple chemical sensitivity, effects of 149
Multiple compartment syndrome 145
Multisystem involvement 74
Muscle rigidity 165
Myalgia 281
Myocardial infarction 29, 34
Myocardial ischemia, signs of 286
Myofascial plane 129

## N

Nasogastric tube 75
National Anesthesia Clinical Outcomes Registry 2, 89
National Anesthesia Societies 316
National Confidential Enquiry into Patient Outcome and Death classification 28
Nausea 10, 129, 165, 179
　compound postoperative 285
Near-infrared spectrometry 139, 153, 265, 267
Neck radiation 45
Neonatal intensive care unit 77
Neonatal thoracoscopic surgery, anesthetic implications of 83
Neuraxial techniques 124
Neuroleptics 180
Neuromuscular blockers 266
Neuromuscular disorders 210
Nitric oxide 61
Nitrofurantoin 175
Nitrous oxide 249, 288
Noncatecholamine vasopressor 139, 139*t*
Noninvasive automatic face-analysis system 46
Noninvasive delivery systems 167
Noninvasive ventilation 204-212
　equipment 205
　failure 210
　physiological effects of 206
Nonoperating room anesthesia 2, 88, 89, 95*t*, 97, 98, 98*t*
　complications of 100*b*
　services 7
Nonspecific tissue esters 158*f*
Nonsteroidal anti-inflammatory drugs 180
Noradrenaline 243, 248
Norepinephrine 61, 63
Normal lung motion, absence of 223

Nostril 164
Nutrition 172
    assessment 177
    risk index 178

## O

Obesity 17
    hypoventilation syndrome 205, 209
Obstetric anesthesiologists 57
Obstructive sleep apnea 17, 21, 34, 209
Ondansetron 20
One-lung ventilation 83, 104, 106, 120
    decision tree 118$f$
    indications for 106
    physiology of 117
Open fracture, treatment of 315
Operation theater 80
    team 328
Opioid 161
    free techniques 19
Optic nerve sheath diameter 234
    measurement 234$f$
Optimal blood pressure target 248
Optimal fluid resuscitation 246
Oral gastric tube in situ 73$f$
Organ
    donation 260
    dysfunction
        attenuate sepsis-related 250
        life-threatening 244
    injuries 324
    system 74
Orogastric tube 73
Oxidative stress 149
Oxygen
    delivery equipment 92
    hemoglobin dissociation curve 278
    partial pressure of 277, 278
    saturation 278
    supplementation 283
    toxicity, risk of 176
    transport changes 280
Oxygenation 262

## P

Pain 124
    acute on chronic 165
    labor 161
    management 161, 176, 295
    postoperative 161
    procedural 165
    relief 179
Palmar burning sensation 281
Pancreatitis 29
Paralytic ileus 29
Paravertebral block 125, 126, 127$f$
Passive leg raise 197, 246
    test 231$f$

Patent ductus arteriosus 74, 98
Patent foramen ovale 286
Pectoral interfascial superficial block 127$f$
Pectoral nerve block 127$f$
Pectoserratus nerve blocks 127
Pediatric
    airway 104, 105
    flexible fiberoptic bronchoscopes sizes 108$f$
    postanesthetic discharge scoring system 101$t$
    procedures, pharmacological considerations for 93
    sedation state scale 94
    thoracic
        anesthesia 104
        surgery 105
Pelvis 220, 236
Perfusion 205
    indices 270
    pressure 245
Pericardial effusion 58$f$, 227, 228$f$
Pericardium 219
Perimortem cesarean delivery 57
Peripheral nerve injury 29
Peripheral venous access 222
Peritoneal catheter placements 8
Personal protective equipment, use of 330
Pharmacodynamics 158
Pharmacokinetics 158
Phenylephrine 61
Phosphodiesterase inhibitors 284
Physiological emergency surgery acuity score 35
Placenta accreta 60
Planning labor analgesia 63
Plasma
    clearance 159
    esterases 156
    free hemoglobin 269
Pleura 219
Pleural effusion 29, 58$f$, 224
    large 224$f$
Pneumonia 76, 180, 207
Pneumothorax 29, 81, 151$f$, 223
    indicators of 223
Point-of-care ultrasound 57, 58$f$, 186, 215, 246
    abdominal 58$f$, 59
    cardiac 58, 226
    gastric 59
    lung 58
    perioperative 185
    protocol-driven 238, 240
    vascular 59
Polymyxin B 251
Polyvinylchloride 47
Portable hyperbaric bag 281, 284, 284$f$
Portable remote robot-assisted intubation system 48

Positive airway pressure 22, 206
Positive end-expiratory pressure 205, 267
Postanesthesia care 100, 101
    unit 101
Postanesthetic discharge scoring system 101
    pediatric adaptation of 88
Postcardiac arrest syndrome 66
Postdural puncture headache, incidence of 290
Postoperative critical care 176
Potassium 35
Power Doppler mode 219
Predictive machine learning model 43
Preeclampsia 65
    cardiopulmonary manifestations of 65
Pregnancy 150, 280
    disorder of 65
Pressure support 206
Prophylactic dose 282, 283
Propofol 11, 95, 118, 178, 266, 289
    bolus dose of 178
Protein
    binding 159
    oxidation of 149
Pulmonary artery 268, 286
    catheter 83, 268, 269
    endarterectomy 137
    pressure 137, 267, 270
Pulmonary capillary wedge pressure 246
Pulmonary endarterectomy 136
    anesthesia for 136
Pulmonary vascular resistance 83, 138, 207
Pulse
    oximetry 97, 153, 317
    pressure variation 197, 199$f$, 246
    wave Doppler 219, 230
Pump failure 269

### Q

Quality assurance team, member of 200

### R

Radiation protection 89
Radical cancer resections 176
Ramsay sedation scale 96$t$
Rapid sequence induction 152
Reactive nitrogen species 150$f$
Reactive oxygen species 150$f$
Real-time carbon monoxide 246
Red blood cell 150$f$
Reflection 217, 218, 305, 308
    artifact 218$f$
Refraction 217
Regional analgesic techniques 104
Remifentanil 156, 157$f$, 159, 159$t$, 160$t$, 161-164, 166, 167, 178
    acid 159$f$
    bolus dose of 178
    crosses placenta 163
    drug 162
    half-life 158, 160
    major metabolites of 159$f$
    metabolism of 158$f$
    minor metabolites of 159$f$
    overview of 156
    pharmacodynamics 158
    suppression 164
    target-controlled infusion pumps 162
    vial strengths 162
Remimazolam 11
Renal bicarbonate excretion 278
Renal disease
    acute 34
    end-stage 34
Renal water losses 286
Respiration
    phase of 229$f$
    spontaneous 229$f$
Respiratory
    care equipment 22
    challenges 286
    complications 82, 100
    disease 165
    distress syndrome 65, 76, 79
    failure 204, 212
        acute 209, 223, 223$fc$
        hypoxic 210
        non-COVID-19 type 1 207
    mechanics 206
    physiology 105
    rate, intermittent 96
Restrictive lung disease 205, 209
Resuscitation 197, 243
    cardiopulmonary 55
Resynchronization therapy device 128
Rib fractures 151$f$
Right atrial pressures 139, 230$t$
Right heart pressures 286
Right ventricle 227, 270
    end-diastolic area 228$f$
Right ventricular failure 61
    severity of 138
Rivaroxaban 175
Robotic surgery 166
Robotic video-assisted thoracic surgery 126$f$
Root cause analysis 325
Royal College of Anesthesiologists 328

### S

Sarcopenia 169, 171, 177
Seashore sign 239$f$
Sedation 88, 93, 94, 164
    holds 161
    levels of 94
    plan of 91
Sedative medication 11
Seizures 281
    eclamptic 65

Selepressin 249
Sensitivity 43
Sepsis 29, 243, 244, 246, 252
Septic shock 243, 244, 248, 250, 252
    management of 243, 245*fc*
Serratus anterior plane 123
    block 125, 127*f*, 128
Serum concentration 66
Severe adult respiratory failure 258
Severe peripheral vascular disease 265
Severe respiratory
    compromise 76
    depression 165
    disease 76
Sevoflurane 288
Shock
    cardiogenic 65
    distributive type of 244
    hemorrhagic 30*t*
    hypovolemic 30*t*
    progressive 244
    resuscitation 245
    septic 243, 244, 248, 250, 252
    state 252
Short nutritional assessment questionnaire 178
Sildenafil 284
Simpson's method 226, 226*f*
Simulation
    exercises 66
    training 305, 308
Single lumen endotracheal tube intubation 109
Single photon emission computed
    tomography 138
Small-caliber arterial cannula 265
Smart infusion pumps 167
Society for Ambulatory Anesthesia Cataract
    guidelines 8
Society of Anesthesia and Sleep Medicine 21
Society of Cardiovascular Anesthesiologists 131
Society of Geriatric Oncology 169
Sodium 35
Sonoanatomy 215, 219
    tracheal 232*f*
Sound wave 216*f*
    properties 216
Spinal anesthesia 290
    setting of 62
Spitz classification 72*t*
Spontaneous breathing trial 211
Spontaneous coronary artery dissection 65
Standard American Society of
    Anesthesiologists 139
Staphylococcus aureus, methicillin-resistant 245
Steep learning curves 256
Stent placement 286
Sternotomy 123
Steroids 250
Stratosphere sign 224*f*, 239*f*

Stroke 180
    hemorrhagic 65
    volume variation 197, 199*f*
Subarachnoid block 290
Subclavian artery 222*f*
Subclavian vein 221, 222*f*
    cannulation 222*f*
Sufentanil 157*f*
Superoxide dismutase 149
Surgery, cardiac 187
Surgical-site infection 331
    prevention of 314
Surviving sepsis campaign guideline 243, 248
Swan–Ganz catheter 268
Systemic vascular resistance 246

# T

Tachyarrhythmia 249
    ventricular 286
Tachycardia 249
Tamponade physiology 227
Target-controlled infusion
    minto model 156
    pumps, use of 166
Team training program, principles for 331*t*
Temperature management 80
Tension pneumothorax 238
Terlipressin 139
Thoracic fascial plane blocks, dermatomal
    distribution of 127*f*
Thoracic surgery 123
    analgesic techniques for 120
Thoracic vascular surgery 106
Thoracodorsal nerve 125
Thoracoscopic procedures 84
Thoracoscopic repair 82
Thoracoscopic surgery 70
Thoracoscopic tracheoesophageal fistula,
    anesthesia for 82
Thoracotomy 130
    incision, site of 126*f*
Thrombocytopenia, heparin-induced 264
Thromboelastography 268
Thromboelastometry, rotational 268
Thromboembolism 138, 182
Thrombosis, chronic pulmonary 137
Thrombus 235, 236*f*
Tissue
    Doppler imaging 219
    hypoperfusion 248
    plasminogen activator 65
Trachea 73, 233*f*
    perforation 81
Tracheal anatomy 232*f*
Tracheal cartilage 232*f*
    longitudinal plane 232*f*
Tracheal extubation 153, 211, 212
Tracheal intubation 48

Tracheobronchial resections 259
Tracheoesophageal fistula 70, 71, 71*t*, 72*t*, 74*t*, 80, 259
    anesthetic management of 70
    classification of 71
    repair 70
Tracheostomy
    percutaneous 231
    tubes 43
Tramadol 180
Transcatheter aortic valve replacement 260, 263
Transducer selection 235
Transient ischemic attack 34
Transversus abdominis plane block 64
Transversus thoracic plane 127*f*
Traumatic brain injury 144, 235
    consequences of 145
    management of 144
    pathophysiology of 147, 150*f*
Tumor
    identification of 43
    necrosis factor 172, 173, 244

## U

Ultrasonography 42
Ultrasound 44, 186, 232, 235, 236
    guided
        line insertion 186
        percutaneous cannulation 258
    modes, basic 218
    physics 215
    renal 215
    scan 237*f*
    tracheal 230
    transducers 216*f*
    visualization 220*f*
United States National Institute of Health 257
Universal Health Coverage 313
Upper extremity pulse oximeter monitoring 77
Urea 35
Uremic toxins 251
Urinary retention, postoperative 285
Urine output 31
US Food and Drug Administration 157
Uterine displacement 55

## V

Vagal nerve injury 82
Vaginal delivery 61
Vaginal laceration 60
Vancomycin 266
Vaporizers 276, 287
Vascular access 56, 215, 220
Vascular system 138
Vasoactive agents 248, 249
Vasodilation 281
    systemic 61, 248
Vasomotor failure 250
Vasopressin 139, 248
Vasopressors 63, 243
Venoarterial extracorporeal membrane oxygenation 259*t*, 260, 266, 267
    central 261
    peripheral 260
Venous thromboembolism, risk of 285
Venovenous extracorporeal membrane oxygenation 266, 267
    femoral-jugular 259
    jugular-bicaval 260
    use of 259*b*
Ventilation 105, 205
    inadequate 79
    perfusion mismatch 117
Ventilatory sensitivity 278
Ventilatory support 76
Ventricular
    fibrillation 258
    septal defect 74, 98
    tachycardia ablation 260, 263
Venturi masks 290
Vertigo 281
Video-assisted
    surgery 104
    thoracic surgery 126*f*
    thoracoscopic surgery 106
    thoracoscopy 125
Videolaryngoscopy 45, 46, 47
Vital capacity 172, 173
Vital tissues 244
Vitamin 139
Vocal cord 45
    abduction 233*f*
    function 233*f*
        evaluation of 233
    movement of 233
    paralysis 233
Vogt classification 71
Volatile anesthetics, partial pressure of 276
Vomiting 10, 129, 165, 179, 281, 285

## W

Waterston classification 72*t*
Wavelength 216
White blood cell 36
World Federation of Societies of Anaesthesiologists 313
World Health Organization Surgical Checklist 326*t*
Wound dehiscence 29